Food, Nutrition, and Mental Health

Food, Nutrition, and Mental Health

Edited by
Michael T. Compton, M.D., M.P.H.

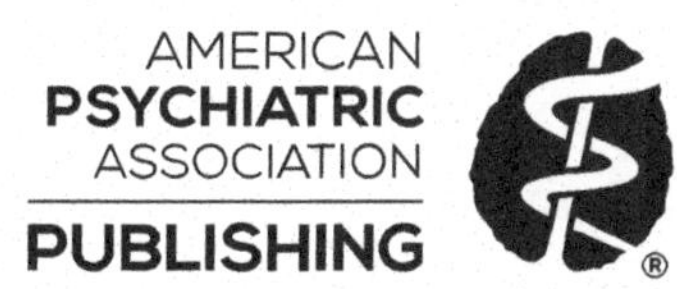

Note: The authors have worked to ensure that all information in this book is accurate at the time of publication and consistent with general psychiatric and medical standards, and that information concerning drug dosages, schedules, and routes of administration is accurate at the time of publication and consistent with standards set by the U.S. Food and Drug Administration and the general medical community. As medical research and practice continue to advance, however, therapeutic standards may change. Moreover, specific situations may require a specific therapeutic response not included in this book. For these reasons and because human and mechanical errors sometimes occur, we recommend that readers follow the advice of physicians directly involved in their care or the care of a member of their family.

First Edition

Manufactured in the United States of America on acid-free paper
29 28 27 26 25 5 4 3 2 1

American Psychiatric Association Publishing
800 Maine Avenue SW, Suite 900
Washington, DC 20024–2812
www.appi.org

Library of Congress Control Number: 2025943145

British Library Cataloguing in Publication DataA CIP record is available from the British Library.

EU GPSR Authorized Representative: LOGOS EUROPE, 9 rue Nicolas Poussin, 17000, LA ROCHELLE, France; E-mail: Contact@logoseurope.eu

Contents

Contributors

Ashley Andreou, M.D., M.P.H.
Psychiatry Resident, New York Presbyterian Hospital-Columbia University Medical Center and New York State Psychiatric Institute, New York, New York

Luigi Attademo, M.D.
Psychiatrist, Department of Mental Health, North West Tuscany Local Health Authority, Cecina, Leghorn, Italy

Francesco Bernardini, M.D.
Psychiatrist, Department of Mental Health, West Friuli Local Health Authority, Pordenone, Italy

Omid Cohensedgh, M.D.
Resident Psychiatrist, New York Presbyterian Hospital-Columbia University Medical Center and New York State Psychiatric Institute, New York, New York

Michael T. Compton, M.D., M.P.H.
Research Psychiatrist, New York State Psychiatric Institute; Professor of Psychiatry, Columbia University Vagelos College of Physicians and Surgeons, New York, New York

Amy Ehntholt, Sc.D.
Research Scientist, New York State Psychiatric Institute; Assistant Professor of Clinical Behavioral Science in Psychiatry, Columbia University Vagelos College of Physicians and Surgeons, New York, New York

Stephanie E. Langlois, M.B.A.
Senior Coordinator, New Hampshire Perinatal Quality Collaborative at Dartmouth Health, Dartmouth Hitchcock Medical Center, Lebanon, New Hampshire

Liana Lau, M.D., M.S.
Child and Adolescent Psychiatrist, Elmhurst Hospital, Brooklyn, New York

Heather Seid, D.C.N., R.D.N.
Bionutrition Research Core Program Manager, Clinical Research Resource, Irving Institute for Clinical and Translational Research, New York, New York

B. Lynette Staplefoote-Boynton M.D., M.P.H.
Internal Medicine and Psychiatry Resident, Duke University Medical Center, Durham, North Carolina

Julie C. Suarez, M.A.
Associate Dean of Land-Grant Affairs, Director of Translational Research Programs, Cornell University College of Agriculture and Life Sciences, Ithaca, New York

Mariam Motunrayo Sulaimon, M.A.
Research Associate, Teachers College, Columbia University, New York, New York

Part 1

An Introduction to Food and Dietary Patterns

1

An Introduction to *Food, Nutrition, and Mental Health*

Michael T. Compton, M.D., M.P.H.

Good nutrition creates health in all areas of our existence.

—T. Colin Campbell, Ph.D.

Food is a basic, continuous human need for health and survival. It is such a routine part of our daily lives that many of us often take it for granted or give it too little thought. The key role of the food we eat is *nutrition*. The type and quality of the food we consume determine its nutritional value and thus our own nutrition, and in turn, our health—our physical health, our emotional or psychological health, and our strength, resilience, and well-being.

This book serves as an overview of multiple aspects of food, nutrition, and mental health. It is written primarily for mental health professionals and other clinicians, but it is informative for a broader audience. This chapter sets the stage for more in-depth examinations of specific content areas.

What We Know

We know, from an enormous body of research in the fields of epidemiology, nutritional sciences, and medicine, that dietary patterns and the types of foods consumed are linked to a multitude of physical health outcomes across physiological systems. We also know that many chronic diseases can be affected (adversely or beneficially) by what one eats: the dietary strategy for achieving type 2 diabetes remission or reversal is just one example (Mozafarri et al. 2024; Panigrahi et al. 2023; Taylor et al. 2021). Unsurprisingly (given the close links between physical health and mental health), dietary patterns are also associated with mental health outcomes (Burgess et al. 2022; Dinan 2023; Ramsey 2021).

Numerous studies document that mental health outcomes are affected by what one eats (Aucoin et al. 2021; Bayes et al. 2022; Eliby et al. 2023; Głąbska et al. 2020; Jacka et al. 2017; Lane et al. 2022). For example, Prevención con Dieta Mediterránea (PREDIMED) was a randomized, controlled trial that tested a Mediterranean diet supplemented with extra-virgin olive oil or nuts for primary prevention of cardiovascular disease (Estruch et al. 2018). The study demonstrated that a Mediterranean diet supplemented with nuts lowers the risk of depression among those with type 2 diabetes (Sánchez-Villegas et al. 2013). Another randomized, controlled trial, Supporting the Modification of Lifestyle in Lowered Emotional States (SMILES) (Jacka et al. 2017), documented that individual nutrition counseling sessions delivered by a clinical dietitian (compared with a social support protocol as the control condition) among adults with clinical depression was associated with fewer depressive symptoms and a greater likelihood of remission. Similarly, the randomized, controlled trial called A Mediterranean Diet in Men With Depression (AMMEND) (Bayes et al. 2022) showed that a Mediterranean diet intervention (compared with befriending therapy as the control condition) among young males with clinical depression was associated with decreased depressive symptoms and increased quality of life.

Although less is known about causality and underlying mechanisms than these associations (Adan et al. 2019), the pathways by which our eating patterns and dietary composition affect our mental health are complex and range from the constellation of our gut microbiome to the social aspects of cooking together and eating together. Mechanisms of action considered most likely to be at play include reduced inflammation, lowered cortisol stress response, greater antioxidant capacity and thus lower oxidative stress, improved blood flow to the brain (providing necessary substrates and cofactors needed to produce neurotransmitters), improvements in the gut microbiome, and increased brain-derived neurotrophic factor (Burgess et al. 2022; Butler and Mörkl 2023).

What We Need to Know

There is strong evidence of how food security, certain nutrients (e.g., vitamin D), and dietary patterns are associated with depression. Other mental health outcomes are less consistently studied (Sparling et al. 2022), and more research is needed. Longitudinal studies would help in sorting out directionality (or bidirectionality, given that just as dietary patterns impact mental well-being, mental well-being also impacts dietary patterns).

In comparison to some of the other social determinants of mental health, food and nutrition insecurity has been somewhat neglected by the mental health field. This is now changing, as routine screening, assessment, and referral processes are improving. To provide dietary recommendations for improving mental health, a major challenge is to advance knowledge from population-based observations toward personalized nutrition (Adan et al. 2019). Mental health professionals and other clinicians need to be equipped to offer nutritional counseling with regard to a rational, balanced diet that maximizes whole foods and minimizes ultraprocessed foods, in conjunction with the consumption of prebiotics (insoluble fiber in plant-based foods such as fruits, vegetables, legumes, and whole grains), probiotics (live microorganisms, typically bacteria or yeasts, found naturally in some foods), and antioxidant and anti-inflammatory phytonutrients from plants. They should also be equipped to make referrals to nutrition professionals (e.g., registered dietitians and lifestyle medicine clinicians). More research is required to make recommendations for specific nutrients vis-à-vis specific mental health concerns or conditions, as the field of *nutritional psychiatry* (incorporating nutrition into the treatment of mental health disorders) is relatively nascent, but growing—especially given the low-risk and potentially high-yield nature of nutritional interventions (Norwitz and Naidoo 2021).

What Is Covered in This Book

Part 1 of this book is an introduction to food and dietary patterns. Chapters 2 and 3 provide brief overviews of macronutrients and micronutrients, respectively, written primarily for clinicians, many of whom learned much of this information during their training, which may have been some years ago. Specifically, Chapter 2 covers carbohydrates, protein, and fat (both healthy and unhealthy), as well as fiber. It summarizes what is known about the intake of these macronutrients with regard to mental health and mental illnesses. Chapter 3 is a primer on vitamins, minerals, and phytonutrients, while also addressing known mental health correlates of specific micronutrient deficiencies. After those reviews of macronutrients and micronutrients, Chapter 4 covers a number of dietary patterns and specific diets. The "Western diet" or "standard American diet" and ultraprocessed foods are described, as are specific types of low-calorie diets, fasting and intermittent fasting, low-carbohydrate (high-protein/high-fat) diets, and low-fat diets. Other topics include the Mediterranean diet, the Blue Zone diet, and plant-predominant eating patterns, as well as portion control and mindful eating practices.

Part 2 of the book is about food insecurity and diet quality, as well as counseling and resources for the clinical setting. Chapter 5 covers the links between food insecurity and mental health. The prevalence of food insecurity in the United States is detailed, and the large literature on food insecurity and mental health—among pregnant and postpartum women, young children, adolescents and young adults, and older adults—is summarized. The chapter also details how to screen for food insecurity and related risk factors in the clinical setting, how clinicians can address food insecurity and related risk factors, and policy approaches to food insecurity as a social determinant of mental health. Chapter 6 describes rating scales and assessments in the clinical setting, regarding not just food insecurity, but also nutrition insecurity, nutritional status/malnutrition, food intake and diet quality, and other food- and nutrition-related constructs. Chapter 7 provides clinical guidance on assessing and addressing food- and nutrition-related issues in the clinical setting, including mental health practice settings. An overview of public health and medical societies' guidelines on nutrition is provided, and the clinical approach—including screening and assessment, nutrition education and dietary counseling (even when time is very limited in clinical encounters), referring to resources, collaborating with registered dietitians, and follow-up throughout the course of treatment—is outlined. Ways to promote cultural humility and include social context in conversations about food insecurity and dietary intake are described. Federally funded programs related to food and nutrition are summarized as well. Chapter 8 gives an overview of emerging "Food Is Medicine" programs, including medically tailored meals, medically tailored groceries, and produce prescription programs, as well as government and private-sector involvement (through federal funding, state Medicaid Section 1115 demonstration waivers, health plans/insurance companies, and public-private partnerships). Chapter 9 details food- and nutrition-related policies and programs, covering a broad array of resources that are important for clinicians to be familiar with: childhood hunger and nutrition programs, farmer-friendly programs incentivizing fresh fruits and vegetables, nutrition education programs, the Dietary Guidelines for Americans, state and local food policy councils, food hubs, and emergency or charitable food assistance programs.

Part 3 of the book addresses special topics on food, nutrition, and mental health. Chapter 10 addresses psychotropic medications associated with increased appetite and iatrogenic weight gain, including antipsychotics, antidepressants, and mood stabilizers. Weight gain prevention and management strategies are described, including weight and metabolic monitoring recommendations, nonpharmacologic interventions to address weight gain, and pharmacologic interventions for weight gain. Chapter 11 is also clinically oriented, focusing on eating disorders and disordered eating patterns. DSM-defined eating disorders are described, including anorexia nervosa and atypical anorexia nervosa, bulimia nervosa, binge eating disorder, avoidant/restrictive food intake disorder, pica, rumination disorder, purging disorder, and night eating syndrome. The chapter also covers screening for eating disorders and clinical considerations, eating disorders in the context of food insecurity, non-DSM disordered eating patterns (emotional eating, food addiction, orthorexia), psychiatric symptoms and disordered eating, and psychiatric medications and disordered eating. Chapter 12 is an overview of what clinicians should know about the gut–brain connection and the microbiome. It addresses the development and maintenance of the gut microbiome, its influences on psychiatric disorders, and considerations around the treatment of psychiatric conditions with the gut microbiome as a mediator. How both nutritional factors and socialization patterns affect the gut microbiome is described.

Finally, Part 4 is about cooking, gardening, and growing food. Chapter 13 is on cooking, cooking together, and eating together and how these activities benefit both physical health and mental health. Therapeutic cooking programs and culinary medicine are also described. Chapter 14 is about gardening and gardening together, as well as the physical health and mental health benefits. Horticultural therapy and therapeutic community gardens are also covered. Finally, Chapter 15 considers potential health implications of how our food is produced, covering large farms and monocultures, genetically modified organism commodity crops, concentrated animal feeding operations, and ultraprocessed foods. Additionally, two eating patterns are described: the local food movement and the slow food movement, as well as the EAT-Lancet Commission's planetary health diet.

What Is Not Covered in This Book

Despite covering a broad array of content areas, this book does not cover specific recommendations (in terms of vitamins and minerals, for example) for specific mental health conditions (e.g., anxiety disorders and schizophrenia). Other sources (Burgess et al. 2022; Dinan 2023) have recently provided this information. Additionally, more research is needed. Mental health professionals and other clinicians should be equipped to provide nutrition counseling with regard to a healthy diet (and working in conjunction with nutrition experts such as registered dietitians and lifestyle medicine clinicians).

The potential mental health–promoting and cognition-beneficial effects of specific herbal remedies and plant species—such as *Crocus sativus* (saffron), *Lavandula angustifolia* (lavender), *Salvia rosmarinus* (rosemary), *Hypericum perforatum* (St. John's wort), *Curcuma longa* (turmeric), *Bacopa monnieri* (water hyssop), *Ginkgo biloba* (ginkgo tree), *Withania somnifera* (ashwagandha), ginseng, lion's mane mushroom, aloe, and others—are not covered here but are addressed in a number of review articles (Lewis et al. 2021; Picheta et al. 2024).

This book is also not a nutrition textbook. It is instead intended to provide the reader—primarily clinicians, and especially mental health clinicians—with an overview of relevant topics at the convergence of food, nutrition, and mental health. Countless facts and findings about nutritional sciences (pertaining to how the body uses specific nutrients; differential bioavailability of nutrients in various food types; specific nutritional needs of infants, children, and older adults; dietary management of various health issues such as diabetes, heart disease, and certain types of cancer; how genes and diet interact to influence health; epigenetics) are beyond the scope of this introductory text.

Although food insecurity, poor diet quality, and related matters are important social determinants of mental health, a number of crucial issues pertaining to food equity and health equity are also beyond the scope of this book. Such issues include food deserts, food swamps, food apartheid, food justice, and food sovereignty.

Although healthy eating and good nutrition is one crucial element of an overall lifestyle promoting physical and mental health, many other elements of lifestyle are not covered here. For example, as pointed out in Chapter 14, physical activity and exercise are known to be beneficial for physical and mental health (e.g., for depression; Pearce et al. 2022), as are the other pillars of the emerging field of lifestyle medicine, and even more recently, lifestyle psychiatry (Merlo and Fagundes 2023; Noordsy 2019). Fortunately, the same health behaviors that are beneficial to physical health (e.g., weight management, prevention of cardiovascular and metabolic diseases) are beneficial to mental health. In addition to nutrition and physical activity, aspects of lifestyle medicine and lifestyle psychiatry include restorative sleep, stress management, avoidance of risky substances, and positive social connections.

References

Adan RAH, van der Beek EM, Buitelaar JK, et al: Nutritional psychiatry: towards improving mental health by what you eat. Eur Neuropsychopharmacol 29(12):1321–1332, 2019 31735529

Aucoin M, LaChance L, Naidoo U, et al: Diet and anxiety: a scoping review. Nutrients 13(12):4418, 2021 34959972

Bayes J, Schloss J, Sibbritt D: The effect of a Mediterranean diet on the symptoms of depression in young males (the "AMMEND: A Mediterranean Diet in MEN with Depression" study): a randomized controlled trial. Am J Clin Nutr 116(2):572–580, 2022 35441666

Burgess J, Robinson-Wright J, Kennedy D: The Culinary Medicine Textbook: Psychiatry, Food, and Mood. Norwich, VT, Culinary Rehab, 2022

Butler MI, Mörkl S: The Mediterranean diet and mental health, in Nutritional Psychiatry: A Primer for Clinicians. Edited by Dinan T. Cambridge, UK, Cambridge University Press, 2023

Dinan T (ed): Nutritional Psychiatry: A Primer for Clinicians. Cambridge, UK, Cambridge University Press, 2023

Eliby D, Simpson CA, Lawrence AS, et al: Associations between diet quality and anxiety and depressive disorders: a systematic review. J Affect Disord Rep 14:100629, 2023

Estruch R, Ros E, Salas-Salvadó J, et al: Primary prevention of cardiovascular disease with a Mediterranean diet supplemented with extra-virgin olive oil or nuts. N Engl J Med 378(25):e34, 2018 29897866

Głąbska D, Guzek D, Groele B, et al: Fruit and vegetable intake and mental health in adults: a systematic review. Nutrients 12(1):115, 2020 31906271

Jacka FN, O'Neil A, Opie R, et al: A randomised controlled trial of dietary improvement for adults with major depression (the 'SMILES' trial). BMC Med 15(1):23, 2017 28137247

Lane MM, Gamage E, Travica N, et al: Ultra-processed food consumption and mental health: a systematic review and meta-analysis of observational studies. Nutrients 14(13):2568, 2022 35807749

Lewis JE, Poles J, Shaw DP, et al: The effects of twenty-one nutrients and phytonutrients on cognitive function: a narrative review. J Clin Transl Res 7(4):575–620, 2021 34541370

Merlo G, Fagundes CP: Lifestyle Psychiatry: Through the Lens of Behavioral Medicine. Boca Raton, FL, CRC Press, 2023

Mozaffari H, Madani Civi R, Askari M, et al: The impact of food-based dietary strategies on achieving type 2 diabetes remission: a systematic review. Diabetes Metab Syndr 18(8):103096, 2024 39163706

Noordsy DL: Lifestyle Psychiatry. Washington, DC, American Psychiatric Publishing, 2019

Norwitz NG, Naidoo U: Nutrition as metabolic treatment for anxiety. Front Psychiatry 12:598119, 2021 33643090

Panigrahi G, Goodwin SM, Staffier KL, et al: Remission of type 2 diabetes after treatment with a high-fiber, low-fat, plant-predominant diet intervention: a case series. Am J Lifestyle Med 17(6):839–846, 2023 38511112

Pearce M, Garcia L, Abbas A, et al: Association between physical activity and risk of depression: a systematic review and meta-analysis. JAMA Psychiatry 79(6):550–559, 2022 35416941

Picheta N, Piekarz J, Daniłowska K, et al: Phytochemicals in the treatment of patients with depression: a systemic review. Front Psychiatry 9(15):1509109, 2024

Ramsey D: Eat to Beat Depression and Anxiety: Nourish Your Way to Better Mental Health in Six Weeks. New York, Harper Wave, 2021

Sánchez-Villegas A, Martínez-González MA, Estruch R, et al: Mediterranean dietary pattern and depression: the PREDIMED randomized trial. BMC Med 20(11):208, 2013

Sparling TM, Deeney M, Cheng B, et al: Systematic evidence and gap map of research linking food security and nutrition to mental health. Nat Commun 13(1):4608, 2022 35941261

Taylor R, Ramachandran A, Yancy WS, et al: Nutritional basis of type 2 diabetes remission. BMJ 374:n1449, 2021 34233884

2

The Macronutrients: An Introduction to Carbohydrates, Protein, Fat, and Fiber

Heather Seid, D.C.N., R.D.N.

To eat is a necessity, but to eat intelligently is an art.

—Seventeenth-century French author
François VI, Duc de La Rochefoucauld

"Count your macros!" You may have heard this saying echoed in fitness blogs or touted by wellness experts as a way to optimize health. What does it mean to *count macros*? Macronutrients—carbohydrates, proteins, and fats—are essential elements of our diet, crucial for physiological functioning and optimal mental health. Each macronutrient has distinct functions: carbohydrates are the body's primary energy source; proteins are crucial for tissue repair, muscle growth, and neurotransmitter production; and fats support brain structure and function (Bremner et al. 2020). According to the USDA's Dietary Guidelines for Americans (U.S. Department of Agriculture 2020), metaboli-

Table 2.1 **Daily nutritional goals and macronutrient distribution for metabolically healthy adults**

Macronutrients	**Female**			**Male**		
Age (y)	**19–30**	**31–50**	**51+**	**19–30**	**31–50**	**51+**
Calories (kcal/d)	2,000	1,800	1,600	2,400	2,200	2,000
Carbohydrates (% kcal)	45–65	45–65	45–65	45–65	45–65	45–65
Protein (% kcal)	10–35	10–35	10–35	10–35	10–35	10–35
Fat (% kcal)	20–35	20–35	20–35	20–35	20–35	20–35
Fiber (g)	28	25	22	34	31	28

Source. Adapted from the USDA's Dietary Guidelines for Americans 2020–2025; U.S. Department of Agriculture 2020.
Note. 1 g carbohydrate or protein = 4 kcal; 1 g fat = 9 kcal.

cally healthy adults (excluding pregnant and lactating women) should aim to consume 45%–65% of daily calories from carbohydrates, 10%–35% of daily calories from protein, and 20%–35% of daily calories from fat (see Table 2.1).

Counting macros involves tracking the total grams of each macronutrient consumed or calculating the percentage of daily calories each macronutrient contributes. What is often missing in the minutiae of macros, however, is the concept of *diet quality*. Optimizing mental health through diet manipulations requires a recipe that is one part macronutrient amount and one part diet quality. This chapter reviews the relationship between macronutrients and mental health with special attention paid to the quality of foods consumed.

Carbohydrates

Monosaccharides, the simplest form of carbohydrate, consist of a single sugar monomer, such as glucose, fructose, or galactose. Complex carbohydrates break down into monosaccharides to generate energy. Disaccharides, or simple sugars, are two monosaccharides joined by a glycosidic linkage and include sucrose, lactose, and maltose. Polysaccharides, also known as complex carbohydrates or starches, are long chains of monosaccharides bound by glycosidic linkages. Polysaccharides are digested more slowly, promoting satiety, and foods that are high in polysaccharides—such as vegetables, fruits, legumes, and whole grains—also contain an array of vitamins and minerals. Each gram of carbohydrate provides four calories, a unit indicating the amount of energy in food and the amount of energy the body needs to function.

High-carbohydrate foods are an important part of a healthy diet, as they provide the main energy substrate to support physiological functioning and physical activity. Overconsumption of ultraprocessed and low-quality carbohydrates has been linked to obesity, diabetes, and metabolic syndrome, as described by the *carbohydrate-insulin model* (Clemente-Suárez et al. 2022; Sievenpiper 2020). Perhaps surprisingly, clinical investigations of the carbohydrate-insulin model have failed to prove the superiority of low-carbohydrate diets on metabolic improvements and weight loss (Sievenpiper 2020). Rather, the evidence suggests that consumption of high-quality carbohydrates, which contain high levels of fiber and micronutrients (e.g., vitamins such as the B vitamins and minerals such as iron), are beneficial for weight management, lowering cardiometabolic risk factors, and improving diversity of the gut microbiome (Sievenpiper 2020).

Generally, high-quality carbohydrates (i.e., complex carbohydrates) are plant-based foods consumed close to their natural form, with minimal processing or refinement. Examples include whole grains such as oats, barley, farro, and brown rice; pseudocereals such as amaranth and quinoa; legumes such as beans, peas, and lentils; most vegetables; and various fruits. In contrast, low-quality carbohydrates undergo extensive refinement during manufacturing and include sugar-sweetened beverages, white bread, commercial desserts, and ultraprocessed snacks such as potato chips, candy, cookies, and crackers.

Carbohydrate Intake and Mental Health

There are scientific limitations to consider when evaluating the relationship between nutritional intake and mental health. First, behavioral health risks are influenced by a complex interplay of environmental, social, biological, and genetic factors (Kirkpatrick et al. 2019). Unsurprisingly, pinpointing any single factor in the investigated relationship is challenging. Second, epidemiological exploration of diet and behavioral health disorders is particularly prone to reverse causation (Kirkpatrick et al. 2019). Likely, a bidirectional relationship exists, in which optimal mental health promotes healthy lifestyle practices, which reinforces and promotes mental health and well-being (Begdache and Patrissy 2021). Conversely, suboptimal lifestyle practices (including poor diet quality) may lead to compromised mental health, in turn leading to future reinforcement of unhealthy lifestyle practices. Therefore, the temporality of the relationship between diet quality and mental health is difficult to establish in observational or cohort studies (Begdache and Patrissy 2021).

In acknowledgment of the limitations of nutritional research, emerging evidence suggests links between carbohydrate intake and mental health (Kirkpatrick et al. 2019). High-quality carbohydrates, rich in fiber, lead to slower glucose release and a tempered insulin response, which has been associated with better mood regulation (Kirkpatrick et al. 2019). By contrast, greater ingestion of simple and refined carbohydrates leads to blood sugar spikes and crashes, which can negatively impact mood and may exacerbate emotional volatility (Kirkpatrick et al. 2019).

Micronutrients in complex carbohydrates, such as vitamin B_6, vitamin B_{12}, and folic acid (folate), are necessary for producing neurotransmitters such as serotonin, dopamine, and norepinephrine, which have key roles in regulating mood and appetite (Sarris et al. 2015). When diet quality is poor, there is an increased risk of nutritional deficiencies and related mood disturbances (Sarris et al. 2015). Increasingly, correcting nutritional deficiencies through supplementation and whole foods as monotherapy or augmentation therapy is showing promise in the treatment of some behavioral health disorders (Sarris et al. 2015).

Mental Illnesses and Carbohydrate Intake

Individuals with mental health conditions such as depression and anxiety may crave carbohydrate-rich foods and simple sugars. These foods may temporarily increase serotonin levels and thus may be unwittingly used as a strategy by patients to improve symptoms. However, this can create a harmful cycle in which the short-term mood improvement ultimately worsens mental health over time because of the low nutritional quality of these foods and the overall diet. Additionally, excessive intake of simple carbohydrate foods can lead to increased weight, obesity, and metabolic syndrome, all of which are associated with increased risk for depression (Varaee et al. 2023).

Depression is specifically believed to be interconnected with obesity in mutually reinforcing cycles of physiological adaptations, biological changes, and behavioral factors (Milaneschi et al. 2019). Interestingly though, research does not support a significant association between low-carbohydrate diets and improvements in depression and anxiety symptoms (Kirkpatrick et al. 2019; Varaee et al. 2023). Rather, there is accumulating evidence from interventional and observational studies regarding the importance of diet quality, rather than rote macronutrient manipulation, in improving and managing mental health conditions throughout the lifespan (Loughman et al. 2021; Sarris et al. 2015).

The focus on diet quality takes on added importance when considering the metabolic effects of many psychiatric medications. Several medications used to treat a variety of psychiatric disorders (including major depression, bipolar disorder, and schizophrenia) carry adverse metabolic consequences (Abosi et al. 2018). Specifically, weight gain is a concern with psychotropic medications that potentially influence weight by interfering with the regulation of leptin and adiponectin (Ricken et al. 2016). Additionally, some antipsychotics and antidepressants may heighten cravings for carbohydrates, which can lead to potential weight gain and further influence mental health in a negative feedback loop (Ricken et al. 2016).

Protein

Amino acids are the building blocks of protein. There are 20 amino acids; 9 are essential and 11 nonessential. The nine essential amino acids are phenylalanine, valine, threonine, tryptophan, isoleucine, methionine, histidine, leucine, and lysine (remembered with the mnemonic PVT TIM HiLL), and these must be supplied from the diet. The nonessential amino acids, which can be produced by the body, are alanine, arginine, asparagine, aspartic acid, cysteine, glutamic acid, glutamine, glycine, proline, serine, and tyrosine. In times of stress and catabolic illness, however, some amino acids (arginine, cysteine, glutamine, glycine, proline, serine, and tyrosine) become conditionally essential and require supplementation from the diet to avoid deficiencies.

Like carbohydrates, proteins provide four calories per gram. Protein is essential for growing and repairing body tissues, producing hormones and enzymes, providing structural support, and producing neurotransmitters. With regard to dietary intake, a *complete protein* contains all nine essential amino acids in sufficient amounts required by the body. Animal-based foods are typically complete protein sources and include foods such as eggs, fish, poultry, meat, and dairy products. Some plant-based foods, such as chia seeds, quinoa, and soy, are also complete proteins. Nuts, seeds, grains, and legumes are excellent sources of protein, even though they may not contain the complete complement of essential amino acids. Individuals who follow a vegetarian or vegan diet should be advised to consume two or more complementary plant-based pro-

Table 2.2 **Plant-based proteins, their specific limited amino acids, and complementary approaches for a complete protein**

Food	Limited amino acid	Complement
Legumes	Methionine	Grains, nuts, seeds
Grains	Lysine, threonine	Legumes
Nuts, seeds	Lysine	Legumes
Vegetables	Methionine	Grains, nuts, seeds
Corn	Tryptophan, lysine	Legumes

Source. Adapted from American Society for Nutrition 2011.

teins to receive the full essential amino acid distribution throughout the day. As shown in Table 2.2, this can be accomplished by combining legumes and grains (e.g., beans and rice, hummus with pita, peanut butter on whole-grain bread), which create complete proteins.

Like carbohydrates, protein can be examined from quantitative and qualitative standpoints. First, adequate intake of dietary protein is requisite for optimal functioning. Healthy adults require 0.8–1.2 g/kg/day, and individuals ≥65 years of age and adults with obesity require ≥1.2 g/kg/day. Individualized protein needs depend on many factors such as age, sex, physical activity level, and comorbidities. The majority of protein intake should be from lean sources (low in saturated fat—see more on this in the next section), such as poultry, fish, low-fat dairy products, and plant-based foods (Clemente-Suárez et al. 2022). Patients should be encouraged to limit high-fat meats (such as fatty cuts of red meat) and those that have undergone considerable processing (such as deli meats, hot dogs/sausages, low-quality protein powder, and ultraprocessed meat substitutions). Additionally, meats prepared using high-fat cooking methods such as deep-frying, pan-frying, and stir-frying should be limited or avoided, regardless of the type of meat. Rather, meats should be prepared by steaming, baking, poaching, and sautéing with small amounts of fat or oil.

Overall, diets that rely on greater consumption of plant-based protein sources are associated with better cardiovascular and metabolic health outcomes compared with animal-based protein diets (Ferrari et al. 2022). As an added bonus, vegetable-based protein sources have a lower environmental impact. Production of plant-based proteins is typically more sustainable, requires fewer natural resources for production, and causes less greenhouse gas emissions than production of animal-based proteins (Ferrari et al. 2022). Recent evidence also suggests that animal-based protein intake is associated with an increased risk of depression, anxiety, and stress, particularly in women; this relationship was not observed in individuals consuming high amounts of plant-based protein (Sheikhi et al. 2023). Shifting toward plant-based proteins can benefit both personal health and the planet, as detailed in Chapter 15, "Food Production and Mental Health."

Protein Intake and Mental Health

Research suggests that adequate protein intake is beneficial for optimal mental health and may improve mood regulation, enhance cognition, and reduce the risk of depression (Sarris et al. 2015). Importantly, consuming a calorically adequate diet with a full complement of amino acids has been shown to reduce the risk of mental health symptoms (Sarris et al. 2015). The amino acids tryptophan, tyrosine, and phenylalanine are used to synthesize neurotransmitters, and studies indicate that these amino acids are significantly lower in patients with depressive symptoms compared with healthy individuals (Jacobs et al. 2000). In interventional trials, tryptophan-depleted diets resulted in lower serotonin levels and reports of poor memory and depressed mood (Biskup et al. 2012; Riedel et al. 1999; Sarris et al. 2015). Including a variety of protein sources in the diet can help ensure that these key amino acids are available for neurotransmitter production and maintenance of optimal emotional and cognitive functioning.

Mental Illnesses and Protein Intake

For individuals with mental illnesses, sufficient protein intake (≥0.8–1.2 g/kg/day) can lessen the severity of symptoms and be an effective tool for managing some side effects of psychiatric medications (Sarris et al. 2015). For example, individuals with schizophrenia or bipolar disorder may also experience decreased cognitive functioning, which contributes to problems with activities of daily living and decreased quality of life (Bremner et al. 2020). In this population, inadequate dietary protein intake is associated with reduced cognitive functioning—particularly in measures of memory and language processing (Biskup et al. 2012; Riedel et al. 1999). Strategies to increase total protein intake from high-quality protein sources should be included as a means to lessen potential cognitive impairment.

Along with cognitive benefits, adequate protein intake may also play a role in managing the weight challenges often faced by individuals with psychiatric conditions. There is a bidirectional relationship between obesity and psychiatric disorders, with obesity being two to three times more prevalent among individuals with psychiatric conditions versus the general population (Loughman et al. 2021). Conversely, individuals with obesity are more likely to experience psychiatric illnesses than those of normal weight (BMI 18–25 kg/m^2) (Loughman et al. 2021). This risk is further compounded by the metabolic side effects of many medications used to treat psychiatric disorders, such as those for major depression, bipolar disorder, and schizophrenia, which often cause or exacerbate weight gain (Abosi et al. 2018). Adequate protein intake may help mitigate weight gain by promoting satiety and reducing sugar cravings. Protein consumption decreases levels of ghrelin (a hormone that plays a key role in regulating appetite and energy balance) while increasing levels of appetite-suppressing hormones such as glucagon-like peptide 1 (GLP-1), cholecystokinin, and peptide YY (Paddon-Jones et al. 2008). Moreover, protein helps stabilize blood sugar levels, preventing drastic fluctuations in glucose that can lead to sugar cravings and overeating (Paddon-Jones et al. 2008).

Fat

Since the 1980s, dietary fat has been widely criticized by both the scientific community and mainstream media, leading to the widespread adoption of low-fat diets as a strategy for promoting weight loss and heart health (La Berge 2008). Supermarket shelves remain filled with low-fat and fat-free products, many of which are counterintuitive (e.g., fat-free coffee creamer, a form of ultraprocessed food). A shift in perspective has emerged, however, with growing recognition of the benefits of Mediterranean and Blue Zone diets, prompting a more balanced and moderate approach to fat intake.

Fats are categorized as either *unsaturated* or *saturated*, which refers to the types of chemical bonds between carbon atoms. Unsaturated fats have at least one (mono) double bond or more (poly) double bonds between carbon atoms. Most *monounsaturated fatty acids* (MUFAs) are omega-9 (e.g., oleic acid), although MUFAs can also belong to other omega families. Nutritionally significant *polyunsaturated fatty acids* (PUFAs) are primarily omega-3 and omega-6 fatty acids. Food sources of these fatty acids are given in Table 2.3. The three main omega-3 fatty acids are

Table 2.3 Sources of dietary fat by category

Fat category	Dietary source
Saturated fat	Red/fatty meats: beef, pork, lamb Full-fat dairy: butter, cheese, whole milk, ghee yogurt Lard, tallow Coconut and palm oil
Polyunsaturated fat (omega-3 and omega-6)	Omega-3 Canola oil (rapeseed oil) Chia seeds Edamame/soybeans Fatty fish (e.g. salmon, tuna, mackerel, herring, trout) Flaxseed and flaxseed oil Hemp seeds Nuts and nut oils: walnuts, pecans, pistachios, macadamia Seaweed and marine algae (e.g. spirulina) Omega-6 Avocado and avocado oil Chicken and chicken skin Egg yolks Nuts and seeds: almonds, cashews, pumpkin seeds, sunflower seeds Peanut butter and peanut oil Oils: almond, cashew, corn, grapeseed, safflower, sunflower, soybean
Monounsaturated fat (omega-9)	Olives Avocados Olive, avocado, and canola oil Sesame seeds Nuts: peanuts, almonds, hazelnuts, cashews
Trans Fat	Processed foods: margarine, shortening, baked goods, fried foods Some processed meat Small amounts naturally occur in dairy products

Note. Foods typically contain a combination of different types of fats, with varying proportions of saturated, monounsaturated, and polyunsaturated fats. Both omega-3 and omega-6 fatty acids are essential for health, but maintaining an appropriate balance between the two (ideally in a 1:1–1:4 ratio of omega-3 to omega-6) is important for reducing inflammation and supporting overall health.

α-linolenic acid, eicosapentaenoic acid, and docosahexaenoic acid. Saturated fatty acids contain only single bonds between carbon atoms. Trans fats, in contrast, are unsaturated fatty acids with at least one double bond in the trans configuration. They occur naturally in small amounts in ruminant products and more commonly through industrial hydrogenation of oils. All fats, regardless of chemical structure, provide nine calories per gram (more than twice as much as the four per gram from carbohydrates and protein) and are vitally important for vitamin and nutrient metabolism, hormone production, energy, energy storage, and cell structure.

A body of evidence explores the relationship between dietary fat intake and disease risk. A recent aggregation of prospective cohort studies mainly found no association of total fat, MUFAs, and PUFAs with risk of chronic diseases when comparing the highest versus lowest intake categories (Schwingshackl et al. 2021). A higher intake of total saturated and trans fats from processed foods (but not from naturally occurring trans fats in dairy products) was associated with an increased risk of cardiovascular disease and mortality (Schwingshackl et al. 2021). Additionally, reviews of randomized, controlled trials performing substitution evaluations found that replacing dietary saturated fats with PUFAs or MUFAs improves blood lipids and glycemic control, with the effect of PUFAs being more pronounced (Schwingshackl et al. 2021). Generally, the available evidence supports dietary strategies to replace saturated fats with MUFAs and PUFAs and avoid consumption of industrial trans fats to improve overall health and well-being.

Fat Intake and Mental Health

The types and amounts of fat consumed are an important risk factor for not only cardiometabolic health but also mental health. The brain contains a high concentration of lipids, and dietary fatty acids influence specific brain regions to regulate processes affecting emotion, behavior, and cognition (Tsuboi et al. 2013). In recent years, research has explored the connections between fatty acids and depression, focusing on the role of inflammation and oxidative stress (Tsuboi et al. 2013). Saturated fats yield greater oxidative stress in vivo. Individuals with higher saturated fat intake have more depressive symptoms and increased rates of irritability, aggression, and cognitive decline versus individuals with lower saturated fat intake (Tsuboi et al. 2013). MUFAs, on the other hand, tend to be inversely associated with depressive symptoms (Wolfe et al. 2009).

When evaluating the relationship between PUFA intake and depression, it is important to evaluate omega-3 and omega-6 fatty acids individually. Omega-3 fatty acids are often reported as being positively associated with improvements in depressive symptoms (Wolfe et al. 2009). Omega-3s have anti-inflammatory properties and enhance neurotransmitter function. Conversely, omega-6 fatty acids have been positively associated with an increased risk of depressive symptoms (Wolfe et al. 2009).

The Western diet has a low ratio of omega-3 to omega-6 fatty acids. The optimal ratio for cardiometabolic health is 1:1–1:4, whereas the typical Western diet has a ratio of about 1:10–15 (Martínez García et al. 2018). The omega-6s in the Western diet primarily come from widespread overconsumption of processed vegetable oils (e.g., corn and soybean) rather than whole food sources such as nuts and seeds. A typical Mediterranean diet, on the other hand, has an omega-3 to omega-6 ratio of 1:5, and the majority of omega-6s are from unprocessed sources (Martínez García et al. 2018). Generally, studies suggest that a Mediterranean dietary pattern may decrease the risk of depression, whereas a Western-style diet may increase the risk of depression (Li et al. 2017). More randomized, controlled trials and cohort studies are required to identify the ideal macronutrient distribution and diet composition to optimize mental health.

Mental Health and Fat Intake

Currently, more than 50% of energy purchased by U.S. households comes from moderately processed to ultraprocessed food (UPF) (Poti et al. 2015). UPF seems to be a dominant and unyielding part of U.S. consumer intake patterns, and unsurprisingly, UPF is known to have higher fat content—specifically in the form of saturated fats (Poti et al. 2015). For numerous reasons, mental health issues are also correlated with higher intake of UPFs and convenience foods (Ejtahed et al. 2024). Increased intake of UPF leads to higher consumption of saturated fats, which can raise inflammation levels and, in turn, heighten the risk of depression and other mental health symptoms and conditions.

The bidirectional relationship between poor mental health and poor diet creates a harmful, reinforcing cycle. However, there is an opportunity for a positive shift. With the right resources and support, individuals who make healthier, high-quality food choices, such as reducing UPF and saturated fat intake and replacing them with more PUFAs and

MUFAs, can experience positive improvements in their mental health (Ejtahed et al. 2024). Working with a registered dietitian is essential for personalized guidance and expert support. As members of the care team, dietitians can help patients develop sustainable and effective nutrition plans for improving health and diet quality.

Fiber

Fiber is a term for the indigestible parts of plant-based foods, primarily carbohydrates, that pass through the digestive system relatively intact. Rather than being treated as a distinct macronutrient category, dietary fiber is classified as a type of carbohydrate and is categorized by solubility, viscosity, and fermentability. Only a small amount of fiber is metabolized in the stomach and small intestine; most dietary fiber is excreted as waste. During transit through the gastrointestinal (GI) tract, fiber serves many beneficial roles.

Soluble fiber attracts water and becomes a gel-matrix during digestion, which slows the transit of *chyme* (partly digested food) through the small intestine and slows nutrient absorption. The soluble fiber gelatinous network traps dietary cholesterol, limiting reabsorption into the bloodstream. Slower digestion and nutrient transit stabilize blood glucose and subsequent insulin response. Additionally, soluble fiber adds fluid and bulk to the stool, which helps to make bowel movements easier and alleviates and prevents constipation. Good sources of soluble fiber are oat bran, barley, beans, lentils, seeds, nuts, and most fruits and vegetables.

Insoluble fiber does not dissolve in water and passes through the GI system relatively intact. Insoluble fiber moves waste through the small intestine and supports healthy digestion. Additionally, insoluble fiber slows the absorption of dietary sugar and carbohydrates and effectively manages blood glucose. Good sources of insoluble fiber include fruits, vegetables, nuts, seeds, and whole grains. Insoluble fiber is naturally more prevalent in the skins and seeds of fruits, so consuming foods with these components intact is helpful for increasing intake of insoluble fiber (e.g., skins of apples and eggplant; seeds of cucumbers and tomatoes).

Both soluble and insoluble fiber play important roles in improving GI motility, managing lipid and glucose levels, promoting satiety, and maintaining stable weight. Arguably, though, one of the most significant health benefits of dietary fiber is its positive impact on intestinal microbiota. Soluble fiber acts as a food source (prebiotic) for beneficial bacteria in the large intestine. When microbiota consume soluble fiber, they release short-chain fatty acids that support gut health and overall well-being. Short-chain fatty acids, particularly butyrate, help to reduce inflammation, maintain the intestinal barrier, and suppress the growth of pathogenic bacteria (Clemente-Suárez et al. 2022). Insoluble fiber is generally poorly fermented by the gut microbiota, but it does reduce waste transit time and thus limits colonic bacterial fermentation time.

According to the 2020–2025 Dietary Guidelines for Americans (U.S. Department of Agriculture 2020), more than 90% of women and 97% of men do not meet the recommended intakes for dietary fiber. This is attributed to underconsumption of whole grains, fruits, and vegetables, which is a dietary pattern observed in more than 85% of U.S. adults. Adult men and women need a minimum of 25–30 g of fiber per day (with no upper limit established). Individuals with suboptimal fiber intake should be encouraged to slowly increase their daily intake—accompanied by increased water intake—until tolerance is established. Increasing fiber too quickly may lead to GI upset, nausea, diarrhea, constipation, gas, bloating, and in some cases, vitamin and mineral deficiencies. Whenever possible, it is recommended to increase fiber through whole foods rather than supplements (for the added benefit of increased vitamins, minerals, and an ideal soluble fiber/insoluble fiber mix). Fiber supplements may be useful, however, for maximizing the health benefits of fiber while working toward improved diet quality.

Fiber Intake and Mental Health

Fiber is a crucial component of a healthy diet. Research suggests inverse associations between dietary fiber intake and depressive symptoms (Swann et al. 2020). The hypothesized mechanisms center around the role dietary fiber plays in attenuating systemic inflammation and oxidative stress. It is possible that adequate fiber intake drives gene expression of the gut microbiome and leads to increased production of neurotransmitters (Swann et al. 2020). Additionally, decreased systemic inflammation may alter some neurotransmitter concentrations and thereby reduce depressive symptoms (Swann et al. 2020).

Interestingly, there appears to be an inverse dose–response relationship between dietary fiber intake and depressive and anxiety symptoms. A recent meta-analysis found that each 5 g increase in fiber intake was associated with a 5% lower risk of depression (Saghafian et al. 2023). Additionally, in adults with overweight or obesity, higher intake of dietary fiber was related to a decreased risk of reported psychological distress (Saghafian et al. 2023). In normal-weight individuals, high dietary fiber intake was associated with a lower risk of anxiety symptoms (Saghafian et al. 2023). Research findings vary depending on the population studied and the type and amount of fiber, and thus additional studies are needed to clarify this relationship and confirm the underlying physiological mechanisms.

Clinical Pearls

- Clinicians should understand that dietary intake of complex carbohydrates (found in vegetables, fruits, and legumes) and healthy fats (especially omega-3s in certain fish, seeds, and nuts) are linked to improvements in mental health symptoms.
- Clinicians should understand that adequate protein intake is essential for neurotransmitter production. Plant-derived proteins are generally richer in fiber and certain vitamins and minerals (such as magnesium and folate), whereas animal proteins provide other nutrients such asvitamin B12, heme iron, and zinc.
- It is important for clinicians to recognize the reinforcing and bidirectional relationship between poor diet quality and poor mental health.
- Clinicians should be aware that psychotropic medications can influence appetite and dietary choices and reinforce unhealthy eating patterns.
- When indicated, clinicians should enlist the support of a registered dietitian early in the treatment plan.

Key Chapter Points

- Macronutrients—carbohydrates, proteins, and fats—are essential components of our diet. All are crucial for optimal physiological functioning and mental health.
- Although not a macronutrient, fiber is an integral component of a healthy diet. Gut health is influenced by fiber intake and has a significant impact on mental well-being. Foods such as whole grains, legumes, fruits, and vegetables, which contain an array of soluble and insoluble fiber, should be consumed daily.
- Individuals with mental health conditions, including serious mental illness, frequently experience poor diet quality influenced by a variety of internal and external factors. Internally, challenges

such as low energy or motivation for meal planning and preparation and appetite changes may negatively impact food choices. Externally, barriers such as limited access to nutritious foods (e.g., residing in a food desert), insufficient skills to obtain and prepare healthy meals, and inadequate awareness of the connection between diet and mental health may further contribute to poor dietary patterns.

- As health care providers, we must work on addressing the factors that influence food choice to help patients improve their diet quality and, ultimately, their health.
- Seeking support from a registered dietitian is an effective strategy for maximizing health benefits associated with optimal dietary intake. Collaborating with a dietitian helps individuals build sustainable eating habits tailored to their unique needs and challenges.

References

Abosi O, Lopes S, Schmitz S, et al: Cardiometabolic effects of psychotropic medications. Horm Mol Biol Clin Investig 36(1):/j/hmbci.2018.36.issue-1/hmbci-2017-0065/hmbci-2017–0065.xml, 2018 29320364

American Society for Nutrition: Protein complementation, 2011. Available at: https://nutrition.org/protein-complementation/. Accessed January 6, 2025.

Begdache L, Patrissy CM: Customization of diet may promote exercise and improve mental wellbeing in mature adults: the role of exercise as a mediator. J Pers Med 11(5):435, 2021 34069663

Biskup CS, Sánchez CL, Arrant A, et al: Effects of acute tryptophan depletion on brain serotonin function and concentrations of dopamine and norepinephrine in C57BL/6J and BALB/cJ mice. PLoS One 7(5):e35916, 2012 22629305

Bremner JD, Moazzami K, Wittbrodt MT, et al: Diet, stress, and mental health. Nutrients 12(8):2428, 2020 32823562

Clemente-Suárez VJ, Mielgo-Ayuso J, Martín-Rodríguez A, et al: The burden of carbohydrates in health and disease. Nutrients 14(18):380, 2022 36145184

Ejtahed HS, Mardi P, Hejrani B, et al: Association between junk food consumption and mental health problems in adults: a systematic review and meta-analysis. BMC Psychiatry 24(1):438, 2024 38867156

Ferrari L, Panaite SA, Bertazzo A, et al: Animal- and plant-based protein sources: a scoping review of human health outcomes and environmental impact. Nutrients 14(23):5115, 2022 36501146

Jacobs BL, van Praag H, Gage FH: Adult brain neurogenesis and psychiatry: a novel theory of depression. Mol Psychiatry 5(3):262–269, 2000 10889528

Kirkpatrick CF, Bolick JP, Kris-Etherton PM, et al: Review of current evidence and clinical recommendations on the effects of low-carbohydrate and very-low-carbohydrate (including ketogenic) diets for the management of body weight and other cardiometabolic risk factors: a scientific statement from the National Lipid Association Nutrition and Lifestyle Task Force. J Clin Lipidol 13(5):689–711.e1, 2019 31611148

La Berge AF: How the ideology of low fat conquered America. J Hist Med Allied Sci 63(2):139–177, 2008 18296750

Li Y, Lv MR, Wei YJ, et al: Dietary patterns and depression risk: a meta-analysis. Psychiatry Res 253:373–382, 2017 28431261

Loughman A, Staudacher HM, Rocks T, et al: Diet and mental health. Mod Trends Psychiatry 32:100–112, 2021 34032648

Martínez García RM, Jiménez Ortega AI, López Sobaler AM, et al: Nutrition strategies that improve cognitive function. Nutr Hosp 35(Spec No6):16–19, 2018 30351155

Milaneschi Y, Simmons WK, van Rossum EFC, et al: Depression and obesity: evidence of shared biological mechanisms. Mol Psychiatry 24(1):18–33, 2019 29453413

Paddon-Jones D, Westman E, Mattes RD, et al: Protein, weight management, and satiety. Am J Clin Nutr 87(5):1558S–1561S, 2008 18469287

Poti JM, Mendez MA, Ng SW, et al: Is the degree of food processing and convenience linked with the nutritional quality of foods purchased by US households? Am J Clin Nutr 101(6):1251–1262, 2015 25948666

Ricken R, Bopp S, Schlattmann P, et al: Leptin serum concentrations are associated with weight gain during lithium augmentation. Psychoneuroendocrinology 71:31–35, 2016 27235637

Riedel WJ, Klaassen T, Deutz NE, et al: Tryptophan depletion in normal volunteers produces selective impairment in memory consolidation. Psychopharmacology (Berl) 141(4):362–369, 1999 10090643

Saghafian F, Hajishafiee M, Rouhani P, et al: Dietary fiber intake, depression, and anxiety: a systematic review and meta-analysis of epidemiologic studies. Nutr Neurosci 26(2):108–126, 2023 36692989

Sarris J, Logan AC, Akbaraly TN, et al: Nutritional medicine as mainstream in psychiatry. Lancet Psychiatry 2(3):271–274, 2015 26359904

Schwingshackl L, Zähringer J, Beyerbach J, et al: Total dietary fat intake, fat quality, and health outcomes: a scoping review of systematic reviews of prospective studies. Ann Nutr Metab 77(1):4–15, 2021 33789278

Sheikhi A, Siassi F, Djazayery A, et al: Plant and animal protein intake and its association with depression, anxiety, and stress among Iranian women. BMC Public Health 23(1):161, 2023 36694166

Sievenpiper JL: Low-carbohydrate diets and cardiometabolic health: the importance of carbohydrate quality over quantity. Nutr Rev 78(Suppl 1):69–77, 2020 32728757

Swann OG, Kilpatrick M, Breslin M, et al: Dietary fiber and its associations with depression and inflammation. Nutr Rev 78(5):394–411, 2020 31750916

Tsuboi H, Watanabe M, Kobayashi F, et al: Associations of depressive symptoms with serum proportions of palmitic and arachidonic acids, and α-tocopherol effects among male population: a preliminary study. Clin Nutr 32(2):289–293, 2013 22901744

U.S. Department of Agriculture: Dietary Guidelines for Americans, 2020–2025 (9th ed.): U.S. Government Printing Office, 2020. Available at: https://www.dietaryguidelines.gov/sites/default/files/2020-12/Dietary_Guidelines_for_Americans_2020-2025.pdf. Accessed January 6, 2025.

Varaee H, Darand M, Hassanizadeh S, et al: Effect of low-carbohydrate diet on depression and anxiety: a systematic review and meta-analysis of controlled trials. J Affect Disord 325:206–214, 2023 36584702

Wolfe AR, Ogbonna EM, Lim S, et al: Dietary linoleic and oleic fatty acids in relation to severe depressed mood: 10 years follow-up of a national cohort. Prog Neuropsychopharmacol Biol Psychiatry 33(6):972–977, 2009 19427349

3

The Micronutrients: An Introduction to Vitamins, Minerals, and Phytonutrients

Michael T. Compton, M.D., M.P.H.

By the proper intakes of vitamins and other nutrients and by following a few other healthful practices from youth or middle age on, you can, I believe, extend your life and years of well-being by twenty-five or even thirty-five years.

—Linus Pauling

Unlike the macronutrients (carbohydrates, proteins, and fats)—which are the essential nutrients that the body needs in large quantities for energy, structural components for various bodily functions, and overall health—the micronutrients (vitamins and minerals) are essential nutrients needed in smaller amounts for diverse physiologic functions. *Vitamins* are organic compounds essential for an organism's health, required for diverse metabolic functions, including normal cell growth and development, building and repairing tissues, energy production, vision, blood clotting, bone health, and immune function. They are not synthesized in sufficient amounts by the body and thus must be obtained through the diet. Similarly, *minerals* (such as calcium, chloride, iron, magnesium, phosphorus, potassium, selenium, sodium, and zinc) are essential nutrients that the body needs to develop and function properly. Like vitamins, they play a crucial role in various physiological processes; unlike vitamins, they are inorganic elements. The body cannot produce them; they are found in the earth and in various types of food. *Phytonutrients*—also known as phytochemicals—are natural compounds found in plants that contribute to their color, flavor, and disease resistance. They are not considered essential or required nutrients like vitamins and minerals, but they play a significant role in promoting health and reducing the risk of chronic diseases. This chapter provides a brief introduction to vitamins, minerals, and phytonutrients, highlighting their relevance to mental health, and aims to increase awareness among mental health practitioners.

Fat-Soluble Vitamins

The fat-soluble vitamins include vitamins A, D, E, and K. They can dissolve in fats and oils and are absorbed along with fats in the diet. The fat-soluble vitamins are stored in the body's fatty tissue and in the liver; as such, they are retained by the body for a longer period than water-soluble vitamins. As a consequence, they can potentially reach toxic levels if intake exceeds the body's ability to store and use them, which would likely only occur through high doses of supplements rather than through routine dietary sources. On the other hand, individuals with fat malabsorption (e.g., Crohn's disease, cystic fibrosis, pancreatic disorders) or those on low-fat diets may be at risk for deficiency. A brief overview of key physiological functions of these four vitamins—along with indications of deficiency and toxicity—is provided in Table 3.1.

Vitamin A (retinol, retinal, retinoic acid) is a group of vital micronutrients that play an essential role in maintaining healthy vision, immune function, and skin health. Some of the most common dietary sources of vitamin A include fish, dairy products, and fruits and vegetables rich in beta-carotene, such as carrots, sweet potatoes, and spinach, among many other fruits and vegetables. Specifically, animal-based food products are a rich source of the retinyl ester form of the vitamin, whereas vegetables and fruits contain carotenoids, most of which are provitamin A (Carazo et al. 2021). Unsurprisingly, given that vitamin A inter-

Table 3.1 Overview of key physiological functions, and indications of deficiency and toxicity, of the four fat-soluble vitamins

Vitamin	Functions and indications	Consequences of deficiency	Consequences of toxicity
A, retinol	Corneal and conjunctival development; normal vision; cellular growth and development; fetal bone and central nervous system development; epithelial, bone, and tooth growth; immune system functioning; formation and maintenance of skin, hair, and mucous membranes; skin health	Night blindness, xerophthalmia (dryness of the eyes, which can potentially lead to corneal damage and blindness), dry and cracked skin, increased susceptibility to infections, delayed growth and development in children, and infertility and reproductive issues	Liver damage, joint pain, and birth defects during pregnancy
D, calciferol	Calcium and phosphorus absorption and metabolism; bone and tooth formation and mineralization; bone health, skeletal homeostasis, and skeletal muscle function; neuromuscular activity; immune system functioning; parathyroid hormone secretion regulation	Fatigue, bone pain, muscle weakness, frequent infections, slow wound healing, depression or anxiety, and hair loss	High blood calcium levels, potentially leading to kidney stones, organ damage, and irregular heartbeat

Table 3.1 Overview of key physiological functions, and indications of deficiency and toxicity, of the four fat-soluble vitamins (*continued*)

Vitamin	Functions and indications	Consequences of deficiency	Consequences of toxicity
E, tocopherol	Antioxidant and anti-inflammatory effects; skin health; immune system functioning; platelet coagulation inhibition; cellular signaling	Muscle weakness, loss of coordination, nerve damage, anemia, skin problems (e.g., dryness, flakiness), impaired immune function, and night blindness	Toxicity can cause impaired blood clotting, leading to hemorrhages and stroke
K, phyllo-quinone	Blood clotting; bone health; cardiovascular health	Easy bruising, bleeding (e.g., nosebleeds, bleeding gums, heavy menstrual bleeding, prolonged bleeding after injuries or surgery, spontaneous hematomas), sleepiness, vomiting, seizures, petechiae, pale skin, and reduced bone strength (and thus increased risk of osteoporosis)	Hemolytic anemia, liver damage, and jaundice

acts with multiple molecular targets, including nuclear receptors, opsin in the retina, and some enzymes (Carazo et al. 2021), a deficiency in vitamin A can lead to serious health issues, including vision problems such as night blindness, increased susceptibility to infections, and skin disorders. Low vitamin A may also affect mental health by contributing to mood disturbances. For example, a meta-analysis that included 25 observational studies (involving 100,955 participants) demonstrated that dietary vitamin A intake was inversely associated with depression (risk ratio [RR] 0.83, 95% CI 0.70–1.00; $P = 0.05$) and that dietary vitamin A intake among individuals with depression was lower than in control subjects; similar findings were observed for dietary beta-carotene in particular (Zhang et al. 2022). Conversely, excessive intake of vitamin A, particularly in the form of supplements, can lead to toxicity, resulting in symptoms such as nausea, headaches, dizziness, and even neurological issues. Because of a teratogenic risk, supplementation should be avoided during pregnancy.

Vitamin D (cholecalciferol) helps regulate calcium and phosphorus in the body, promoting healthy bone and tooth formation, among other physiologic functions. Major dietary sources of vitamin D include fatty fish such as salmon, fortified dairy products, and egg yolks. Another source is exposure to sunlight, which stimulates the synthesis of vitamin D in the skin. Deficiencies in vitamin D can lead to health issues such as rickets in children, osteomalacia in adults, and increased risk of osteoporosis; it has also been associated with mood disorders such as depression and anxiety. Some populations may be at elevated risk for vitamin D deficiency, such as people with darker skin tones, those with limited sun exposure (such as in the lower or higher latitudes), individuals with obesity, and older adults. Vitamin D plays a neuroprotective role, by influencing serotonin synthesis and brain plasticity, for example—physiologic processes that are relevant for diverse mental health conditions such as depression and anxiety. Vitamin D supplementation has been shown to reduce the incidence of depression and improve depressive symptoms in adults with primary depression (Mikola et al. 2023; Musazadeh et al. 2023; Wang et al. 2024; Xie et al. 2022); most studies involve individuals who are not vitamin D deficient, although supplementation may be even more beneficial among those who are. Studies have also shown potential positive effects of vitamin D on mental health in children (Głąbska et al. 2021), and deficiency in vitamin D has been associated with an increased risk of ADHD, anxiety, and suicide. It should be noted that excessive levels of vitamin D can result in hypercalcemia, which can cause nausea, weakness, and cognitive impairments; as such, maintaining normal levels of vitamin D is essential.

Vitamin E (tocopherol) is a powerful antioxidant that plays a crucial role in protecting cells from oxidative damage and supporting immune function. Dietary sources of vitamin E include nuts, seeds, broccoli, peppers, tomatoes, and leafy green vegetables such as spinach, Swiss chard, beet greens, turnip greens, mustard greens, and collard greens, as well as plant oils such as sunflower and olive oil. Deficiency in vitamin E can lead to neurological problems, as it may cause issues with coordination and sensory functions and may also negatively impact mental health. Because inflammatory and oxidative pathways are now known to play a role in depression and anxiety, lower serum levels of antioxidants such as vitamin E have been implicated in both disorders (Lee et al. 2022), although more research is needed. Excessive intake of vitamin E, particularly through supplements, may increase risk of bleeding and other adverse effects.

Vitamin K (phylloquinone) is vital for proper blood clotting and plays an essential role in bone metabolism and cardiovascular health. Key dietary sources of vitamin K include leafy green vegetables, fermented foods (menaquinones, a form of vitamin K), and certain vegetable oils. A deficiency in vitamin K can lead to easy bruising and excessive bleeding, and it may also contribute to bone weakness, potentially increasing the risk of fractures. Higher dietary vitamin K intake may be associated with a lower prevalence of depressive symptoms (Bolzetta et al. 2019; Zhang et al. 2023), although further research is warranted.

Water-Soluble Vitamins

The body does not store these vitamins, so excess amounts are usually excreted, although some toxicity can occur with high levels of supplementation. With regard to the eight B vitamins, although they are chemically diverse compounds, they all play important roles in cell metabolism and synthesis; each is either a cofactor/coenzyme for key metabolic processes (such as energy metabolism and biosynthetic pathways) or a precursor needed to make one.

Vitamin B1 (thiamine) is essential for energy metabolism and the proper functioning of diverse bodily systems. Dietary sources of thiamine include whole grains, legumes, nuts, seeds, many fruits and vegetables, fish, and pork. A deficiency in vitamin B1—referred to as beriberi or thiamine deficiency disorders—presents many challenges to clinicians, in part due to the array of potential clinical manifestations, including those in metabolic, neurologic, cardiovascular, respiratory, gastrointestinal, and musculoskeletal systems (Smith et al. 2021). The brain is highly vulnerable to thiamine deficiency—especially during rapid growth (i.e., during perinatal periods and in children)—owing to its heavy reliance on mitochondrial adenosine triphosphate (ATP) production. Thiamine deficiency contributes to a number of conditions spanning from mild neurological and psychiatric symptoms (confusion, reduced memory, and sleep disturbances) to severe encephalopathy, ataxia, congestive heart failure, muscle atrophy, and even death (Dhir et al. 2019). Focal thalamic degeneration due to thiamine deficiency—known as Wernicke's encephalopathy or Wernicke–Korsakoff syndrome—is most commonly attributable to alcohol abuse (Mrowicka et al. 2023). As is true of most other water-soluble vitamins that are excreted in urine, excesses are unlikely to cause toxicity.

Vitamin B2 (riboflavin) plays a critical role in energy production and the metabolism of fats, drugs, and steroids. Good dietary sources of riboflavin include milk and dairy products, eggs, leafy green vegetables, and fish and lean meats. A deficiency in vitamin B2 can lead to ariboflavinosis, which presents with symptoms such as sore throat, redness and swelling of the lining of the mouth and throat, and potential mental health symptoms such as fatigue and mood swings. Among older adults, vitamin B2 intake may be positively associated with cognitive performance (Ji et al. 2024).

Vitamin B3 (niacin/nicotinic acid) is vital for DNA repair, energy production, the synthesis of cholesterol and fatty acids, and neuronal development and survival. It can be found in foods such as meat, poultry, fish, nuts, seeds, legumes, and whole grains. A deficiency in niacin can lead to pellagra, characterized by diarrhea, dermatitis, and dementia (Prabhu et al. 2021). Excessive intake through supplements can lead to flushing, skin irritation, gastrointestinal issues, and in extreme cases, liver damage. *Vitamin B5 (pantothenic acid)* is necessary for the synthesis of coenzyme A, which is essential for fatty acid metabolism and energy production. Dietary sources include beef, poultry, mushrooms, avocados, eggs, milk, whole grains, legumes, and some vegetables. A deficiency in vitamin B5 is very rare, as the vitamin is found in so many types of foods.

Vitamin B6 (pyridoxine) is involved in amino acid metabolism, neurotransmitter synthesis, and immune function. It can be found in foods such as fish, poultry, starchy vegetables, chickpeas, and bananas. A deficiency in vitamin B6 may lead to anemia, skin conditions, and neurological disorders, often manifesting as depression or confusion.

Conversely, excessive supplementation can result in nerve damage or sensory neuropathy. *Vitamin B7 (biotin)* plays a crucial role in macronutrient metabolism. Dietary sources of biotin include egg yolks, fish, legumes, nuts, seeds, and an array of vegetables. A deficiency in biotin can cause hair loss, skin rashes, and neurological/psychiatric symptoms such as fatigue.

Vitamin B9 (folate) is essential for DNA synthesis and repair and is particularly important during periods of rapid growth such as gestation/pregnancy. Dietary sources include dark green leafy vegetables, legumes, nuts and seeds, and a variety of fruits. A deficiency in folate in developing fetuses can lead to neural tube defects; in adults, deficiency can lead to megaloblastic anemia and fatigue. Folic acid, used as a supplement during pregnancy and in other circumstances, as well as in fortified foods, is a synthetic form of vitamin B9; it has higher bioavailability than folate and is readily converted to the active form of folate. Regarding folate and depression, a meta-analysis suggested that individuals with depression have lower serum levels of folate and lower dietary folate intake than those without depression (Bender et al. 2017). Folate supplementation may be considered as a means of improving the efficacy of antidepressant medications (Gao et al. 2024), although evidence has been mixed (Liwinski and Lang 2023).

Vitamin B12 (cobalamin) is crucial for red blood cell formation, neurological function, and DNA synthesis. It is primarily found in animal products, including meat, fish, egg yolks, and dairy products; therefore, vegetarians and vegans need to rely on fortified foods or supplements to ensure adequate intake. Vitamin B12 deficiency can lead to anemia, fatigue, and neurological problems such as memory loss and mood changes. Despite some positive reports, a meta-analysis involving 16 randomized, controlled trials with 6,276 participants found vitamin B12 supplementation to be ineffective for improving cognitive function or depressive symptoms (without overt vitamin B12 deficiency) (Markun et al. 2021). Thus, although severe vitamin B12 deficiency can lead to serious neuropsychiatric symptoms, the link between milder vitamin B12 deficiency and common mental health conditions is not consistently substantiated. On the other hand, another meta-analysis (Tan et al. 2023) suggested a correlation between mental health or mental health disorders and vitamin B12 levels or intake in children and adolescents.

Vitamin C (ascorbic acid) is a powerful antioxidant that plays a vital role in collagen synthesis, immune function, and the absorption of iron from plant-based foods. Rich dietary sources of vitamin C include citrus fruits, strawberries, kiwi, other fruits, peppers, and a number of vegetables. A deficiency in vitamin C can lead to scurvy, characterized by symptoms such as fatigue, joint pain, and skin issues, as well as increased susceptibility to infections. Although dietary vitamin C intake among individuals with depression may be lower than in control subjects (Ding and Zhang 2022), and vitamin C supplementation may be associated with improved mental vitality (Sim et al. 2022) and mood improvement among individuals with subclinical depression (Yosaee et al. 2021), findings have been equivocal.

Minerals

Dietary minerals are essential inorganic nutrients that play crucial roles in various physiological functions. They are divided into two categories: macrominerals, which are needed in larger amounts (calcium, phosphorus, magnesium, potassium, sodium, chloride, and sulfur), and trace minerals, which are required in smaller quantities (iron, zinc, iodine, cobalt, copper, fluoride, manganese, and selenium). The various dietary minerals are found in a wide array of food types; for example, calcium is predominantly found in dairy products and leafy green vegetables, while iron can be sourced from meat, seafood, beans, lentils, and dark green leafy vegetables. A well-balanced diet that includes a variety of food types can ensure adequate mineral intake.

Each mineral serves specific functions that contribute to the body's metabolic processes and are critical for maintaining overall health. For example, calcium and phosphorus are essential for bone health, potassium and sodium are needed for fluid balance and neuronal function, magnesium plays a role in muscle function and energy production, zinc is vital for immune function and wound healing, iron is integral to oxygen transport in the blood, and selenium acts as an antioxidant, helping protect cells from damage. As such, deficiencies in essential minerals can lead to a variety of health issues, both physical and mental. For example, calcium deficiency is linked to osteoporosis and increased risk of fractures; magnesium deficiency may lead to muscle cramps, migraines, and heightened anxiety; and iron deficiency can result in anemia, characterized by fatigue, weakness, mood disturbances, and cognitive impairments such as reduced concentration. Given the large number of dietary minerals, many clinicians may not know if someone is at risk for a specific deficiency. As such, partnering with a registered dietitian who is skilled in nutrition-focused physical exams and obtaining a nutrition history may be beneficial.

Deficiencies in select dietary minerals have been linked to mental health outcomes. Deficiencies in magnesium, zinc, and selenium have been associated with depression (Zielińska et al. 2023), for example. Table 3.2 lists examples of potential and postulated mental health correlates of specific micronutrient deficiencies; additional information is provided elsewhere (Baik 2024; Zielińska et al. 2023). Given the diversity of minerals, broad-spectrum micronutrients (a formulation that includes at least 10 different vitamins or minerals), as opposed to a single-nutrient approach, may be ideal (Villagomez et al. 2023) for adults with regard to depression and anxiety, as well as children with regard to aggression, autism-spectrum disorder, ADHD, and emotional dysregulation (Rucklidge et al. 2021; 2023; 2025).

Phytonutrients

Phytonutrients, also known as phytochemicals, are natural compounds found in plants that contribute to their color, flavor, and disease resistance. These compounds are not considered essential nutrients like vitamins and minerals, yet they play a significant role in promoting health and reducing the risk of chronic disease. The various fruits and vegetables that we commonly eat contain thousands of different phytochemicals—cruciferous vegetables (like cabbage) alone contain up to 100. Across all plants, more than 10,000 different phytochemicals have been identified, with many more yet to be discovered.

The physiological functions of phytonutrients in fruits and vegetables are diverse, as they often act as antioxidants, anti-inflammatory agents, and immune system enhancers. Compounds such as flavonoids, carotenoids, and polyphenols can help neutralize free radicals in the body, thereby reducing oxidative stress, which is linked to aging and various diseases. Sulforaphane, found in cruciferous vegetables such as cabbage, broccoli, and Brussels sprouts, can activate detoxification enzymes and may promote the elimination of harmful compounds from the body. Anthocyanins found in blueberries, blackberries, and certain other fruits and vegetables reduce inflammation and improve heart health by enhancing blood vessel function. Similarly, lycopene in tomatoes may support heart health and may be associated with a reduced risk of prostate cancer. Plant sterols and stanols are plant compounds that can help lower low-density lipoprotein (LDL) cholesterol levels. They are structurally similar to cholesterol and reduce absorption of cholesterol in the gut, which then leads to more cholesterol being

Table 3.2 Examples of potential and postulated mental health correlates of specific micronutrient deficiencies

Vitamin or mineral	Effect
Substantial (but not unequivocal) evidence	
Vitamin D (calciferol)	Depression, especially during the winter months when sun exposure is low (reduced vitamin D synthesis in the skin); anxiety; cognitive decline and increased risk of dementia
Zinc	Depression and anxiety; potentially also bipolar disorder, Alzheimer's disease, schizophrenia, and ADHD
Vitamin B12 (cobalamin)	Psychiatric symptoms such as depression and cognitive dysfunction; psychotic symptoms in the context of severe deficiency
Emerging evidence, with more research needed	
Vitamin A (retinol)	Depression
Vitamin B1 (thiamine)	Depression
Vitamin B6 (pyridoxine)	Depression
Vitamin B9 (folate)	Depression; prenatal depression
Vitamin C (ascorbic acid)	Depression
Vitamin E (tocopherol)	Depression; anxiety
Vitamin K (phylloquinone)	Depression
Magnesium	Depression
Selenium	Depression
Copper	Depression (elevated copper may also be associated with depression risk)
Iron	Depression; postpartum depression
Calcium	Depression
Manganese	Depression

excreted. Additionally, phytonutrients can influence gene expression and modulate hormonal balance, underscoring their complexity and importance in overall health maintenance. Table 3.3 gives a sampling of the types of phytonutrients found in several vegetables across eight families of plants.

With regard to mental health, certain phytonutrients, such as curcumin in turmeric, have demonstrated potential in reducing symptoms of anxiety and depression by modulating neurotransmitter levels and reducing neuroinflammation. Flavonoids found in dark chocolate and green tea have been associated with enhanced memory and cognitive performance, potentially owing to their ability to improve blood flow to the brain. Despite countless phytonutrients with antioxidant and anti-inflammatory properties, little is known about their specific potential impacts on mental health and mental illnesses.

Clinical Pearls

- Clinicians should encourage a food-first approach to help clients receive a diverse complement of vitamins and minerals.
- Clinicians can consider supplementation of specific B vitamins (including vitamin B12 [cobalamin], and vitamin B9 [folate]), or B vitamin supplementation more broadly, as an adjunctive treatment for some clients with depressive disorders. Individuals adhering to a vegetarian or vegan eating pattern may need vitamin B12–fortified foods or supplements to ensure adequate intake, given that most dietary vitamin B12 comes from animal-based foods.
- In light of the large number of micronutrients and the mixed findings with regard to specific micronutrients and mental health outcomes, clinicians should recommend a rational, balanced diet that maximizes whole foods and minimizes ultraprocessed foods, in conjunction with the consumption of prebiotics (insoluble fiber in plant-based foods such as fruits, vegetables, legumes, and whole grains), probiotics (live microorganisms, typically bacteria or yeasts, found naturally in some foods such as yogurt, sauerkraut, and kimchi), and antioxidant and anti-inflammatory phytonutrients from plants.
- Clinicians should recognize the likely beneficial effects of diverse phytonutrients (many of which have antioxidant and anti-inflammatory properties) on mental health, given the links

Table 3.3 Examples of phytonutrients from several vegetables across eight families of plants

Vegetables	Phytonutrients
Broccoli, Brussels sprouts, cabbage, collards, kale	Glucosinolates that are converted into isothiocyanates such as sulforaphane
Garlic, leeks, onions, scallions, shallots	Organosulfur compounds, such as allicin in garlic
Beans, lentils	Phenolic compounds, saponins, and phytosterols
Beets, Swiss chard	Betalains and flavonoids
Curly endive, escarole	Sesquiterpene lactones (e.g., costunolide), phenolic compounds such as chicoric acid, caftaric acid, and quercetin
Celery, Florence fennel, parsley	Flavonoids (e.g., apigenin and luteolin), coumarins, and essential oils
Pumpkins, winter squash	Carotenoids (e.g., beta-carotene), polyphenols
Peppers, tomatoes	Phenolic compounds, capsaicinoids in peppers, lycopene in tomatoes

between depressive disorders (and other psychiatric illnesses) and oxidative stress and inflammatory processes.

- Clinicians serving individuals with mental illnesses should be interested in a healthy diet not only for potential mental health benefits, but also for physical health benefits; this is crucial given the high rates of physical health comorbidities.

Key Chapter Points

- Vitamins are organic compounds—not synthesized (or not synthesized in sufficient amounts) by the body, and thus obtained through the diet—essential for a multitude of physiologic and metabolic functions.
- Minerals are inorganic elements, also needed in small amounts for diverse bodily functions, which must be obtained from food.
- Deficiencies in, or reduced intake of, a number of vitamins—including all four fat-soluble vitamins, as well as vitamin B12

(cobalamin), vitamin B1 (thiamine), vitamin B6 (pyridoxine), vitamin B9 (folate), and vitamin C (ascorbic acid)—have been associated with poor mental health outcomes, with depression being most commonly studied. In many cases, however, findings have not been entirely consistent.
- Thousands of phytonutrients exist within plant-based foods. Although they are not considered essential nutrients like vitamins and minerals, they affect physiological functions, serving as antioxidants, anti-inflammatory agents, and immune system enhancers.
- Broad-spectrum micronutrient supplementation may be beneficial, but optimizing micronutrient and phytonutrient intake can be achieved through a balanced diet that maximizes whole foods and minimizes ultraprocessed foods.

References

Baik HW: Mental health and micronutrients: a narrative review. Ann Clin Nutr Metab 16(3):112–119, 2024

Bender A, Hagan KE, Kingston N: The association of folate and depression: a meta-analysis. J Psychiatr Res 95:9–18, 2017 28759846

Bolzetta F, Veronese N, Stubbs B, et al: The relationship between dietary vitamin K and depressive symptoms in late adulthood: a cross-sectional analysis from a large cohort study. Nutrients 11(4):787, 2019 30959758

Carazo A, Macáková K, Matoušová K, et al: Vitamin A update: forms, sources, kinetics, detection, function, deficiency, therapeutic use and toxicity. Nutrients 13(5):1703, 2021 34069881

Dhir S, Tarasenko M, Napoli E, et al: Neurological, psychiatric, and biochemical aspects of thiamine deficiency in children and adults. Front Psychiatry 10:207, 2019 31019473

Ding J, Zhang Y: Associations of dietary vitamin C and E intake with depression: a meta-analysis of observational studies. Front Nutr 9:857823, 2022 35464032

Gao S, Khalid A, Amini-Salehi E, et al: Folate supplementation as a beneficial add-on treatment in relieving depressive symptoms: a meta-analysis of meta-analyses. Food Sci Nutr 12(6):3806–3818, 2024 38873435

Głąbska D, Kołota A, Lachowicz K, et al: The influence of vitamin D intake and status on mental health in children: a systematic review. Nutrients 13(3):952, 2021 33809478

Ji K, Sun M, Li L, et al: Association between vitamin B2 intake and cognitive performance among older adults: a cross-sectional study from NHANES. Sci Rep 14(1):21930, 2024 39304710

Lee ARYB, Tariq A, Lau G, et al: Vitamin E, alpha-tocopherol, and its effects on depression and anxiety: a systematic review and meta-analysis. Nutrients 14(3):656, 2022 35277015

Liwinski T, Lang UE: Folate and its significance in depressive disorders and suicidality: a comprehensive narrative review. Nutrients 15(17):3859, 2023 37686891

Markun S, Gravestock I, Jäger L, et al: Effects of vitamin B12 supplementation on cognitive function, depressive symptoms, and fatigue: a systematic review, meta-analysis, and meta-regression. Nutrients 13(3):923, 2021 33809274

Mikola T, Marx W, Lane MM, et al: The effect of vitamin D supplementation on depressive symptoms in adults: a systematic review and meta-analysis of randomized controlled trials. Crit Rev Food Sci Nutr 63(33):11784–11801, 2023 35816192

Mrowicka M, Mrowicki J, Dragan G, et al: The importance of thiamine (vitamin B1) in humans. Biosci Rep 43(10):BSR20230374, 2023 37389565

Musazadeh V, Keramati M, Ghalichi F, et al: Vitamin D protects against depression: evidence from an umbrella meta-analysis on interventional and observational meta-analyses. Pharmacol Res 187:106605, 2023 36509315

Prabhu D, Dawe RS, Mponda K: Pellagra a review exploring causes and mechanisms, including isoniazid-induced pellagra. Photodermatol Photoimmunol Photomed 37(2):99–104, 2021 33471377

Rucklidge JJ, Bruton A, Welsh A, et al: Annual research review: micronutrients and their role in the treatment of paediatric mental illness. J Child Psychol Psychiatry 66(4):477–497, 2025 39703999

Rucklidge JJ, Johnstone JM, Kaplan BJ: Nutrition provides the essential foundation for optimizing mental health. Evid Based Pract Child Adolesc Ment Health 6(1):131–154, 2021 1875342

Rucklidge JJ, Johnstone JM, Villagomez A, et al: Broad-spectrum micronutrients and mental health, in Nutritional Psychiatry: A Primer for Clinicians. Edited by Dinan T. Cambridge, UK, Cambridge University Press, 2023

Sim M, Hong S, Jung S, et al: Vitamin C supplementation promotes mental vitality in healthy young adults: results from a cross-sectional analysis and a randomized, double-blind, placebo-controlled trial. Eur J Nutr 61(1):447–459, 2022 34476568

Smith TJ, Johnson CR, Koshy R, et al: Thiamine deficiency disorders: a clinical perspective. Ann N Y Acad Sci 1498(1):9–28, 2021 33305487

Tan Y, Zhou L, Gu K, et al: Correlation between vitamin B12 and mental health in children and adolescents: a systematic review and meta-analysis. Clin Psychopharmacol Neurosci 21(4):617–633, 2023 37859436

Villagomez A, Cross M, Ranjbar N: Broad spectrum micronutrients: a potential key player to address emotional dysregulation. Front Child Adolesc Psychiatry 2:1295635, 2023 39839581

Wang R, Xu F, Xia X, et al: The effect of vitamin D supplementation on primary depression: a meta-analysis. J Affect Disord 344:653–661, 2024 37852593

Xie F, Huang T, Lou D, et al: Effect of vitamin D supplementation on the incidence and prognosis of depression: an updated meta-analysis based on randomized controlled trials. Front Public Health 10:903547, 2022 35979473

Yosaee S, Keshtkaran Z, Abdollahi S, et al: The effect of vitamin C supplementation on mood status in adults: a systematic review and meta-analysis of randomized controlled clinical trials. Gen Hosp Psychiatry 71:36–42, 2021 33932734

Zhang Y, Ding J, Liang J: Associations of dietary vitamin A and beta-carotene intake with depression: a meta-analysis of observational studies. Front Nutr 9:881139, 2022 35548582

Zhang Y, Tan W, Xi X, et al: Association between vitamin K intake and depressive symptoms in US adults: data from the National Health and Nutrition Examination Survey (NHANES) 2013–2018. Front Nutr 10:1102109, 2023 37032783

Zielińska M, Łuszczki E, Dereń K: Dietary nutrient deficiencies and risk of depression (review article 2018–2023). Nutrients 15(11):2433, 2023 37299394

4

An Introduction to Dietary Patterns and Specific Diets

Michael T. Compton, M.D., M.P.H.

If it came from a plant, eat it; if it was made in a plant, don't.

—Michael Pollan

Understanding the content and potential benefits of specific diets or eating patterns is of interest to clinicians, to some extent as related to mental health and specific mental illnesses, but perhaps more importantly in relation to the physical health of individuals served, including those with mental illnesses. Here, a number of specific diets and eating patterns are summarized briefly; the term *eating patterns* refers to the combination of all foods and beverages a person habitually consumes over time. Diets specific to medical conditions, including the Dietary Approaches to Stop Hypertension (DASH) diet, the carbohydrate-controlled diet (for diabetes), the gluten-free diet, the ketogenic diet, and others, are not covered. Additionally, diets or eating patterns linked to religious or personal belief systems, such as the kosher diet and the halal diet, are not considered.

The Western Diet or "Standard American Diet" and Ultraprocessed Food

Before describing a number of specific diets and eating patterns, I review the Western diet (also called the standard American diet), given that it is the typical eating pattern in many developed countries and the United States in particular. The Western diet is characterized by a high intake of red and processed meats, refined grains, sugar-sweetened beverages, high-fat dairy products, and ultraprocessed foods (as noted in Chapter 2, "The Macronutrients", more than 50% of energy purchased by U.S. households comes from moderately processed to ultraprocessed foods; Poti et al. 2015). This eating pattern typically includes large amounts of saturated fats, added sugars, and salt and is low in fruits, vegetables, legumes, whole grains, seeds, and nuts. The ease and availability of ultraprocessed foods (in fast foods, convenience foods, snacks, sweets, and ready-to-eat meals) make the Western diet highly appealing, but it is also linked to numerous health problems. Research consistently associates the Western diet with an increased risk of overweight, obesity, insulin resistance, type 2 diabetes, metabolic syndrome, cardiovascular disease, inflammatory processes, certain cancers, and other chronic conditions (Clemente-Suárez et al. 2023). It has also been linked to poor mental health (Zhang et al. 2023).

The high-calorie but nutrient-poor profile of the Western diet can contribute to metabolic syndrome and inflammatory diseases, making it a significant factor in the global rise of lifestyle-related health issues, including among individuals with mental illnesses. The imbalance in this diet—marked by excessive intake of saturated fats, added sugars, and salt—coupled with a lack of essential nutrients and fiber, poses significant risks for chronic physical diseases as well as poor mental health. Given its prevalence and health consequences, multiple health and nutrition experts and guidelines (including the Dietary Guidelines for Americans) recommend a shift toward more balanced and nutrient-dense dietary patterns, such as the Mediterranean diet or plant-predominant diets centered around whole, minimally processed foods (fruits, vegetables, whole grains, and plant-based or lean-meat proteins), which offer better nutritional profiles and health benefits.

The Western diet contains large amounts of ultraprocessed foods, which are industrially manufactured products that contain multiple ingredients, including additives such as preservatives, flavorings, col-

Table 4.1 Characteristics of ultraprocessed foods

Ultraprocessed foods feature formulations of ingredients, mostly of exclusive industrial use, that are made by a series of industrial processes, many requiring sophisticated equipment and technology. Such processes include the fractioning of whole foods into substances that are further chemically modified. For example, corn kernels and soybeans are processed into oils that are refined, bleached, deodorized, hydrogenated, and interesterified; proteins that are hydrolyzed; and starches that are modified. The modified food fractions are then combined with additives and assembled using industrial techniques. In the most basic terms, these ingredients are industrial and cannot be found in a person's kitchen.
Convenient: time-saving and/or ready-to-consume
Inexpensive: low cost, with little risk of spoilage/waste
Highly profitable: low-cost ingredients and long shelf-life
Aggressively marketed: emphatic branding (often with health claims, which healthy foods usually do not include)
Designed to make us consume in excess, by tapping into innate reward and motivation systems. We crave foods with taste/flavor profiles signaling that they are high in calories (sugars and fats). Fiber is stripped out of ultraprocessed foods, and they are digested more rapidly. They tend to be high in both rapidly absorbed refined carbohydrates and fat, which is not true of naturally occurring foods (e.g., fruits are high in sugars but not fats, nuts are high in fats but not sugars).

orings, and emulsifiers—ingredients that are not typically found in home kitchens and pantries. As detailed in Table 4.1, the manufacturing process for ultraprocessed foods often involves significant alteration of the original food components, which can strip away natural nutrients and replace them with artificial ingredients to enhance taste, texture, and shelf life. This processing makes these foods highly convenient and appealing, but they are usually low in essential nutrients such as vitamins, minerals, and fiber while being high in calories, sugars, unhealthy fats, and sodium. Such foods are engineered to trigger reward pathways, thus subconsciously encouraging repeat purchases. Furthermore, the low nutrient density and high caloric content of these foods can displace healthier, more nutrient-rich options from the plate, exacerbating nutritional deficiencies and increasing the risk of diet-related diseases.

Common Weight-Loss and Short-Term Diets

Clearly, the Western diet, replete with ultraprocessed foods, is not recommended from either a physical health or a mental health perspective. Yet it is perhaps the most common eating pattern of most Americans—including individuals with mental illness—in part because of its convenience and affordability; extensive marketing; and the food environment in which we live. In this section, I briefly describe a sampling of weight-loss diets and short-term diets; many others could be enumerated. They are somewhat artificially placed into several general conceptual categories here, although other categorizations could be used. The purpose in describing these diets is not to recommend them, but to provide a brief overview for clinicians who may have clients using or considering these diets. Many are not sustainable over the long term, and most have no evidence base for physical health or mental health benefits—some are likely to be quite unhealthy. In the next section, I describe eating patterns known to be healthy, and thus recommended—such as the Mediterranean diet—based on their reliance on whole foods (as opposed to processed and ultraprocessed foods), with an emphasis on a plant-predominant food profile (as opposed to a high reliance on animal-derived foods).

Low-Calorie Diets

Low-calorie diets are designed to reduce daily caloric intake and promote weight loss. Typically, these diets restrict calorie consumption to fewer than 1,200–1,500 calories per day for women and 1,500–1,800 calories per day for men, depending on individual factors such as age, weight, and activity level. The principle behind a low-calorie diet is to create a caloric deficit, in which the number of calories consumed is less than the number of calories burned by the body (calories are burned through the basal metabolic rate, the thermic effect of food, nonexercise activity thermogenesis, and exercise). The caloric deficit forces the body to use stored fat for energy, leading to weight loss. Low-calorie diets often emphasize nutrient-dense foods such as fruits, vegetables, lean proteins, and whole grains to ensure that, despite reduced caloric intake, essential nutrients are still provided. Randomized, controlled trials using partial meal replacement plans or reduced calorie diets for weight management suggest that these types of interventions can safely and effectively produce significant and sometimes sustainable weight loss and improve weight-related disease risk factors (Heymsfield et al. 2003).

Although low-calorie diets can be effective for weight loss, they come with potential challenges and risks. Reducing caloric intake too drastically can lead to nutrient deficiencies, decreased energy levels, and loss of muscle mass. It is important for those following low-calorie diets to ensure that their eating plan is balanced and includes a variety of foods to meet nutritional needs. Long-term adherence to low-calorie diets can be difficult and may lead to feelings of deprivation or increased hunger, which can affect overall satisfaction and sustainability.

Because a low-calorie diet is a tool to rapidly reduce weight, combining it with physical activity can enhance weight loss and improve overall health outcomes. A registered dietitian can help individuals create a tailored eating plan that meets their specific health needs and goals while maintaining proper nutrition and well-being.

Commercial, membership-based weight loss programs such as Jenny Craig and Nutrisystem provide prepackaged, portion-controlled meals designed to simplify the process of managing caloric intake and achieving weight-loss goals. Participants follow a structured plan that includes a variety of meals and snacks, which are designed to be nutritionally balanced and convenient. Some emphasize low-calorie, high-protein foods and controlled portions to help manage hunger and promote steady weight loss. Commercial weight loss programs such as these also offer support through online tools and resources to help participants stay motivated and adhere to the program. Although these programs have been effective for many in achieving weight loss, some people may find the reliance on prepackaged foods (which are not free of diverse ultraprocessed ingredients) challenging or unappealing, and long-term success often depends on transitioning to a more sustainable eating pattern after completing some duration of the program. It should be noted that weight losses reported in testimonials usually exceed those achieved in randomized, controlled trials or other studies.

WeightWatchers is a popular weight management program that helps members create nutrition and meal plans. It focuses on flexible, long-term lifestyle changes rather than restrictive eating. The program operates on a points-based system, in which foods and beverages are assigned points associated with their nutritional value, and participants are allocated a daily and weekly points budget. This approach allows individuals to choose foods within their point limits, promoting balanced eating and portion control. WeightWatchers emphasizes sustainable weight loss and healthy habits, incorporating regular physical activity, behavioral strategies, and support through meetings or online communities. Online tools, workshops, consultation with a registered dietitian, and other member benefits are designed to offer support and motivation.

Very-low-calorie diets are not covered here. They provide a high degree of dietary structure, typically provide ≤800 kcal/day, are designed to produce rapid weight loss, are commonly consumed as liquid shakes, and are generally only appropriate for patients with BMI ≥30 (Tsai and Wadden 2006). Additionally, detox diets, liquid diets, and short-term "crash diets" for rapid weight loss are not covered here; their health value is highly questionable. Common characteristics of such fad diets include 1) they make claims of rapid weight loss or exaggerated health benefits with little scientific support, 2) they often eliminate entire food groups (e.g., carbohydrates, fats) or severely restrict calories, 3) they lack long-term sustainability and can lead to nutritional deficiencies, 4) they rely on gimmicks or trendy concepts rather than evidence-based guidelines, 5) they are usually not supported by major health organizations, 6) they may include expensive products such as supplements or special foods, and 7) they tend to resurface in cycles, rebranded under new names.

Intermittent Fasting and Time-Restricted Eating

Fasting and intermittent fasting focus on cycling between periods of eating and fasting, rather than strictly limiting caloric intake on a daily basis. Fasting involves abstaining from food for a set period, which can range from several hours to several days, and intermittent fasting involves a structured pattern of eating and fasting within a specified time frame (generally defined as >60% energy restriction 2–3 days per week, or on alternate days). One form of intermittent energy restriction is time-restricted feeding, referring to limiting the daily period of food intake to 8–10 hours or less on most days of the week. These eating patterns are based on the idea that periodic fasting brings about improved metabolic function, weight loss, and thus reduced risk of chronic diseases; they may also enhance insulin sensitivity, which can help regulate blood glucose levels and reduce the risk of type 2 diabetes. Weight loss is another common outcome, as fasting periods typically lead to reduced calorie consumption and increased fat oxidation. Available evidence suggests that intermittent energy restriction paradigms produce weight loss equivalent to that of continuous energy restriction using low-calorie diets (Rynders et al. 2019). Some findings also suggest that intermittent fasting may improve cardiovascular health by lowering blood pressure, cholesterol levels, and inflammatory markers, although research is limited.

Fasting and intermittent fasting may not be suitable for everyone, however, and can present certain challenges. Individuals with specific health conditions such as diabetes should approach fasting with caution and seek medical advice before starting. Additionally, fasting can sometimes lead to issues such as nutrient deficiencies, decreased energy levels, and difficulties with adherence. It is important to focus on balanced, nutrient-dense foods during eating periods and to stay hydrated throughout fasting periods to mitigate potential adverse effects. As with any dietary approach, it is crucial to consider personal health goals and consult with health care professionals to determine the most appropriate and sustainable strategy.

Low-Carbohydrate (High-Protein/High-Fat) Diets

Low-carbohydrate diets have gained in popularity in recent years owing to claims of benefits regarding weight loss and metabolic health. These diets focus on reducing the intake of carbohydrates, especially foods such as bread, pasta, rice, and sugary snacks. By limiting carbohydrates, the body is encouraged to use stored fat for energy, leading to weight loss. Low-carbohydrate diets can vary in their strictness. Some, such as the ketogenic diet, reduce carbohydrate intake to very minimal levels; others, such as the Atkins diet and the paleo diet, allow for moderate amounts of carbohydrates. An emphasis on whole foods and high-protein, high-fat sources also helps stabilize blood sugar levels and reduce cravings, making it easier for many to adhere to these otherwise difficult eating patterns. A high intake of branched-chain amino acids (leucine, isoleucine, and valine) from animal-derived foods, in combination with a Western diet, may increase the risk of metabolic disease, pose a significant acid load to the kidneys, and when energy demand is low, contribute to a positive energy balance (as excess protein can be converted to glucose [via gluconeogenesis] or ketone bodies), which is undesirable if weight loss is the goal (Pesta and Samuel 2014).

Several potential health benefits are associated with low-carbohydrate diets, beyond weight loss. Some research suggests that these diets can improve markers of heart health, such as lowering triglycerides and increasing high-density lipoprotein (HDL) cholesterol levels. They may also improve insulin sensitivity and reduce blood sugar levels in the context of type 2 diabetes, and they may reduce the risk of metabolic syndrome. Benefits for glycemic control need to be balanced with impacts on nonglycemic outcomes such as low-density lipoprotein (LDL) cholesterol, the microbiome, and inflammation (Landry et al. 2021). Furthermore, restricting carbohydrate intake can sometimes lead to nutrient deficiencies, particularly if the diet lacks variety and adequate sources of fiber, vitamins, and minerals. Some people may also experience side effects such as constipation, headache, and fatigue, particularly in the early stages of the diet, as the body adjusts to a lower intake of carbohydrates. Long-term adherence to a low-carbohydrate diet can be challenging because of the restrictions on many common and culturally significant foods.

The Atkins diet is a low-carbohydrate diet designed to promote weight loss and improve metabolic health by reducing carbohydrate intake and increasing protein and fat consumption. Developed by Dr. Robert Atkins in the 1970s (Atkins 1972), the diet is structured in four phases: induction, balancing, premaintenance, and lifetime maintenance. The induction phase is the most restrictive, allowing only 20–25 g of carbohydrates per day to jump-start fat burning by forcing the body into ketosis, using fat as the primary energy source. As individuals progress through the phases, they gradually increase their carbohydrate intake while monitoring their body's response to find a sustainable level of carbohydrate consumption that supports weight maintenance and overall health. The Atkins diet emphasizes high-protein foods such as meat, fish, eggs, and cheese while restricting high-carbohydrate foods such as bread, pasta, and sugary snacks. Although the Atkins diet has been effective for many in achieving weight loss and improving certain health markers such as blood sugar and cholesterol levels, it may not be suitable for everyone, particularly those with specific health conditions. Other similar high-protein, low-carbohydrate diets have been described and popularized, such as the Stillman diet developed by Dr. Alfred Stillman (Stillman and Baker 1974) and the Dukan diet, created by French nutritionist Dr. Pierre Dukan (Dukan 2011).

The South Beach diet is a popular low-carbohydrate diet that focuses on improving overall health while promoting weight loss through a balanced approach to eating. Created by cardiologist Dr. Arthur Agatston in the early 2000s, the South Beach diet is designed to help stabilize blood sugar levels and reduce cravings by emphasizing the consumption of lean proteins, healthy fats, and low-glycemic-index carbohydrates (Agatston 2003). The diet is divided into three phases. Phase 1 is the most restrictive, lasting 2 weeks and eliminating most carbohydrates to help kick-start weight loss and curb cravings for sugary and starchy foods. Phase 2 gradually reintroduces healthy carbohydrates such as whole grains, fruits, and certain vegetables, focusing on those with a low glycemic index to maintain steady blood sugar levels. Phase 3 is a maintenance phase, encouraging a long-term healthy eating pattern that includes a variety of nutrient-dense foods. The South Beach diet differs from other low-carbohydrate diets by allowing a more moderate intake of carbohydrates, especially from nutrient-rich sources, which may make the diet easier to follow in the long term. The diet is often praised for its heart-healthy approach, emphasizing the quality of the fats and carbohydrates consumed, but it may still require careful planning to ensure that all nutritional needs are met.

The paleo diet, also known as the paleolithic or "caveman" diet, is based on the idea of eating in a way that mimics the dietary patterns of our prehistoric ancestors (Cordain 2010). It emphasizes whole, unprocessed foods that would have been available to early humans, such as lean meats, fish, fruits, vegetables, nuts, and seeds, while excluding foods that are the products of modern agriculture, such as grains, legumes, dairy products, and refined sugars, as well as processed foods. Proponents of the paleo diet argue that this approach aligns more closely with human evolutionary biology, potentially leading to improved digestion, better metabolic health, and reduced risk of chronic disease. The diet encourages high-quality protein sources and healthy fats while minimizing carbohydrate intake, particularly from refined and processed sources. Although the paleo diet has been praised for its emphasis on whole foods and its potential benefits for weight management and blood sugar control, critics point out that it can be restrictive and may lead to deficiencies in certain nutrients, such as calcium and fiber, if not carefully planned.

Low-Fat Diets

Low-fat diets emphasize reducing the intake of fats, particularly saturated fats, to promote overall health and weight loss. The concept of low-fat dieting gained popularity in the 1980s and 1990s, as research suggested a link between high fat consumption and an increased risk of overweight, obesity, and heart disease. Low-fat diets typically recommend that fat intake should comprise no more than 30% of total daily calories, focusing primarily on reducing foods high in saturated and trans fats, such as butter, fatty cuts of meat, full-fat dairy products, and fried foods. Instead, these diets encourage the consumption of fruits, vegetables, whole grains, lean proteins, and low-fat or fat-free dairy options that are lower in fat and calories. By lowering fat intake, the goal is to reduce overall calorie consumption and lose weight or maintain a healthy weight. Data regarding the long-term success (in terms of weight loss or weight regain/reduced weight maintenance) of low-carbohydrate versus low-fat diets are inconclusive (Seid and Rosenbaum 2019).

There are several potential health benefits of low-fat diets. For one, reducing the intake of saturated and trans fats can help lower LDL cholesterol levels, which reduces the risk of cardiovascular disease. Additionally, low-fat diets often promote the consumption of nutrient-dense, high-fiber foods such as fruits, vegetables, and whole grains, which can improve digestive health, enhance satiety, and provide essential vitamins and minerals. Low-fat diets may also benefit individuals with certain health conditions, such as gallbladder disease or pancreatitis, in which fat intake needs to be carefully controlled to manage symptoms. However, while low-fat diets can offer these benefits, they are most effective when they focus on the quality of the foods consumed, rather than simply the reduction of fat.

Despite their potential advantages, low-fat diets are not without criticism. Some research suggests that very-low-fat diets, which limit fat intake to less than 20% of total daily calories, may lead to deficiencies in essential fatty acids and fat-soluble vitamins (A, D, E, and K). Moreover, there is growing recognition that not all fats are detrimental to health—unsaturated fats, such as those found in avocados, nuts, seeds, and olive oil, are beneficial and important for brain health, hormone production, and the absorption of certain nutrients. Additionally, some individuals may find low-fat diets difficult to maintain long term, especially if they substitute fats with high-carbohydrate processed foods, which can lead to unintended weight gain. Therefore, although low-fat diets can be effective for some, a balanced approach that includes healthy fats in moderation may be a more sustainable and health-promoting option.

A number of low-fat, high-fiber (i.e., predominantly whole-food, plant-based, nutrient-dense) diets have been described and popularized for chronic disease prevention or reversal, including the Pritikin diet (Pritikin and McGrady 1979), the McDougall diet (McDougall and McDougall 1990), and the Ornish diet (Ornish 1992).

The Mediterranean Diet, the Blue Zone Diet, and Plant-Predominant Eating Patterns

Increasing fruits and vegetables is a dietary change that can reduce energy density, enhance satiety, and decrease overall energy intake. Such dietary improvements often come with other replacements and reductions that are beneficial to health. For example, a diet may reduce ultraprocessed food and replace sugar-sweetened beverages with noncaloric beverages (diet beverages) or water, which may be an effective weight-loss strategy (Peters et al. 2014; Tate et al. 2012).

The Mediterranean diet is a way of eating inspired by the traditional dietary patterns of countries bordering the Mediterranean Sea, such as Greece, Italy, and Spain. The diet emphasizes whole, minimally processed foods, including a variety of fruits, vegetables, whole grains, legumes, nuts, and seeds. Healthy fats, particularly olive oil, are a cornerstone of the Mediterranean diet, replacing less-healthy fats such as butter. Fish and seafood are recommended as primary protein sources, to be consumed at least twice a week, whereas poultry, eggs, cheese, and yogurt are eaten in moderation. Red meat and sweets are limited, and meals are often accompanied by moderate wine consumption (usually red wine), for those who choose to drink. The Mediterranean diet is known not only for its rich flavors and flexibility but also for its numerous health benefits, which include reduced risk of heart disease, stroke, type 2 diabetes, and certain cancers. It also encourages interpersonal relationships through family or community dining and engagement. Its emphasis on fresh, whole foods, healthy fats, and a balanced lifestyle has made the Mediterranean diet a popular and sustainable approach to healthy eating. Table 4.2 shows common ingredients in the Mediterranean diet.

The Mediterranean diet has received substantial research attention with regard to its potential impacts on mental health (Butler and Mörkl 2023). Growing evidence from cohort studies documents associations between the Mediterranean diet and reduced risk of depression (Shafiei et al. 2023) and alleviated depressive symptoms in people experiencing major or mild depression (Bizzozero-Peroni et al. 2025). The diet's anti-inflammatory properties, attributed to its high levels of omega-3 fatty acids and plant-based whole foods, are thought to contribute to beneficial effects on mental health by modulating neuroinflammation and oxidative stress, which are linked to mood disorders.

Table 4.2 Common ingredients in the Mediterranean diet

Ingredient	Examples
Fruits	Oranges, grapes, cherries, and berries
Vegetables	Leafy greens, peppers, tomatoes, cucumbers, eggplants, and artichokes
Legumes	Lentils, chickpeas, and various beans
Whole grains	Whole-wheat pasta, brown rice, and barley, as well as pseudograins such as quinoa
Nuts and seeds	Almonds, walnuts, pistachios, and sunflower seeds
Olive oil	Particularly extra virgin olive oil, used as a primary fat source
Fish and seafood	Salmon, sardines, mackerel, and other fatty fish
Poultry and lean meats	Chicken and turkey in moderate amounts
Dairy	Primarily in the form of yogurt and cheese, consumed in moderation
Herbs and spices	Such as basil, oregano, and rosemary for seasoning, preferred over salt

The Blue Zone diet (Buettner 2015) is inspired by the dietary patterns of the world's longest-lived people, residing in regions known as "blue zones"; examples include Okinawa in Japan, the Nicoya Peninsula in Costa Rica, Sardinia in Italy, and Ikaria in Greece. This dietary approach emphasizes the consumption of whole, plant-based foods, including a variety of vegetables, fruits, legumes, whole grains, nuts, and seeds, while minimizing processed foods, sugars, and animal products. Key components of this eating pattern include maintaining a balanced caloric intake, practicing portion control, and fostering social connections around meals, which contribute to overall well-being. The Blue Zone diet not only supports longevity but also enhances quality of life by promoting heart health, reducing the risk of chronic diseases, and encouraging a holistic approach to nutrition that intertwines physical health with emotional and social aspects. Like the Mediterranean diet, the Blue Zone diet can be considered a lifestyle philosophy.

A vegetarian diet is a dietary pattern that excludes meat and fish but typically includes other animal products such as dairy and eggs, depending on the specific type of vegetarianism followed. This diet emphasizes plant-based foods, including fruits, vegetables, whole grains, legumes, nuts, and seeds, while avoiding animal flesh. Variations of the vegetarian diet include lacto-ovo-vegetarianism, which includes dairy products and eggs; lacto-vegetarianism, which includes dairy but not eggs; and ovo-vegetarianism, which includes eggs but not dairy. (Those who predominantly eat a plant-based diet but occasionally eat meat are sometimes referred to as "flexitarian.") Adopting a vegetarian diet that also limits processed meat substitutes can offer several health benefits, such as reduced risk of chronic diseases (heart disease, hypertension, and certain cancers), as well as improved digestion and weight management. However, it is important for vegetarians to carefully plan their diet to ensure that they obtain adequate amounts of essential nutrients such as protein, iron, calcium, vitamin B12, and omega-3 fatty acids, which are commonly found in animal products. With thoughtful dietary choices and supplementation if necessary, a vegetarian diet can support overall health and well-being.

The vegan diet is a plant-based eating pattern that excludes all animal products, including meat, dairy, eggs, and honey. It focuses on consuming a variety of fruits, vegetables, whole grains, legumes, nuts, and seeds. Adherents of the vegan diet often cite its potential to reduce the risk of chronic diseases such as heart disease, type 2 diabetes, and certain cancers, as well as its positive environmental impact because of reduced reliance on animal agriculture. Vegans, like vegetarians, must be mindful of obtaining adequate levels of nutrients that are commonly found in animal products. This often requires careful planning, supplementation, and the inclusion of fortified foods to ensure a balanced and nutrient-rich diet.

The pescatarian diet includes fish and seafood as the primary sources of animal protein, excluding other meats such as poultry, beef, and pork. This diet focuses on incorporating a variety of fish, shellfish, fruits, vegetables, whole grains, legumes, nuts, and seeds into daily meals. By including fish, which is rich in omega-3 fatty acids, the pescatarian diet offers potential cardiovascular benefits and supports overall heart health. It also provides a good source of high-quality protein and essential nutrients such as vitamin B12 and iodine. Although the pescatarian diet offers many health benefits, it is important to choose sustainably sourced seafood to avoid exposure to harmful contaminants such as mercury. Additionally, those following a pescatarian diet should ensure a well-rounded intake of nutrients by including a variety of plant-based foods.

The locavore diet focuses on consuming food that is locally sourced, emphasizing ingredients grown and produced within a specific geographic region (typically 100–250 miles from one's home). This dietary approach supports local farmers and reduces the environmental impacts associated with long-distance food transportation. By prioritizing fresh, seasonal produce, meats, dairy, and other local products, the locavore diet promotes sustainability and encourages a deeper connection to the food supply and the local agricultural community (see Chapter 15, "Food Production and Mental Health"). Additionally, it often results in a diet rich in seasonal fruits and vegetables, which can enhance flavor and nutritional value. Among its numerous benefits is reducing the carbon footprint of food production and supporting local economies; unfortunately, the locavore diet may pose challenges in terms of food variety and availability, especially in regions with short growing seasons or a limited diversity of agricultural products.

The climatarian diet is a dietary approach designed to minimize environmental impact and combat climate change by focusing on foods with a lower carbon footprint. This diet emphasizes the consumption of plant-based foods, such as fruits, vegetables, whole grains, legumes, and nuts, while reducing or avoiding foods associated with higher greenhouse gas emissions, particularly red meats and dairy products. By prioritizing sustainably sourced and locally produced foods, the climatarian diet aims to reduce food-related carbon emissions and promote more sustainable agricultural practices. In addition to environmental benefits, this diet can also align with health goals by encouraging the intake of nutrient-dense, whole foods and reducing reliance on processed and high-calorie options. The climatarian diet seeks to balance ecological responsibility with personal health, offering a way to make a positive impact on the planet through everyday food choices.

Similarly, the Planetary Health diet is a comprehensive dietary approach designed to improve human health while minimizing environmental impact. Developed by the EAT-Lancet Commission, this diet emphasizes a shift toward a predominantly plant-based eating pattern, incorporating a variety of fruits, vegetables, whole grains, legumes, nuts, and seeds. More detail is given in Chapter 15, "Food Production and Mental Health." The Planetary Health diet advocates for reduced consumption of red meat and processed foods and encourages moderate intake of poultry, fish, and dairy products. It aims to balance nutritional needs with sustainable food production practices, thereby addressing both the rising rates of diet-related health conditions and the urgent need to reduce greenhouse gas emissions and preserve natural resources. By promoting a diet that supports both individual health and planetary sustainability, it seeks to create a healthier future for people and the planet.

Portion Control and Mindful Eating Practices

Portion control is a crucial aspect of maintaining a balanced diet and plays a significant role in enhancing diet quality, nutrition, and overall physical health. Encouraging clients to consider portion control may be especially relevant today, given the food environment in which we live—replete with high-calorie prepared meals and processed foods, as well as large restaurant portions. By regulating portion sizes, individuals can better manage their caloric intake, avoiding excessive consumption of unhealthy foods that can lead to weight gain and related health issues such as obesity, diabetes, and cardiovascular disease. By focusing on portion sizes, one can improve dietary habits, enhance nutritional intake, and support long-term physical well-being.

Somewhat relatedly, mindful eating encourages individuals to pay full attention to the experience of eating, promoting a deeper awareness of food choices, flavors, and the body's hunger and satiety signals. This practice involves savoring each bite, acknowledging the sensory aspects of food, and recognizing emotional triggers that may lead to overeating or unhealthy eating habits. By cultivating mindfulness around meals, individuals can break the cycle of disordered eating patterns and develop a healthier relationship with food. In essence, mindful eating transforms eating from a mindless activity into a nourishing and enriching experience.

Future Research Directions

Although research on the Mediterranean diet and associated physical and mental health outcomes is accumulating, research is needed on other eating patterns and diets. Additionally, diverse mental health outcomes, beyond depressive symptoms, should be examined. Ideally, studies should be longitudinal rather than cross-sectional, allowing enough time for changes in dietary patterns to exert their full influence on the physical and mental health outcomes being studied. More research is also needed on adherence to dietary changes being used as an adjunctive or alternative treatment, as well as factors associated with improved adherence. Finally, given that enhanced nutrition is just one element of lifestyle optimization, other aspects of lifestyle should be evaluated and intervened on in study designs, alongside dietary changes.

Clinical Pearls

- Clinicians should recommend a balanced and varied diet that includes a high intake of fruits, vegetables, legumes, whole grains, seeds and nuts, fatty fish, lean meats, and low-fat dairy products, while limiting red and processed meats as well as foods and beverages high in added sugars, saturated fats, and sodium.
- The Mediterranean diet should be considered as an adjunctive, if not alternative, treatment for mild to moderate depressive symptoms, as accumulating research supports its efficacy.
- Clinicians should be aware that in addition to what one eats (content), how one eats (process) is important. Portion control and mindful eating practices support healthy weight management and reduce the risk of diet-related health conditions.
- Dietary recommendations and counseling should be accompanied by physical activity recommendations as a crucial component of a healthy lifestyle, advocating for at least 150 minutes of moderate-intensity exercise per week.
- For clients interested in more intensive guidance around healthy eating, weight loss, or physical and mental health promotion through healthy diet, clinicians should consider referrals to registered dietitians or lifestyle medicine clinicians.

Key Chapter Points

- The Western diet—associated with an increased risk of overweight, obesity, insulin resistance, type 2 diabetes, other metabolic disturbances, cardiovascular disease, inflammatory processes, certain cancers, and other chronic conditions—is characterized by a high intake of processed and ultraprocessed foods, red and processed meats, refined grains, high-fat dairy products, and sugar-sweetened beverages, while being low in fruits, vegetables, legumes, whole grains, seeds, and nuts.

- Multiple types of weight-loss and short-term diets have been popularized over the past five decades, including low-calorie diets, low-carbohydrate (high-protein/high-fat) diets, and low-fat diets.
- The Mediterranean diet has been linked to improved physical and mental health outcomes, especially with regard to depressive symptoms.
- In addition to the composition of one's diet, portion control is important, especially in a food environment that promotes overly large meal portions.
- Mindful eating encourages individuals to pay full attention to the experience of eating, promoting a deeper awareness of food choices, flavors, and the body's hunger and satiety signals.

References

Agatston A: The South Beach Diet: The Delicious, Doctor-Designed, Foolproof Plan for Fast and Healthy Weight Loss. New York, Rodale Books, 2003

Atkins RC: Dr. Atkins' Diet Revolution: The High Calorie Way to Stay Thin Forever: The Famous Vogue Superdiet Explained in Full. Philadelphia, D. McKay Co., 1972

Bizzozero-Peroni B, Martínez-Vizcaíno V, Fernández-Rodríguez R, et al: The impact of the Mediterranean diet on alleviating depressive symptoms in adults: a systematic review and meta-analysis of randomized controlled trials. Nutr Rev 83(1):29–39, 2025 38219230

Buettner D: The Blue Zones Solution: Eating and Living Like the World's Healthiest People. Washington, DC, National Geographic, 2015

Butler MI, Mörkl S: The Mediterranean Diet and Mental Health, in Nutritional Psychiatry: A Primer for Clinicians. Edited by Dinan T. Cambridge, UK, Cambridge University Press, 2023

Clemente-Suárez VJ, Beltrán-Velasco AI, Redondo-Flórez L, et al: Global impacts of Western diet and its effects on metabolism and health: a narrative review. Nutrients 15(12):2749, 2023 37375654

Cordain L: The Paleo Diet: Lose Weight and Get Healthy by Eating the Food You Were Designed to Eat. Boston, Houghton Mifflin, 2010

Dukan P: The Dukan Diet: 2 Steps to Lose the Weight, 2 Steps to Keep It Off Forever. New York, Crown Archetype, 2011

Heymsfield SB, van Mierlo CA, van der Knaap HC, et al: Weight management using a meal replacement strategy: meta and pooling analysis from six studies. Int J Obes Relat Metab Disord 27(5):537–549, 2003 12704397

Landry MJ, Crimarco A, Gardner CD: Benefits of low carbohydrate diets: a settled question or still controversial? Curr Obes Rep 10(3):409–422, 2021 34297345

McDougall JA, McDougall M: The McDougall Program: Twelve Days to Dynamic Health. New York, Dutton Adult, 1990

Ornish D: Dr. Dean Ornish's Program for Reversing Heart Disease: The Only System Scientifically Proven to Reverse Heart Disease Without Drugs or Surgery. New York, Ballantine Books, 1992

Pesta DH, Samuel VT: A high-protein diet for reducing body fat: mechanisms and possible caveats. Nutr Metab (Lond) 11(1):53, 2014 25489333

Peters JC, Wyatt HR, Foster GD, et al: The effects of water and non-nutritive sweetened beverages on weight loss during a 12-week weight loss treatment program. Obesity (Silver Spring) 22(6):1415–1421, 2014 24862170

Poti JM, Mendez MA, Ng SW, et al: Is the degree of food processing and convenience linked with the nutritional quality of foods purchased by US households? Am J Clin Nutr 101(6):1251–1262, 2015 25948666

Pritikin N, McGrady PM: The Pritikin Program for Diet and Exercise. New York, Putnam Publishing Group, 1979

Rynders CA, Thomas EA, Zaman A, et al: Effectiveness of intermittent fasting and time-restricted feeding compared to continuous energy restriction for weight loss. Nutrients 11(10):2442, 2019 31614992

Seid H, Rosenbaum M: Low carbohydrate and low-fat diets: what we don't know and why we should know it. Nutrients 11(11):2749, 2019 31726791

Shafiei F, Salari-Moghaddam A, Larijani B, et al: Mediterranean diet and depression: reanalysis of a meta-analysis. Nutr Rev 81(7):889–890, 2023 36928725

Stillman IM, Baker SS: Dr. Stillman's 14-Day Shape-Up Program: An Amazing New Diet with Exercises. New York, Delacorte Press, 1974

Tate DF, Turner-McGrievy G, Lyons E, et al: Replacing caloric beverages with water or diet beverages for weight loss in adults: main results of the Choose Healthy Options Consciously Everyday (CHOICE) randomized clinical trial. Am J Clin Nutr 95(3):555–563, 2012

Tsai AG, Wadden TA: The evolution of very-low-calorie diets: an update and meta-analysis. Obesity (Silver Spring) 14(8):1283–1293, 2006 16988070

Zhang H, Li M, Mo L, et al: Association between western dietary patterns, typical food groups, and behavioral health disorders: an updated systematic review and meta-analysis of observational studies. Nutrients 16(1):125, 2023 38201955

Part 2

Food Insecurity, Nutrition, Diet Quality, and Counseling and Resources for the Clinical Setting

5

Food Insecurity and Mental Health

Michael T. Compton, M.D., M.P.H.
Amy Ehntholt, Sc.D.

One cannot think well, love well, sleep well, if one has not dined well.
—Virginia Woolf

Far too many people in low- and middle-income countries—and even in developed, high-income countries, including the United States—are not sure they will have enough food to last through the month or the week (or are unsure where their food will come from or how they will get it). This uncertainty is known as *food insecurity,* a condition in which the availability of nutritionally adequate and safe foods, or the ability to acquire such foods in socially acceptable ways, is limited or uncertain, most often because of constrained financial resources. Unfortunately, many Americans cannot afford or do not have ready access to enough nutritious foods. In addition to provoking anxiety, food insecurity is a tremendous burden on one's capacity to thrive and succeed at anything in life or to even have an active mental life beyond the confines of securing food or facing the other related social challenges with which those who are hungry have to cope.

Food Insecurity: An Overview

Food insecurity is a multidimensional construct involving deficiencies in quantity, quality, and access to nutritious and safe foods, which can be understood at both the societal level and the individual level. The causes of food insecurity are complex, and its consequences are diverse and interrelated. For individuals, food insecurity is a socio-environmental risk factor that is usually intertwined with other risk factors, such as poverty, unemployment, housing instability, violence and trauma, and limited education (poor education in general and poor health and food literacy in particular), as well as poor social support, social isolation, and loneliness.

Food insecurity affects not only the individual but also the community. Its impact on communities may compound other community-level risks, such as area-level poverty. At the societal level, food insecurity is a root cause of individual-level risk factors, linked to income inequality and other social determinants of health. In a land of abundant food like the United States, the inability to access sufficient nutritious food reveals powerlessness, social exclusion, and unjust distribution of the most basic needs and opportunities. It also is evidence of market failure—a mismatch between demand and supply (i.e., insufficient demand due to insufficient money to buy) and thus an inability of the market to deliver a needed commodity. These circumstances have profound effects on individuals and communities alike.

The anxiety-provoking uncertainty as to whether a person, household, or community will have enough nutritious food is a clinical, public health, and social justice problem of sufficient importance, even in the United States, to deserve heightened scrutiny. Despite the known links between food insecurity and poor mental health outcomes and mental illnesses, food insecurity is too often neglected by both clinicians (perhaps especially by mental health professionals) and policymakers. Nonetheless, research linking food insecurity and mental health has rapidly accumulated in recent years (see Figure 5.1).

Food security is one of several conditions necessary for a population to be physically and mentally healthy and well nourished (Coleman-Jensen et al. 2012). Because health is a state of physical, emotional, behavioral, and social well-being and not merely the absence of disease, food security is, by definition, a social determinant of both physical health and mental health.

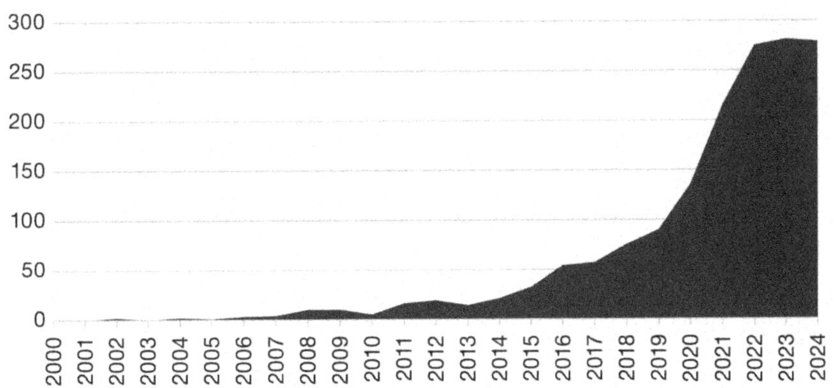

Figure 5.1 **Food insecurity and mental health–related publications over time, 2000–2024.**

Note. Search query used on pubmed.gov (January 7, 2025): ("food secur*"[Title/Abstract] OR "food insecur*"[Title/Abstract] AND "mental health" [Title/Abstract]).

Prevalence of Food Insecurity in the United States

Food insecurity is a major problem affecting low-income countries and famine areas, leading to hunger, nutritional deficiencies, malnutrition, medical and social problems, and excesses in morbidity and mortality. Food insecurity also occurs in high-income countries, including the United States. Since 1995, to supplement the nationally representative Current Population Survey of the U.S. Census Bureau, the U.S. Department of Agriculture (USDA) has conducted annual surveys on food access and adequacy, food spending, and sources of food assistance for the U.S. population. Survey items are summed to derive useful cut points for defining levels of food security or insecurity; for example, *low food security* indicates reduced quality, variety, or desirability of diet but little or no indication of reduced food intake, whereas *very low food security* refers to multiple indications of disrupted eating patterns and reduced food intake.

In 2023, 18 million U.S. households (13.5%) were food insecure at some time during the year, and 6.8 million households (5.1%) had very low food security (Rabbitt et al. 2024). Because the impact of food insecurity may be most profound when it occurs in childhood, it is par-

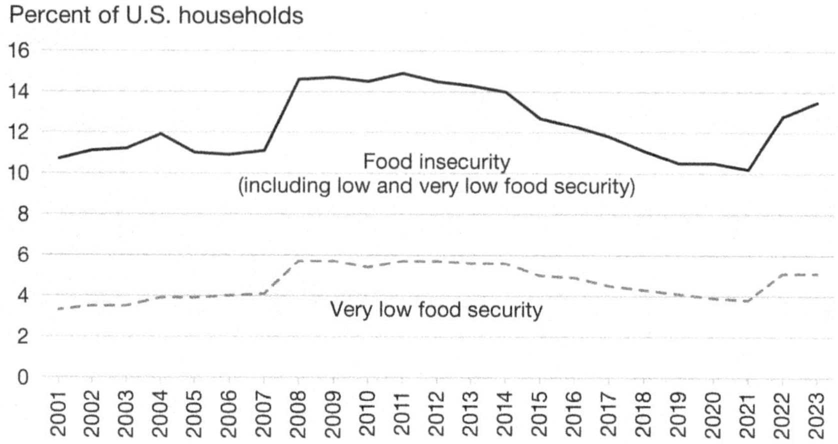

Figure 5.2 Trends in the prevalence of food insecurity and very low food insecurity in U.S. households, 2001–2023.

Note. "Food insecure—At times during the year, these households were uncertain of having or unable to acquire enough food to meet the needs of all their members because they had insufficient money or other resources for food. Food-insecure households include those with low food security and very low food security." (Economic Research Service, https://www.ers.usda.gov/topics/food-nutrition-assistance/food-security-in-the-us/key-statistics-graphics).

Source. USDA, Economic Research Service, using data from U.S. Department of Commerce, U.S. Census Bureau, Current Population Survey Food Security Supplements.

ticularly noteworthy that 17.9% of all U.S. households with children were food insecure at some time during that year, and although adults commonly protect children from the effects of household food insecurity by diverting food to them, in about half of these households, the children themselves were food insecure. Trends in the national prevalence of average household food insecurity from 2012 through 2023 are shown in Figure 5.2, along with trends in states categorized as politically "blue" or "red" in Figure 5.3, exposing the consequences of state-level policies and other compositional and contextual factors.

The prevalence of food insecurity varies substantially across the United States. Using combined data from 2021–2023 (allowing for more stable estimates), the USDA documents that some states have rates of household food insecurity of less than 10% (e.g., New Hampshire, 7.4%; North Dakota, 8.6%; South Dakota, 9.0%), whereas others have rates in excess of 16% (e.g., Louisiana and Mississippi, 16.2%; Texas, 16.9%;

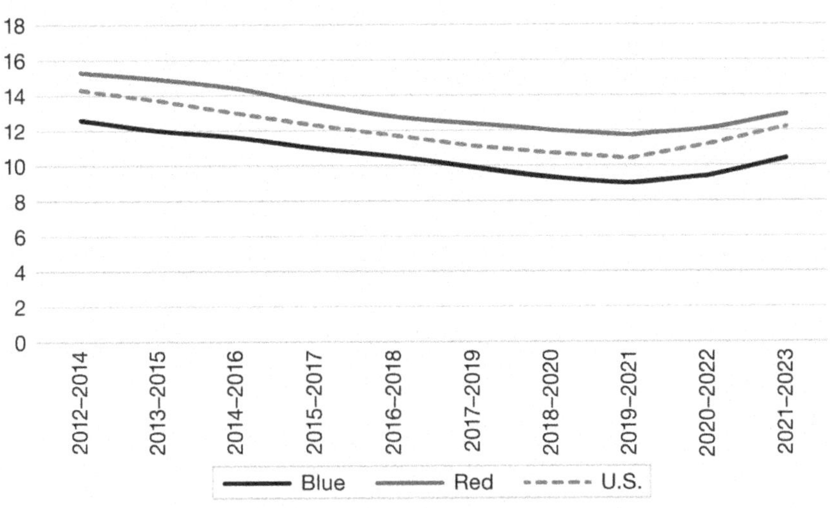

Figure 5.3 **Average prevalence of household food insecurity in red versus blue states (categorized by statewide results in the last four presidential elections).**

Note. Red = won by the Republicans in all four elections; blue = won by the Democrats in all four elections. States were removed from analysis if they were won by the Republicans in three of the four elections; won by each party twice in the four elections; and won by the Democrats in three of the four elections.

Source. USDA, Economic Research Service using data from U.S. Department of Commerce, U.S. Census Bureau, Current Population Survey Food Security Supplements.

Arkansas, 18.9%) (Rabbitt et al. 2024); see Table 5.1. Between-state variations in the prevalence of food insecurity are driven by differences in states' populations (e.g., pertaining to education and employment) and differences in tax policies, employment-related policies, and the nature of participation in federal food and nutrition assistance programs. It is also noteworthy that in general, the states with the highest rates of food insecurity tend to correspond to the states with the greatest degree of income inequality among their citizens, consistent with the observation across nations that a more equal distribution of resources equates to fewer people with food insecurity (Wilkinson and Pickett 2009).

In addition to state-to-state variation, the prevalence of food insecurity varies across demographic groups or circumstances. Rates of food insecurity are substantially higher than the national average in Black and Hispanic families, in households with incomes near or below the

Table 5.1 States with the highest and lowest prevalence of food insecurity (2021–2023)

State	Prevalence (%)
Highest	
Arkansas	18.9
Texas	16.9
Louisiana	16.2
Mississippi	16.2
Oklahoma	15.4
Kentucky	14.5
South Carolina	14.4
West Virginia	13.7
Wyoming	13.1
Michigan	13.0
Lowest	
New Hampshire	7.4
North Dakota	8.6
District of Columbia	8.8
South Dakota	9.0
Minnesota	9.1
Vermont	9.2
Massachusetts	9.3
Washington	9.5
Hawaii	9.6
Rhode Island	9.7

Source. Rabbitt et al. 2024. Available at: https://www.ers.usda.gov/topics/food-nutrition-assistance/food-security-in-the-u-s/interactive-charts-and-highlights/#States. Accessed January 7, 2025.

federal poverty level, in households with children (especially households headed by a single mother), and in large cities or rural areas compared with suburban areas. Furthermore, food insecurity is much more prevalent in households containing a working-age adult with a disability, including a mental health disability (Reed-Jones 2024). Many such households face other risks for poor mental health (e.g., housing instability), again reinforcing that such social risks tend to cluster together among the most socially and economically disadvantaged individuals, families, and communities. Attention to *food deserts*, or areas characterized by poor access to healthy and affordable foods, emphasizes that community-level social and spatial disparities in food access and diet quality likely contribute to health inequities (Walker et al. 2010). Modern methods for measuring the food environment (e.g., geospatial analysis) hold promise for identifying community-level predictors of individual diet quality and for informing policy pertaining to the food environment.

Food Insecurity as a Social Determinant of Health

Diet is one of the principal determinants of many common health conditions, including the most prevalent chronic diseases affecting individuals in developed countries, such as cardiovascular disease, type 2 diabetes, and cancer (Hamilton et al. 2024; Hu 2024; Wang et al. 2019). Food insecurity is associated with poorer self-reported health status (Leung et al. 2020a), which is linked to many adverse health outcomes, and also with objectively measured health indicators such as hypertension and diabetes (Levi et al. 2023). Food insecurity may also be associated with increased inflammatory responses (Gowda et al. 2012), which in turn are tied to diverse morbidities, including cardiovascular diseases. Food insecurity is related not only to incidence of many chronic diseases but also to the course of those diseases. For example, food insecurity is predictive of poorer glycemic control among those with diabetes (Walker et al. 2021); evidence suggests that this association may be partly driven by emotional distress and difficulty following a healthy diet (Seligman et al. 2012). Even short but repeated periods of food insecurity and hunger can have a cumulative adverse effect on health (Kirkpatrick et al. 2010).

One reason for the connection with chronic diseases is that food insecurity is related to diet quality. Individuals and families in the United

States with constrained financial resources tend to spend more of their limited food dollars on sugar-sweetened beverages and energy-dense but nutritionally barren foods that are high in refined sugars, saturated fats, and salt. Overreliance on processed foods and fast food—and the resulting reduced dietary variety, low consumption of fresh fruits and vegetables, and insufficient intake of micronutrients such as the B complex vitamins—is associated with chronic diseases that are the leading causes of death in the United States. Thus, although food insecurity can cause hunger and reduced food intake, in the United States and other high-income countries where certain types of foods are generally available beyond the population's needs but others are not (which is a market failure and policy failure, as noted above), food insecurity is paradoxically associated with overweight and obesity (Carvajal-Aldaz et al. 2022; Dinour et al. 2007; Institute of Medicine 2011; Larson and Story 2011).

Food insecurity has profound effects on the physical health of children. Sufficient and nutritious food is a requirement for optimal physical, cognitive, social, and emotional growth and development (Stang et al. 2006). Children from food-insecure households have an increased prevalence of many illnesses and higher hospitalization rates (Abraham et al. 2023; Pai and Bahadur 2020). Affected children are at increased risk for iron deficiency anemia, developmental delays, stunted growth, compromised immune function and infections, impaired attainment of social skills, learning delays, poor school performance, and behavioral and emotional problems.

Food Insecurity as a Social Determinant of Mental Health

There can be little doubt that food insecurity (and hunger, when present) leads to psychological stress—anxiety, frustration, a sense of powerlessness, and disconnection from others—which in turn triggers diverse physiological responses that elevate the risk for mental illness. As noted above, the link between food insecurity and mental illness was not given much attention at the start of this century. Only a handful of research articles investigating the association were indexed in PubMed between 2000 and 2005 (none in 2000 and 2001; see Figure 5.1). The number began to grow after 2010, with a steep incline around 2019 and a subsequent ballooning during the COVID-19 pandemic (jumping from 135 papers in 2020 to 215 in 2021, with close to 300 in each ensuing year). Among these studies was a 2020 systematic review and meta-analysis that pooled data from 19 studies involving 372,143 individual participants from 10 countries (Pourmotabbed et al. 2020), which found a positive relationship between food insecurity and risk of depression (odds ratio [OR] = 1.40) and stress (OR = 1.34); subgroup analyses showed the risk of depression to be greater among men than women and greater among those ≥65 years old. Other highlights of recent research follow, grouped into the broad categories that emerge on examination of the literature.

Food Insecurity and Mental Health Among Pregnant and Postpartum Women

The link between food insecurity and adverse mental health outcomes, especially perinatal depression, has been repeatedly documented around the world: in multiple and diverse countries classified by the World Bank (World Bank 2024) as "low-income economies" (Mark et al. 2021; Natamba et al. 2017; Woldetensay et al. 2018), in "lower-middle-income economies" (Ayyub et al. 2018; Decaro et al. 2016; Hasan et al. 2021; Khoshgoo et al. 2020; Piperata et al. 2016), and in "upper-middle-income economies" (Abrahams et al. 2018; Harmel and Höfelmann 2022; Weigel et al. 2016).

High-income economies such as the United States (Richards et al. 2020; Siefert et al. 2001; 2004; Wu et al. 2018), the United Kingdom (Melchior et al. 2009; Power et al. 2017), and Canada (Tarasuk et al. 2020) are not immune to the adverse mental health impacts of food insecurity on perinatal depression and related adverse behavioral health outcomes. In the United States, perinatal and maternal depression has been linked to food insecurity in nationally representative surveys (Johnson and Markowitz 2018) and prospective cohort studies (Laraia et al. 2006; 2015) among low-income African American mothers (Laraia et al. 2009), low-income pregnant Latinas (Hromi-Fiedler et al. 2011), and migrant Latino farmworker families (Pulgar et al. 2016). Supplemental Nutrition Assistance Program (SNAP) participation may reduce distress and depression (Munger et al. 2016), and losing such benefits is associated with maternal depression (Casey et al. 2004).

The effects of food insecurity extend beyond the perinatal period; for example, data from 19,127 mothers of a nationally representative sample of U.S. children ages 0–5 from the 2016–2017 National Survey of Children's Health revealed links between food insecurity and mothers' poor mental health after controlling for multiple other variables (Linares et al. 2020). Mental health impacts can persist long-term (Daundasekara et al. 2022) and are greater at more serious levels of food insecurity (Liebe et al. 2022). The causal relationship between household food insecurity and maternal depression has been shown to be bidirectional (Huddleston-Casas et al. 2009; Reesor-Oyer et al. 2021). Some studies suggest a potential moderating role of various forms of social support (e.g., Natamba et al. 2017; Piperata et al. 2016; Tsai et al. 2016; Woldetensay et al. 2018)—such support reduces the impact of food insecurity on adverse mental health outcomes.

Food Insecurity and Mental Health Among Young Children

Household food insecurity affects not just mothers, but their infants and young children as well. It has been linked to poorer mental health among young children, even in models adjusting for demographics, other social adversities, and parental mental health (Dean et al. 2023). Specifically, associations have been seen between food insecurity and both externalizing and internalizing behavior problems (Hayati Rezvan et al. 2021; Hobbs and King 2018; Kimbro and Denney 2015; King 2017; Nagata et al. 2019; Slopen et al. 2010; Whitaker et al. 2006). Such associations may be mediated by poor sleep (King 2017); developmental risk (Rose-Jacobs et al. 2008); anxiety and depression (Weinreb et al. 2002; Zheng et al. 2021); psychosocial dysfunction, including attention problems (Melchior et al. 2012; Spencer et al. 2020); and severe emotional dysregulation (Hatsu et al. 2022). Research suggests that food insecurity may be associated with preterm birth (an important cause of neonatal mortality and long-term complications) (Dolatian et al. 2018) and prenatal alcohol use (which is associated with fetal alcohol syndrome among offspring) (Eaton et al. 2014). Qualitative work has highlighted the different forms of psychological distress reported by children experiencing food insecurity, which include worrying about food availability, embarrassment, and sadness (Leung et al. 2020b). Outside of the United States, Chen and colleagues (2009) analyzed a large longitudinal dataset from the Taiwan National Health Insurance scheme (N = 764,526) and found that imputed measures of food insecurity predicted mental disorders among elementary school–aged children. Another study, of children ages 6–12 in a low-income region in Quito, Ecuador, revealed an association between household food insecurity and poorer psychosocial function (Weigel et al. 2018).

Attention has been drawn to the interactive nature of other factors at play in the relationship between food insecurity and mental health among young children (e.g., the role of caregivers and the impact of their mental health), as well as the possible long-term repercussions. A study conducted at 26 Head Start centers in Arkansas found that children of mothers with high-level symptoms of maternal depression had nearly eight times the odds of food insecurity (adjusted OR = 7.81; 95% CI 3.71–16.45) compared with children whose mothers had no symptoms of maternal depression (Ward et al. 2019). From Children's HealthWatch, among 26,950 caregiver-child pairs surveyed in 2000–2010 (Black et al. 2012), food insecurity was present in 24% of households, and the presence of both caregiver depressive symptoms and household food insecurity increased the likelihood of multiple negative child health indicators, such as hospitalizations and developmental risk, which is consistent with cumulative stress models.

As with other adverse childhood experiences, the consequences of experiencing food insecurity as a child may be seen later in life. For example, data from the Estonian Health Interview Survey 2006 revealed that going to bed hungry in childhood was associated with significantly increased odds of depressive symptoms in adulthood (in a sample of n = 5,095; Stickley and Leinsalu 2018), and significantly increased odds of thoughts of death or suicide in adults ages 60 and older (in a sample of n = 2,455; Stickley and Leinsalu 2018). A longitudinal study of Canadian children found that child hunger predicted depression and suicidal ideation in late adolescence and young adulthood (McIntyre et al. 2013). Along with experiencing persistent childhood food insecurity, having caregivers who themselves experienced psychological distress placed children at greater risk for psychological distress in young adulthood (Pryor et al. 2023); access to SNAP benefits lowered the risk. Shielding children from food insecurity was found in one study to be associated with reduced risks of common psychiatric outcomes and poor mental health in youth and adults, possibly owing to its association with less severe food insecurity (Ovenell et al. 2022).

Food Insecurity and Mental Health Among Older Children, Adolescents, and Young Adults

Studies finding a significant association between food insecurity and common mental health disorders among older children and adolescents have spanned the globe, from Canada (Men et al. 2021) and the United States (McLaughlin et al. 2012; Poole-Di Salvo et al. 2016) to several countries in Africa (Jebena et al. 2016; Jesson et al. 2021; McRell et al. 2022; Tetteh et al. 2024), China (Yang et al. 2021), Taiwan (Lee et al. 2021), Ecuador (Romo et al. 2016), the Caribbean (Pengpid and Peltzer, 2023), and India (Rani et al. 2018). Specific mental health outcomes linked to food insecurity for this age group include depression and anxiety disorders (Bradette-Laplante et al. 2020; Goldman-Hasbun et al. 2019; Jesson et al. 2021; McIntyre et al. 2017; McLaughlin et al. 2012; Pengpid and Peltzer 2023); suicidality (Brinkman et al. 2021; Pengpid and Peltzer 2023; Romo et al. 2016; Tetteh et al. 2024); problematic substance use (McLaughlin et al. 2012; Pengpid and Peltzer 2023; Tetteh et al. 2024); negative behavioral outcomes (e.g., bullying, truancy) (Pengpid and Peltzer 2023); and eating pathology and unhealthy eating behaviors (Hooper et al. 2020; Kim et al. 2021; Kent et al. 2022). Food insecurity's relationship with adverse mental outcomes in this age group may be stronger among females than among males (Hammami et al. 2020). Several studies offer evidence of a gradient in association (Goldman-Hasbun et al. 2019; Romo et al. 2016); for example, in their analysis of several mental illnesses, Men and colleagues (2021) found that the relative risks of suicidal thoughts among youth with marginal, moderate, and severe food insecurity were 1.77, 2.44, and 6.49, respectively.

Effects of food insecurity in childhood and adolescence linger. In their investigation of longitudinal trajectories of food insecurity during the first 13 years of life, Paquin et al. (2021) found that persistent high-risk food insecurity was associated with psychosocial problems in later adolescence. A longitudinal study of the effect of hunger self-reported by Canadian youth across 6 years found that depression in ever-hungry youth remained elevated over time, unlike the findings for never-hungry youth (McIntyre et al. 2017). Lee et al. (2021) examined the trajectory of food insecurity over time and its association with mental health and sleep outcomes in Taiwanese youth ages 12–18 years and found an association between persistent moderate food insecurity and mental health problems and sleep disturbances. Social support (Hammami et al. 2020) and interpersonal connections (Brinkman et al. 2021) might alleviate the relationship in this age group. However, participation in the National School Lunch Program (NSLP) was not shown to buffer the relationship between food insecurity and depression (Frank and Sato 2023). Similarly, in a separate study, the association between household food insecurity and parent-reported adolescent mental health problems was not changed by receiving a free or reduced-price lunch at school (Poole-Di Salvo et al. 2016).

Unsurprisingly, the majority of studies on college-aged individuals or young adults have been conducted in university or college settings, including in the United States: at an Appalachian university (Hagedorn and Olfert 2018); the California public university system (Martinez et al. 2020); a large, public university in Mississippi (Reeder et al. 2020); schools in the Southwest (Coakley et al. 2022; Umeda et al. 2020); and other institutions of higher education (Becerra and Becerra 2020; Bruening et al. 2018; Hagedorn et al. 2021). Studies from outside the United States reveal associations between experiences of food insecurity at this age and worse mental health among varied groups: Canadian students transitioning to university (Howard and Barker 2021); youth in Arab countries (Asfahani et al. 2019); a community sample of young adults in France (Pryor et al. 2016); university students in Malaysia (Ahmad et al. 2021); medical students in Iran (Amin et al. 2022); and college students in Lebanon (Itani et al. 2022). Results from analyses of these and other populations of the same age link food insecurity to academic performance through poorer mental health (Martinez et al. 2020) and find direct connections between food insecurity and psychological distress (Becerra and Becerra 2020; Guzman et al. 2022; Marmolejo et al. 2024); stress (Ahmad et al. 2021; Bruening et al. 2018; Darling et al. 2017); depression and anxiety (Amin et al. 2022; Coakley et al. 2022; Coffino et al. 2021; Itani et al. 2022; Neal and Zigmont 2022; Oh et al. 2022; Umeda et al. 2020); suicidal ideation (Nagata et al. 2019; Pryor et al. 2016); substance use (Baer et al. 2015; Becerra and Becerra 2020; Neal and Zigmont 2022; Oh et al. 2022; Pryor et al. 2016); coping strategies (Hagedorn and Olfert 2018); poorer sleep health (Hagedorn et al. 2021; Nagata et al. 2019); and disordered eating (Darling et al. 2017; Royer et al. 2021).

The prevalence of food insecurity among this age group has been shown to be high, and the relationship with adverse mental health outcomes is strong. Of a sample of graduate students at a northeastern U.S. university (n = 263), for example, almost half reported food insecurity, and 21.8% reported very low food security (Coffino et al. 2021). A separate study found disparities in prevalence by race, with African American students having more than three times the odds of food insecurity compared with their White counterparts (OR = 3.50; 95% CI 1.38–8.90) (Reeder et al. 2020); students reporting very low food security had 4.52 times the odds of depression compared with their food-secure peers. Differences by gender have been noted in the relationship between food insecurity and psychological distress. Among study participants at a minority-serving institution (n = 302), food-insecure students had 3.65 times the odds of reporting psychological distress and 2.69 times the odds of poor self-perceived mental health compared with food-secure students (Becerra and Becerra 2020).

Food Insecurity, Poor Mental Health, Psychological Distress, Depression, and Suicidality

Across the various mental health outcomes, those most consistently studied in relation to food insecurity are stress- and depression-related outcomes, including poor mental health and psychological distress, depressive symptoms and major depressive disorder, and suicidality.

Associations between food insecurity and poor mental health, psychological distress, and depressive symptoms have been documented around the world (Frongillo et al. 2017, 2019; Jones 2017), in countries from low and lower-middle income economies such as Ethiopia (Birhanu and Tadesse 2019; Hadley et al. 2008; Maes et al. 2010), Pakistan (Jafree 2020), Uganda (Perkins et al. 2018), and Zambia (Cole and Tembo 2011); upper-middle income economies such as South Africa (Tomita et al. 2019, 2020); and high-income economies such as Canada (Pound and Chen 2021; Shafiee et al. 2021), Panama (Maupin and Hackman 2022), and the United States (Adynski et al. 2023; Ciciurkaite and Brown 2022; Sharkey et al. 2011; Stuff et al. 2004; Willis et al. 2020). Diverse samples have been studied—female caretakers in Tanzania (Hadley and Patil 2006; Hadley et al. 2008); ultra-poor women in Bangladesh (Jalal et al. 2015); heads of households (Atuoye and Luginaah 2017) and older adults in Ghana (Gyasi et al. 2020a; Gyasi et al. 2020b); refugees and immigrants in South Africa (Maharaj et al. 2017); and women in conflict-affected areas of Syria (Falb et al. 2019), to name a few. All studies document significant associations.

In the United States, food insecurity has been linked to psychological distress among Hispanic respondents to the California Health Interview Survey (n = 10,966) (Becerra et al. 2015), as well as African American respondents to the same survey (n = 4,003) (Allen et al. 2018). Also in the United States, associations with depressive symptoms or depression have been documented among low-income women in an urban county in Michigan (Heflin et al. 2005); injection drug users (Anema et al.

2010); homebound older adults in North Carolina (Johnson et al. 2011); National Health and Nutrition Examination Survey (2011–2014) respondents with prediabetes or diabetes (Montgomery et al. 2017) and other groups with diabetes (Silverman et al. 2015); both fathers and mothers in food-insecure homes (Tseng et al. 2017); individuals on probation (Dong et al. 2018); low-wage nursing home employees (Okechukwu et al. 2012) and early care and education workers (Loh et al. 2020); Asian Americans (Lai et al. 2021); adult digestive cancer survivors (Madigan et al. 2021); and U.S. foreign-born immigrants (Li et al. 2023).

Several studies suggest that the association between food insecurity and poor mental health may be moderated or attenuated by increased levels of social support (Kollannoor-Samuel et al. 2011; Na et al. 2019) and greater proximate access to vegetables and fruits (Bergmans et al. 2019). A number of studies indicate that adverse mental health outcomes are more strongly linked to food insecurity than to other forms of material hardship, such as having a major financial difficulty, unmet health needs, or inadequate housing (Johnson et al. 2011). Finally, links between food insecurity and suicidal ideation have been documented, such as among respondents to the 2007 Canadian Community Health Survey (n = 5,270) (Davison et al. 2015) and among 2,630 U.S. veterans participating in the National Health and Nutrition Examination Survey (2007–2016). Veterans with low or very low food security had significantly increased odds for suicidal ideation compared with food-secure veterans (Kamdar et al. 2021).

Food Insecurity and Substance Use

Although relatively little research has explored a possible link between food insecurity and substance use, at least 14 published studies—mainly focused on tobacco use, alcohol use, or substance use more broadly—have revealed strong associations. Researchers using data from the 2015 U.S. Panel Study of Income Dynamics (N = 9,048) created a four-category variable based on responses to questions about psychological distress and food insecurity and found smoking prevalence to be highest among individuals who reported psychological distress with food insecurity (39%) (Kim-Mozeleski et al. 2021). Those reporting only food insecurity had higher smoking prevalence (33%) than respondents reporting only psychological distress (20%). A relationship between food insecurity and smoking cessation has also been noted: analyses of the 2015 California Health Interview Survey of 3,007 lower-income adults who had ever smoked showed a quit ratio that was lower for ever-smokers who reported food insecurity with distress (41%) compared with ever-smokers who reported food security without distress (63%) (Kim-Mozeleski and Tsoh 2019). Among a cross-sectional, representative sample of adults in Wisconsin (*N* = 1,616), food insecurity was associated with cigarette smoking in men and women (OR = 3.0; 95% CI 2.1–4.4), but only among men was food insecurity associated with heavy alcohol use (OR = 1.5; 95% CI 1.0–2.2) and dual substance use (OR = 5.2; 95% CI 1.5–18.6) (Bergmans et al. 2019). A link between food insecurity and alcohol use has also been found among women, however (Eaton et al. 2014).

Associations between food insecurity and substance use have also been found across different age groups and other subpopulations, with outcomes including an increased odds of alcohol use and related problematic and risky behaviors (Nagata et al. 2021); a higher prevalence of binge drinking, current marijuana use, and lifetime opioid use among U.S. high school students (Turner et al. 2022); illicit drug use and risky sexual behavior (Zlotorzynska and Sanchez 2022); unhealthy drug or alcohol use among a random sample (*n* = 2,312) of emergency department public hospital patients (Gerber et al. 2020); and an increased odds of sharing injection equipment among injection drug users (Strike et al. 2012).

Food Insecurity and Mental Health Among Older Adults and Those with Cognitive Decline

A growing body of research documents the relationship between food insecurity and mental health among older adults and those with cognitive decline. The majority of studies to date in this area have focused on depression, cognitive impairment, or dementia. Estimates for proportions of adults age 60+ in the United States with depressive symptoms by food security status suggest a gradient in depression by severity: marginal food insecurity (12.3%); low food insecurity (16.3%); and very low food insecurity (25.2%) (Brooks et al. 2019). A significant link between food insecurity and depression in older populations has been seen among welfare recipients in Israel (German et al. 2011); low-income adults in Alabama (Jung et al. 2019); urban elderly Malaysians (Mesbah et al. 2020); American participants in the Health and Retirement Study

(Bergmans and Wegryn-Jones 2020); urban older adults in Mexico City (Vilar-Compte et al. 2016); and older adults in India (Muhammad et al. 2022; Sampaio et al. 2022; Selvamani and Elgar 2023). Meta-analyses of adults age ≥50 in six low- and middle-income countries (China, Ghana, India, Mexico, Russia, and South Africa) (*N* = 34,129), found that the experience of severe food insecurity was associated with 2.43 times the odds of depression, but no association was seen between moderate food insecurity and depression (Smith et al. 2021). Results of a study of low-income adults in Alabama (*N* = 372) suggested that food insecurity and nutritional status were significantly associated indirectly through depressive symptoms (Jung et al. 2019).

Food insecurity has been linked to cognitive impairment among older adults in South Africa (Koyanagi et al. 2019), with higher magnitudes seen among those ≥65 with severe food insecurity (OR 3.87; 95% CI 2.20–6.81), as well as among a sample of Puerto Ricans ages 45–75 in Massachusetts (Gao et al. 2009). Evidence of even more pronounced cognitive impairment was seen for those with very low food security in one longitudinal study (Wong et al. 2016). In India, in a nationally representative sample age ≥60 (*N* = 31,464), those reporting not having enough food of their choice had higher odds (adjusted OR 1.24; 95% CI 1.14–1.35) of cognitive impairment than their peers; those who reported being hungry but not eating also had higher odds of cognitive impairment (adjusted OR 1.30; 95% CI 1.02–1.73) (Srivastava and Muhammad 2022). Recent longitudinal analysis by Lu and colleagues (2023) of changes in food insecurity status found that worse cognition was predicted by persistent food insecurity as well as by a change to food-insecure status, compared with persistent food-secure status, with evidence of mediation by depressive symptoms. Dementia has also been associated with food insecurity. In adjusted models in one study, for example, individuals age ≥60 in Malaysia (*n* = 2,745) who reported a food-insecure childhood had 1.81 times the odds of developing dementia in old age (Momtaz et al. 2014). A longitudinal study in Japan examining neighborhood food environments (availability of food stores within a certain distance of residence that sold fruits and vegetables) found that among adults age ≥65, lower food store availability was associated with higher dementia incidence (Tani et al. 2019).

A few studies have also looked at the possible role of physical health in this relationship. In one study, overweight/obese individuals had a higher prevalence of food insecurity compared with their peers, but multivariate analysis showed that mental illness was a predictor of food insecurity while weight status was not (Brostow et al. 2019). Among a population of older adults age ≥60 with multiple chronic conditions in primary care, those with food insecurity were more likely to be female, disabled, and African American and more likely to report at least one behavioral diagnosis (i.e., alcohol or drug abuse, psychosis, or depression): 67% of food-insecure compared with 26% of food-secure individuals (Jih et al. 2020). Data from the Veterans Aging Cohort Study (N = 6,709) revealed that 24% of participants reported being food insecure and that food insecurity was associated with being African American, using marijuana, having depression, and having worse control of depression (Wang et al. 2015). Meal assistance programs may be effective in alleviating food insecurity's relationship with adverse mental health outcomes among this older population, especially for the homebound (Kim and Frongillo 2007; Ross et al. 2022; Wright et al. 2015).

Food Insecurity Among Individuals With Serious Mental Illness

Although extant research is limited, the prevalence of food insecurity among individuals with serious mental illness appears to be very high. Mangurian et al. (2013) found that 71% of patients with serious mental illness in mental health clinics in San Diego were food insecure; similarly, Compton and Ku (2023) showed that 69% of 300 outpatients with serious mental illness in Washington, DC, were food insecure. Reports from Israel (Kaufman et al. 2013), Ethiopia (Tirfessa et al. 2019, 2020), and Australia (Teasdale et al. 2020) also document very high rates of food insecurity in those with serious mental illness.

In a study of 188 community-dwelling individuals with serious mental illness (85% with schizophrenia) receiving clozapine or a long-acting injectable antipsychotic medication in three mental health services in Sydney, Australia, food insecurity was present in 31%, and tobacco smoking (but not other demographic, diagnostic, or clinical variables) was higher among those who were food insecure (Tripodi et al. 2022). Among 314 adults with serious mental illness living in supportive housing in New York City and Philadelphia, 52% reported low or very low food security (Cunningham et al. 2022), and among 156 adults with both a serious mental illness and type 2 diabetes, 25% had food insecurity (and they had greater psychiatric symptom severity than those who were food secure; Michels et al. 2022). Although the increased prevalence of food insecurity in this population may not be surprising, as it is known that the presence of a disability is a strong risk factor for food insecurity (Coleman-Jensen and Nord 2013; Reed-Jones 2024), the magnitude of the increased prevalence is substantial.

Food Insecurity and Mental Health in Other Populations

Associations between food insecurity and adverse mental health outcomes have been repeatedly documented in other populations, although a review is beyond the purview of this chapter. Such populations include individuals with HIV or at risk of HIV, those who are homeless or unstably housed, and individuals exhibiting clinical or subclinical eating disorder pathology. Additionally, beyond the studies noted above, multiple epidemiologic reports on food insecurity and poor mental health have come from population-based studies involving large, nationally representative surveys, including the National Health and Nutrition Examination Survey (NHANES); the National Health Interview Survey (NHIS); the Behavioral Risk Factor Surveillance System (BRFSS); the National Comorbidity Survey-Replication; the National Longitudinal Study of Adolescent to Adult Health; the Korean National Health and Nutrition Examination Survey; New Zealand's Survey of Families, Income and Employment; Australia's Household, Income and Labour Dynamics Survey; the Indonesia Family Life Survey; the Mexican National Health and Nutrition Survey; and the South African Stress and Health Study, among others.

Assessing Food Insecurity and Related Risk Factors in the Clinical Setting

Food insecurity affects individuals, families, communities, and society at large. The social determinants of mental health must be addressed at the individual level (in the clinical setting), at the family level (through social services and local programs), and at the community and societal level (through local, state, and federal policy initiatives).

Health care teams can routinely use a set of brief, standardized questions to screen for food insecurity. Although questionnaires used in national surveys of food insecurity typically take only a few minutes to administer, even more abbreviated versions have been developed for the screening of food insecurity in clinical settings. Examples of two-item and even one-item screening questions are given in Chapter 6 ("Food- and Nutrition-Related Rating Scales and Assessment in the Clinical Setting"). These questions screen only for food insecurity; other screening is required for nutrition security and diet quality. Screening can be performed by nonphysician health care team members, or screening questions can be added to intake surveys completed by clients or caregivers before the clinical encounter. For those screening affirmatively, additional assessment of possible food insecurity is warranted (Shim and Compton 2020).

How Clinicians Can Address Food Insecurity and Related Risk Factors

The crucial initial step in addressing food insecurity in the clinical setting is to begin routinely asking about it, which need not add excessive time to the typical clinical encounter. Addressing food insecurity (and similarly, hunger, poor diet quality, and nutritional deficiencies) can be thought of as comprising four key elements.

First, if a food-related risk factor is detected through screening, a more extensive evaluation is warranted. This evaluation entails determining the underlying causes; for example, is food insecurity stemming from restricted financial resources alone, or do limited transportation, insufficient local availability (e.g., food deserts), or psychiatric symptoms (e.g., negative symptoms of schizophrenia, depressive symptoms, anxiety symptoms associated with agoraphobia) create barriers? Second, because food insecurity is commonly experienced as a household risk, rather than solely an individual risk, family involvement in assessing and intervening on food insecurity is essential. Third, addressing food insecurity (which might partly begin to attend to poor diet quality and any nutritional deficiencies also present in the context of food insecurity) requires familiarity with local food resources including food pantries. Becoming acquainted with local resources is easy and at the health care team's fingertips, given the extensive information and resources available online. For example, Feeding America's website (www.feedingamerica.org) has a locator that identifies local resources in every state. Finally, the health care team can become more familiar with federal food and nutrition assistance programs (the administration of which varies somewhat across states), such as the Supplemental Nutrition Assistance Program (SNAP) and Special Supplemental Nutrition Program for Women, Infants, and Children (WIC), among many others (see Chapter 7, "Assessing and Addressing Food- and Nutrition-Related Issues in the Clinical Setting," and Chapter 9, "Food- and Nutrition-Related Policies and Programs"). Food-insecure families underuse available assistance programs (Kleinman et al. 2007), although families referred to such programs by health care providers are more likely to contact the recommended agencies and find them beneficial (Fleegler et al. 2007). Some clients might also be eligible for Food Is Medicine programs such as medically tailored groceries and produce prescription programs, as detailed in Chapter 8 ("Food Is Medicine").

Assessing for and ameliorating food insecurity among adults with mental illnesses will have favorable mental health effects for the entire family. Although some clinicians might not feel comfortable stepping into the role of nutritional consultant, dietitians or nutritionists in team-based practice settings can help clients plan meals that are inexpensive yet nutritious. Even if a nutritionist or dietary counselor is not routinely available, dietary counseling need not be burdensome during the standard clinical encounter (see Chapter 7). Federally produced dietary guidance, such as the *Dietary Guidelines for Americans* (U.S. Department of Agriculture and U.S. Department of Health and Human Services 2010), can help health professionals in their dietary counseling.

Because mental health clinicians might not be accustomed to asking about food insecurity and diet quality when assessing other socioenvironmental risks, additional training would be beneficial. Models have been developed to train pediatric residents to screen for psychosocial risk factors, including food insecurity (Burkhardt et al. 2012; Feigelman et al. 2011), but routine monitoring of food insecurity is underused by health care professionals (Hoisington et al. 2012). Furthermore, training in this area is largely missing in psychiatry residencies and other training programs for mental health professionals.

In addition to assessing food-related social determinants of mental health in the clinical setting, truly addressing the problem of food insecurity will require primary care physicians, psychiatrists, other mental health professionals, and other clinicians to step outside of traditional professional boundaries to influence social welfare and economic policy initiatives (Siefert et al. 2001).

Policy Approaches to Food Insecurity as a Social Determinant of Mental Health

Politicians and policymakers have more potent influence over a society's physical and mental health than do doctors in clinical settings. Although policy solutions to food insecurity are more powerful for the overall population than individual-level interventions delivered in the clinic, health care providers (including mental health professionals) often have limited training and confidence in their ability to influence policy. But clinicians, along with public health and policy professionals, have a role, if not a duty, in learning about and taking part in policy approaches to address the underlying causes of poor physical and mental health, including food and nutrition insecurity.

Supporting good nutrition (healthy food in terms of both quantity and quality) across the lifespan from infancy through old age will improve the mental health of individuals, families, and communities and reduce the risk of mental illnesses. Although the particularly detrimental impact of food insecurity in childhood and adolescence has been emphasized in this chapter, many older adults are at risk for food insecurity and hunger (and thus malnutrition, which exacerbates chronic and acute health conditions), in part because of limited incomes, impaired mobility, and poor health (Wolfe et al. 1998). In addition to a focus on food security and nutrition across the lifespan, special attention is needed for vulnerable groups such as racial and ethnic minorities and those who are homeless or marginally housed. Clinical- and policy-level interventions to prevent and ameliorate food insecurity across the life course could help reduce the incidence and prevalence of mental illnesses such as major depressive disorder (Heflin et al. 2005), and researchers, the private and corporate sector, and citizens at large also have a role.

Clinical Pearls

- Clinicians should be aware of the high prevalence of food and nutrition insecurity, living in a food desert, and resulting poor diet quality among individuals with mental illnesses.
- Clinicians should understand the links between food and nutrition insecurity and poor mental health outcomes and poor phys-

ical health outcomes, especially among individuals with mental illnesses.
- Clinicians should screen for food and nutrition insecurity, and among clients screening positive, should conduct a more thorough evaluation of food- and nutrition-related issues.
- Clinicians should make appropriate referrals to local resources such as food pantries, as well as federal food and nutrition support programs such as the Supplemental Nutrition Assistance Program (SNAP).
- Clinicians have a role in advocating for community-level programs as well as state and federal policies that reduce food and nutrition insecurity.

Key Chapter Points

- Food and nutrition security is necessary for good mental health, and good mental health is important to one's ability to maintain food security. Yet food and nutrition insecurity are social determinants of mental health too often neglected in clinical practice settings.
- Despite an abundant food supply, food insecurity is common in the United States. In 2023, 18 million U.S. households (13.5%) were food insecure at some time during the year; furthermore, 17.9% of all U.S. households with children were food insecure at some time during that year. Rates of food insecurity vary widely across the states.
- Food insecurity is driven prominently by poverty or constrained financial resources. In the United States, food insecurity commonly results in reduced diet quality: low consumption of fresh fruits and vegetables and other micronutrient-rich foods and increased intake of inexpensive, energy-dense, and nutritionally barren foods (thus leading to the association between food insecurity and overweight and obesity).
- Multiple studies link food insecurity to various adverse mental health outcomes among pregnant and postpartum women; young children; older children, adolescents, and young adults; older adults and those with cognitive decline; individuals with serious mental illness; and in other populations including individuals with HIV or at risk of HIV, those who are homeless or

unstably housed, and individuals exhibiting clinical or subclinical eating disorder pathology.

- In addition to individual- and clinical-level interventions, policy approaches to food insecurity have a powerful effect on reducing food insecurity at the community and population levels.

References

Abraham S, Breeze P, Sutton A, et al: Household food insecurity and child health outcomes: a rapid review of mechanisms and associations. Lancet 402(Suppl 1):S16, 2023 37997055

Abrahams Z, Lund C, Field S, et al: Factors associated with household food insecurity and depression in pregnant South African women from a low socio-economic setting: a cross-sectional study. Soc Psychiatry Psychiatr Epidemiol 53(4):363–372, 2018 29445850

Adynski H, Schwartz TA, Santos HP: Does participation in food benefit programs reduce the risk for depressive symptoms? J Am Psychiatr Nurses Assoc 29(1):25–37, 2023 33393431

Ahmad NSS, Sulaiman N, Sabri MF: Food insecurity: is it a threat to university students' well-being and success? Int J Environ Res Public Health 18(11):5627, 2021 34070321

Allen NL, Becerra BJ, Becerra MB: Associations between food insecurity and the severity of psychological distress among African-Americans. Ethn Health 23(5):511–520, 2018 28140616

Amin N, Akbari H, Jafarnejad S: Food security, mental health, and socioeconomic status: a cross-sectional study among medical college students in central part of Iran, Kashan. Health Sci Rep 5(1):e476, 2022 35036577

Anema A, Wood E, Weiser SD, et al: Hunger and associated harms among injection drug users in an urban Canadian setting. Subst Abuse Treat Prev Policy 5(1):20, 2010 20796313

Asfahani F, Kadiyala S, Ghattas H: Food insecurity and subjective wellbeing among Arab youth living in varying contexts of political instability. J Adolesc Health 64(1):70–78, 2019 30580768

Atuoye KN, Luginaah I: Food as a social determinant of mental health among household heads in the upper west region of Ghana. Soc Sci Med 180:170–180, 2017 28360010

Ayyub H, Sarfraz M, Mir K, et al: Association of antenatal depression and household food insecurity among pregnant women: a cross-sectional study from slums of Lahore. J Ayub Med Coll Abbottabad 30(3):366–371, 2018 30465367

Baer TE, Scherer EA, Fleegler EW, et al: Food insecurity and the burden of health-related social problems in an urban youth population. J Adolesc Health 57(6):601–607, 2015 26592328

Becerra BJ, Sis-Medina RC, Reyes A, et al: Association between food insecurity and serious psychological distress among Hispanic adults living in poverty. Prev Chronic Dis 12:E206, 2015 26605706

Becerra MB, Becerra BJ: Psychological distress among college students: role of food insecurity and other social determinants of mental health. Int J Environ Res Public Health 17(11):4118, 2020 32526990

Bergmans RS, Coughlin L, Wilson T, et al: Cross-sectional associations of food insecurity with smoking cigarettes and heavy alcohol use in a population-based sample of adults. Drug Alcohol Depend 205:107646, 2019 31677489

Bergmans RS, Wegryn-Jones R: Examining associations of food insecurity with major depression among older adults in the wake of the great recession. Soc Sci Med 258:113033, 2020 32535473

Birhanu TT, Tadesse AW: Food insecurity and mental distress among mothers in rural Tigray and SNNP regions, Ethiopia. Psychiatry J 2019:7458341, 2019 31321225

Black MM, Quigg AM, Cook J, et al: WIC participation and attenuation of stress-related child health risks of household food insecurity and caregiver depressive symptoms. Arch Pediatr Adolesc Med 166(5):444–451, 2012 22566545

Bradette-Laplante M, Courtemanche Y, Desrochers-Couture M, et al: Food insecurity and psychological distress in Inuit adolescents of Nunavik. Public Health Nutr 23(14):2615–2625, 2020 32456742

Brinkman J, Garnett B, Kolodinsky J, et al: Intra- and interpersonal factors buffer the relationship between food insecurity and mental well-being among middle schoolers. J Sch Health 91(2):102–110, 2021 33314273

Brooks JM, Petersen CL, Titus AJ, et al: Varying levels of food insecurity associated with clinically relevant depressive symptoms in U.S. adults aged 60 years and over: results from the 2005–2014 National Health and Nutrition Survey. J Nutr Gerontol Geriatr 38(3):218–230, 2019 31074705

Brostow DP, Gunzburger E, Abbate LM, et al: Mental illness, not obesity status, is associated with food insecurity among the elderly in the health and retirement study. J Nutr Gerontol Geriatr 38(2):149–172, 2019 30794096

Bruening M, van Woerden I, Todd M, et al: Hungry to learn: the prevalence and effects of food insecurity on health behaviors and outcomes over time among a diverse sample of university freshmen. Int J Behav Nutr Phys Act 15(1):9, 2018 29347963

Burkhardt MC, Beck AF, Conway PH, et al: Enhancing accurate identification of food insecurity using quality-improvement techniques. Pediatrics 129(2):e504–e510, 2012 22250022

Carvajal-Aldaz D, Cucalon G, Ordonez C: Food insecurity as a risk factor for obesity: a review. Front Nutr 9:1012734, 2022 36225872

Casey P, Goolsby S, Berkowitz C, et al: Maternal depression, changing public assistance, food security, and child health status. Pediatrics 113(2):298–304, 2004 14754941

Chen L, Wahlqvist ML, Teng NC, et al: Imputed food insecurity as a predictor of disease and mental health in Taiwanese elementary school children. Asia Pac J Clin Nutr 18(4):605–619, 2009 19965355

Ciciurkaite G, Brown RL: The link between food insecurity and psychological distress: the role of stress exposure and coping resources. J Community Psychol 50(3):1626–1639, 2022 34735724

Coakley KE, Cargas S, Walsh-Dilley M, et al: Basic needs insecurities are associated with anxiety, depression, and poor health among university students in the State of New Mexico. J Community Health 47(3):454–463, 2022 35124789

Coffino JA, Spoor SP, Drach RD, et al: Food insecurity among graduate students: prevalence and association with depression, anxiety and stress. Public Health Nutr 24(7):1889–1894, 2021 32792027

Cole SM, Tembo G: The effect of food insecurity on mental health: panel evidence from rural Zambia. Soc Sci Med 73(7):1071–1079, 2011 21852028

Coleman-Jensen A, Nord M: Food insecurity among households with working-age adults with disabilities (Economic Research Report No ERR-144). Washington, DC, U.S. Department of Agriculture, Economic Research Service, January 2013. Available at: https://www.ers.usda.gov/publications/pub-details?pubid=45040. Accessed March 29, 2025.

Coleman-Jensen A, Nord M, Andrews M, et al: Household food security in the United States in 2011 (Economic Research rep. no. ERR-141). Washington, DC, U.S. Department of Agriculture, Economic Research Service, September 2012. Available at: https://www.ers.usda.gov/publications/pub-details?pubid=45021. Accessed March 29, 2025.

Compton MT, Ku BS: Prevalence of food insecurity and living in a food desert among individuals with serious mental illnesses in public mental health clinics. Community Ment Health J 59(2):357–362, 2023 35963919

Cunningham A, Weinstein L, Stefancic A, et al: The association between food insecurity and physical activity in adults with serious mental illness living in supportive housing. Prev Med Rep 30:102008, 2022 36237836

Darling KE, Fahrenkamp AJ, Wilson SM, et al: Physical and mental health outcomes associated with prior food insecurity among young adults. J Health Psychol 22(5):572–581, 2017 26464054

Daundasekara SS, Schuler BR, Hernandez DC: A latent class analysis to identify socio-economic and health risk profiles among mothers of young children predicting longitudinal risk of food insecurity. PLoS One 17(8):e0272614, 2022 36001540

Davison KM, Marshall-Fabien GL, Tecson A: Association of moderate and severe food insecurity with suicidal ideation in adults: national survey data from three Canadian provinces. Soc Psychiatry Psychiatr Epidemiol 50(6):963–972, 2015 25652592

Dean G, Vitolins MZ, Skelton JA, et al: The association of food insecurity with mental health in preschool-aged children and their parents. Pediatr Res 94(1):290–295, 2023 36599944

Decaro JA, Manyama M, Wilson W: Household-level predictors of maternal mental health and systemic inflammation among infants in Mwanza, Tanzania. Am J Hum Biol 28(4):461–470, 2016 26593149

Dinour LM, Bergen D, Yeh MC: The food insecurity-obesity paradox: a review of the literature and the role food stamps may play. J Am Diet Assoc 107(11):1952–1961, 2007 17964316

Dolatian M, Sharifi N, Mahmoodi Z: Relationship of socioeconomic status, psychosocial factors, and food insecurity with preterm labor: a longitudinal study. Int J Reprod Biomed (Yazd) 16(9):563–570, 2018 30643863

Dong KR, Must A, Tang AM, et al: Food insecurity, morbidities, and substance use in adults on probation in Rhode Island. J Urban Health 95(4):564–575, 2018 30030685

Eaton LA, Cain DN, Pitpitan EV, et al: Exploring the relationships among food insecurity, alcohol use, and sexual risk taking among men and women living in South African townships. J Prim Prev 35(4):255–265, 2014 24806889

Falb KL, Blackwell A, Stennes J, et al: Depressive symptoms among women in Raqqa Governorate, Syria: associations with intimate partner violence, food insecurity, and perceived needs. Glob Ment Health (Camb) 6:e22, 2019 31662877

Feigelman S, Dubowitz H, Lane W, et al: Training pediatric residents in a primary care clinic to help address psychosocial problems and prevent child maltreatment. Acad Pediatr 11(6):474–480, 2011 21959095

Fleegler EW, Lieu TA, Wise PH, et al: Families' health-related social problems and missed referral opportunities. Pediatrics 119(6):e1332–e1341, 2007 17545363

Frank ML, Sato AF: Food insecurity and depressive symptoms among adolescents: does federal nutrition assistance act as a buffer? J Dev Behav Pediatr 44(1):e41–e48, 2023 36563345

Frongillo EA, Nguyen HT, Smith MD, et al: Food insecurity is associated with subjective well-being among individuals from 138 countries in the 2014 Gallup World Poll. J Nutr 147(4):680–687, 2017 28250191

Frongillo EA, Nguyen HT, Smith MD, et al: Food insecurity is more strongly associated with poor subjective well-being in more-developed countries than in less-developed countries. J Nutr 149(2):330–335, 2019 30597047

Gao X, Scott T, Falcon LM, et al: Food insecurity and cognitive function in Puerto Rican adults. Am J Clin Nutr 89(4):1197–1203, 2009 19225117

Gerber E, Gelberg L, Rotrosen J, et al: Health-related material needs and substance use among emergency department patients. Subst Abus 41(2):196–202, 2020 31368863

German L, Kahana C, Rosenfeld V, et al: Depressive symptoms are associated with food insufficiency and nutritional deficiencies in poor community-dwelling elderly people. J Nutr Health Aging 15(1):3–8, 2011 21267514

Goldman-Hasbun J, Nosova E, DeBeck K, et al: Food insufficiency is associated with depression among street-involved youth in a Canadian setting. Public Health Nutr 22(1):115–121, 2019 30305193

Gowda C, Hadley C, Aiello AE: The association between food insecurity and inflammation in the US adult population. Am J Public Health 102(8):1579–1586, 2012 22698057

Guzman PG, Lange JE, McClain AC: The association between food security status and psychological distress and loneliness among full-time undergraduate students at a minority-serving institution. Int J Environ Res Public Health 19(22):15245, 2022 36429963

Gyasi RM, Obeng B, Yeboah JY: Impact of food insecurity with hunger on mental distress among community-dwelling older adults. PLoS One 15(3):e0229840, 2020a 32231372

Gyasi RM, Peprah P, Appiah DO: Association of food insecurity with psychological disorders: results of a population-based study among older people in Ghana. J Affect Disord 270:75–82, 2020b 32275223

Hadley C, Patil CL: Food insecurity in rural Tanzania is associated with maternal anxiety and depression. Am J Hum Biol 18(3):359–368, 2006 16634017

Hadley C, Tegegn A, Tessema F, et al: Food insecurity, stressful life events and symptoms of anxiety and depression in east Africa: evidence from the Gilgel Gibe growth and development study. J Epidemiol Community Health 62(11):980–986, 2008 18854502

Hagedorn RL, Olfert MD: Food insecurity and behavioral characteristics for academic success in young adults attending an Appalachian university. Nutrients 10(3):361, 2018 29547533

Hagedorn RL, Olfert MD, MacNell L, et al: College student sleep quality and mental and physical health are associated with food insecurity in a multi-campus study. Public Health Nutr 24(13):4305–4312, 2021 33745495

Hamilton A, Beneke AA, Meisel E, et al: Associations between social determinants of health and outcomes of chronic medical conditions. Cureus 16(8):e67528, 2024 39310648

Hammami N, Leatherdale ST, Elgar FJ: Does social support moderate the association between hunger and mental health in youth? A gender-specific investigation from the Canadian health behaviour in school-aged children study. Nutr J 19(1):134, 2020 33278886

Harmel B, Höfelmann DA: Mental distress and food insecurity in pregnancy. Cien Saude Colet 27(5):2045–2055, 2022 35544830

Hasan SMT, Hossain D, Ahmed F, et al: Association of household food insecurity with nutritional status and mental health of pregnant women in rural Bangladesh. Nutrients 13(12):4303, 2021 34959855

Hatsu IE, Eiterman L, Stern M, et al: Household food insecurity is associated with symptoms of emotional dysregulation in children with attention deficit hyperactivity disorder: the MADDY study. Nutrients 14(6):1306, 2022 35334963

Hayati Rezvan P, Tomlinson M, Christodoulou J, et al: Intimate partner violence and food insecurity predict early behavior problems among South African children over 5-years post-birth. Child Psychiatry Hum Dev 52(3):409–419, 2021 32683574

Heflin CM, Siefert K, Williams DR: Food insufficiency and women's mental health: findings from a 3-year panel of welfare recipients. Soc Sci Med 61(9):1971–1982, 2005 15927331

Hobbs S, King C: The unequal impact of food insecurity on cognitive and behavioral outcomes among 5-year-old urban children. J Nutr Educ Behav 50(7):687–694, 2018 29753634

Hoisington AT, Braverman MT, Hargunani DE, et al: Health care providers' attention to food insecurity in households with children. Prev Med 55(3):219–222, 2012 22710141

Hooper L, Telke S, Larson N, et al: Household food insecurity: associations with disordered eating behaviours and overweight in a population-based sample of adolescents. Public Health Nutr 23(17):3126–3135, 2020 32466815

Howard AL, Barker ET: Mental health of students reporting food insecurity during the transition to university. Can J Diet Pract Res 82(3):125–130, 2021 33876989

Hromi-Fiedler A, Bermúdez-Millán A, Segura-Pérez S, et al: Household food insecurity is associated with depressive symptoms among low-income pregnant Latinas. Matern Child Nutr 7(4):421–430, 2011 20735732

Hu FB: Diet strategies for promoting healthy aging and longevity: an epidemiological perspective. J Intern Med 295(4):508–531, 2024 37867396

Huddleston-Casas C, Charnigo R, Simmons LA: Food insecurity and maternal depression in rural, low-income families: a longitudinal investigation. Public Health Nutr 12(8):1133–1140, 2009 18789167

Institute of Medicine: Hunger and obesity: understanding a food insecurity paradigm. Washington, DC, National Academies Press, 2011. Available at: https://nap.nationalacademies.org/catalog/13102/hunger-and-obesity-understanding-a-food-insecurity-paradigm-workshop-summary. Accessed March 29, 2025.

Itani R, Mattar L, Kharroubi S, et al: Food insecurity and mental health of college students in Lebanon: a cross-sectional study. J Nutr Sci 11:e68, 2022 36106091

Jafree SR: Determinants of depression in women with chronic disease: evidence from a sample of poor loan takers from Pakistan. J Community Psychol 48(7):2238–2251, 2020 32696988

Jalal CS, Frongillo EA, Warren AM: Food insecurity mediates the effect of a poverty-alleviation program on psychosocial health among the ultra-poor in Bangladesh. J Nutr 145(8):1934–1941, 2015 26108542

Jebena MG, Lindstrom D, Belachew T, et al: Food insecurity and common mental disorders among Ethiopian youth: structural equation modeling. PLoS One 11(11):e0165931, 2016 27846283

Jesson J, Dietrich J, Beksinska M, et al: Food insecurity and depression: a cross-sectional study of a multi-site urban youth cohort in Durban and Soweto, South Africa. Trop Med Int Health 26(6):687–700, 2021 33666301

Jih J, Nguyen TT, Jin C, et al: Food insecurity is associated with behavioral health diagnosis among older primary care patients with multiple chronic conditions. J Gen Intern Med 35(12):3726–3729, 2020 31808129

Johnson AD, Markowitz AJ: Food insecurity and family well-being outcomes among households with young children. J Pediatr 196:275–282, 2018 29703363

Johnson CM, Sharkey JR, Dean WR: Indicators of material hardship and depressive symptoms among homebound older adults living in North Carolina. J Nutr Gerontol Geriatr 30(2):154–168, 2011 21598164

Jones AD: Food insecurity and mental health status: a global analysis of 149 countries. Am J Prev Med 53(2):264–273, 2017 28457747

Jung SE, Kim S, Bishop A, et al: Poor nutritional status among low-income older adults: examining the interconnection between self-care capacity, food insecurity, and depression. J Acad Nutr Diet 119(10):1687–1694, 2019 29921540

Kamdar NP, Horning ML, Geraci JC, et al: Risk for depression and suicidal ideation among food insecure US veterans: data from the National Health and Nutrition Examination Study. Soc Psychiatry Psychiatr Epidemiol 56(12):2175–2184, 2021 33770225

Kaufman R, Mirsky J, Witztum E, et al: Food insecurity among psychiatric patients and welfare clients in Israel. Isr J Psychiatry Relat Sci 50(3):188–192, 2013 24622478

Kent K, Murray S, Visentin D, et al: High occurrence of food insecurity in young people attending a youth mental health service in regional Australia. Nutr Diet 79(3):364–373, 2022 35796179

Khoshgoo M, Eslami O, Khadem Al-Hosseini M, et al: The relationship between household food insecurity and depressive symptoms among pregnant women: a cross sectional study. Iran J Psychiatry 15(2):126–133, 2020 32426008

Kim BH, Ranzenhofer L, Stadterman J, et al: Food insecurity and eating pathology in adolescents. Int J Environ Res Public Health 18(17):9155, 2021 34501745

Kim K, Frongillo EA: Participation in food assistance programs modifies the relation of food insecurity with weight and depression in elders. J Nutr 137(4):1005–1010, 2007 17374668

Kim-Mozeleski JE, Poudel KC, Tsoh JY: Examining reciprocal effects of cigarette smoking, food insecurity, and psychological distress in the U.S. J Psychoactive Drugs 53(2):177–184, 2021 33143564

Kim-Mozeleski JE, Tsoh JY: Food insecurity and psychological distress among former and current smokers with low income. Am J Health Promot 33(2):199–207, 2019 29950100

Kimbro RT, Denney JT: Transitions into food insecurity associated with behavioral problems and worse overall health among children. Health Aff (Millwood) 34(11):1949–1955, 2015 26526254

King C: Soft drinks consumption and child behaviour problems: the role of food insecurity and sleep patterns. Public Health Nutr 20(2):266–273, 2017 27573974

Kirkpatrick SI, McIntyre L, Potestio ML: Child hunger and long-term adverse consequences for health. Arch Pediatr Adolesc Med 164(8):754–762, 2010 20679167

Kleinman RE, Murphy JM, Wieneke KM, et al: Use of a single-question screening tool to detect hunger in families attending a neighborhood health center. Ambul Pediatr 7(4):278–284, 2007 17660098

Kollannoor-Samuel G, Wagner J, Damio G, et al: Social support modifies the association between household food insecurity and depression among Latinos with uncontrolled type 2 diabetes. J Immigr Minor Health 13(6):982–989, 2011 21789561

Koyanagi A, Veronese N, Stubbs B, et al: Food insecurity is associated with mild cognitive impairment among middle-aged and older adults in South Africa: findings from a nationally representative survey. Nutrients 11(4):749, 2019 30935047

Lai S, Huang D, Bardhan I, et al: Associations between food insecurity and depression among diverse Asian Americans. Asian Pac Isl Nurs J 5(4):188–198, 2021 33791406

Laraia BA, Siega-Riz AM, Gundersen C, et al: Psychosocial factors and socioeconomic indicators are associated with household food insecurity among pregnant women. J Nutr 136(1):177–182, 2006 16365079

Laraia BA, Borja JB, Bentley ME: Grandmothers, fathers, and depressive symptoms are associated with food insecurity among low-income first-time African-American mothers in North Carolina. J Am Diet Assoc 109(6):1042–1047, 2009 19465186

Laraia B, Vinikoor-Imler LC, Siega-Riz AM: Food insecurity during pregnancy leads to stress, disordered eating, and greater postpartum weight among overweight women. Obesity (Silver Spring) 23(6):1303–1311, 2015 25959858

Larson NI, Story MT: Food insecurity and weight status among U.S. children and families: a review of the literature. Am J Prev Med 40(2):166–173, 2011 21238865

Lee SJ, Lee KW, Cho MS: Association of food insecurity with nutrient intake and depression among Korean and US adults: data from the 2014 Korea and the 2013–2014 US National Health and Nutrition Examination Surveys. Int J Environ Res Public Health 18(2):506, 2021 33435492

Leung CW, Kullgren JT, Malani PN, et al: Food insecurity is associated with multiple chronic conditions and physical health status among older US adults. Prev Med Rep 20:101211, 2020a 32983850

Leung CW, Stewart AL, Portela-Parra ET, et al: Understanding the psychological distress of food insecurity: a qualitative study of children's experiences and related coping strategies. J Acad Nutr Diet 120(3):395–403, 2020b 31959490

Levi R, Bleich SN, Seligman HK: Food insecurity and diabetes: overview of intersections and potential dual solutions. Diabetes Care 46(9):1599–1608, 2023 37354336

Li Y, Chang JJ, Xian H, et al: Racial/ethnic differences in the association between food security and depressive symptoms among adult foreign-born immigrants in the US: a cross-sectional study. J Immigr Minor Health 25(2):339–349, 2023 36083380

Liebe RA, Adams LM, Hedrick VE, et al: Understanding the relationship between food security and mental health for food-insecure mothers in Virginia. Nutrients 14(7):1491, 2022 35406104

Linares DE, Azuine RE, Singh GK: Social determinants of health associated with mental health among U.S. mothers with children aged 0–5 years. J Womens Health (Larchmt) 29(8):1039–1051, 2020 32456536

Loh IH, Oddo VM, Otten J: Food insecurity is associated with depression among a vulnerable workforce: early care and education workers. Int J Environ Res Public Health 18(1):170, 2020 33383668

Lu P, Kezios K, Yaffe K, et al: Depressive symptoms mediate the relationship between sustained food insecurity and cognition: a causal mediation analysis. Ann Epidemiol 81:6–13.e1, 2023 36822280

Madigan KE, Leiman DA, Palakshappa D: Food insecurity is an independent risk factor for depressive symptoms in survivors of digestive cancers. Cancer Epidemiol Biomarkers Prev 30(6):1122–1128, 2021 33849966

Maes KC, Hadley C, Tesfaye F, et al: Food insecurity and mental health: surprising trends among community health volunteers in Addis Ababa, Ethiopia during the 2008 food crisis. Soc Sci Med 70(9):1450–1457, 2010 20189698

Maharaj V, Tomita A, Thela L, et al: Food insecurity and risk of depression among refugees and immigrants in South Africa. J Immigr Minor Health 19(3):631–637, 2017 26984226

Mangurian C, Sreshta N, Seligman H: Food insecurity among adults with severe mental illness. Psychiatr Serv 64(9):931–932, 2013 24026843

Mark TE, Latulipe RJ, Anto-Ocrah M, et al: Seasonality, food insecurity, and clinical depression in post-partum women in a rural Malawi setting. Matern Child Health J 25(5):751–758, 2021 33231821

Marmolejo C, Banta JE, Siapco G, et al: Examining the association of student mental health and food security with college GPA. J Am Coll Health 72(3):819–825, 2024 35417289

Martinez SM, Frongillo EA, Leung C, et al: No food for thought: food insecurity is related to poor mental health and lower academic performance among students in California's public university system. J Health Psychol 25(12):1930–1939, 2020 29939096

Maupin J, Hackman J: Food insecurity, morbidity, and *susto*: factors associated with depression severity in Guatemala measured with the personal health questionnaire 9. Int J Soc Psychiatry 68(8):1654–1662, 2022 34558338

McIntyre L, Williams JVA, Lavorato DH, et al: Depression and suicide ideation in late adolescence and early adulthood are an outcome of child hunger. J Affect Disord 150(1):123–129, 2013 23276702

McIntyre L, Wu X, Kwok C, et al: The pervasive effect of youth self-report of hunger on depression over 6 years of follow up. Soc Psychiatry Psychiatr Epidemiol 52(5):537–547, 2017 28285453

McLaughlin KA, Green JG, Alegría M, et al: Food insecurity and mental disorders in a national sample of U.S. adolescents. J Am Acad Child Adolesc Psychiatry 51(12):1293–1303, 2012 23200286

McRell AS, Fram MS, Frongillo EA: Adolescent-reported household food insecurity and adolescents' poor mental and physical health and food insufficiency in Kenya. Curr Dev Nutr 6(8):nzac117, 2022 35957739

Melchior M, Caspi A, Howard LM, et al: Mental health context of food insecurity: a representative cohort of families with young children. Pediatrics 124(4):e564–e572, 2009 19786424

Melchior M, Chastang JF, Falissard B, et al: Food insecurity and children's mental health: a prospective birth cohort study. PLoS One 7(12):e52615, 2012 23300723

Men F, Elgar FJ, Tarasuk V: Food insecurity is associated with mental health problems among Canadian youth. J Epidemiol Community Health 75(8):741–748, 2021 33579754

Mesbah SF, Sulaiman N, Shariff ZM, et al: Does food insecurity contribute towards depression? a cross-sectional study among the urban elderly in Malaysia. Int J Environ Res Public Health 17(9):3118, 2020 32365772

Michels C, Hallgren KA, Cole A, et al: The relationship among social support, food insecurity and mental health for adults with severe mental illness and type 2 diabetes: a survey study. Psychiatr Rehabil J 45(3):212–218, 2022 35511510

Momtaz YA, Haron SA, Hamid TA, et al: Does food insufficiency in childhood contribute to dementia in later life? Clin Interv Aging 10:49–53, 2014 25565786

Montgomery J, Lu J, Ratliff S, et al: Food insecurity and depression among adults with diabetes: results from the National Health and Nutrition Examination Survey (NHANES). Diabetes Educ 43(3):260–271, 2017 28436293

Muhammad T, Debnath P, Srivastava S, et al: Childhood deprivations predict late-life cognitive impairment among older adults in India. Sci Rep 12(1):12786, 2022 35896620

Munger AL, Hofferth SL, Grutzmacher SK: The role of the supplemental nutrition assistance program in the relationship between food insecurity and probability of maternal depression. J Hunger Environ Nutr 11(2):147–161, 2016 27482302

Na M, Miller M, Ballard T, et al: Does social support modify the relationship between food insecurity and poor mental health? Evidence from thirty-nine sub-Saharan African countries. Public Health Nutr 22(5):874–881, 2019 30394250

Nagata JM, Gomberg S, Hagan MJ, et al: Food insecurity is associated with maternal depression and child pervasive developmental symptoms in low-income Latino households. J Hunger Environ Nutr 14(4):526–539, 2019 31673300

Nagata JM, Palar K, Gooding HC, et al: Food insecurity, sexual risk, and substance use in young adults. J Adolesc Health 68(1):169–177, 2021 32682597

Natamba BK, Mehta S, Achan J, et al: The association between food insecurity and depressive symptoms severity among pregnant women differs by social support category: a cross-sectional study. Matern Child Nutr 13(3):e12351, 2017 27507230

Neal L, Zigmont VA: Undergraduate food insecurity, mental health, and substance use behaviors. Nutr Health 2601060221142669, 2022 36448202

Oh H, Smith L, Jacob L, et al: Food insecurity and mental health among young adult college students in the United States. J Affect Disord 303:359–363, 2022 35157947

Okechukwu CA, El Ayadi AM, Tamers SL, et al: Household food insufficiency, financial strain, work-family spillover, and depressive symptoms in the working class: the work, family, and health network study. Am J Public Health 102(1):126–133, 2012 22095360

Ovenell M, Azevedo Da Silva M, Elgar FJ: Shielding children from food insecurity and its association with mental health and well-being in Canadian households. Can J Public Health 113(2):250–259, 2022 35025102

Pai S, Bahadur K: The impact of food insecurity on child health. Pediatr Clin North Am 67(2):387–396, 2020 32122567

Paquin V, Muckle G, Bolanis D, et al: Longitudinal trajectories of food insecurity in childhood and their associations with mental health and functioning in adolescence. JAMA Netw Open 4(12):e2140085, 2021 34928352

Pengpid S, Peltzer K: Food insecurity and health outcomes among community-dwelling middle-aged and older adults in India. Sci Rep 13(1):1136, 2023 36670204

Perkins JM, Nyakato VN, Kakuhikire B, et al: Food insecurity, social networks and symptoms of depression among men and women in rural Uganda: a cross-sectional, population-based study. Public Health Nutr 21(5):838–848, 2018 28988551

Piperata BA, Schmeer KK, Rodrigues AH, et al: Food insecurity and maternal mental health in León, Nicaragua: potential limitations on the moderating role of social support. Soc Sci Med 171:9–17, 2016 27855323

Poole-Di Salvo E, Silver EJ, Stein REK: Household food insecurity and mental health problems among adolescents: what do parents report? Acad Pediatr 16(1):90–96, 2016 26530851

Pound CM, Chen Y: Female sex and food insecurity in relation to self-reported poor or fair mental health in Canadian adults: a cross-sectional study using national survey data. CMAJ Open 9(1):E71–E78, 2021 33514600

Pourmotabbed A, Moradi S, Babaei A, et al: Food insecurity and mental health: a systematic review and meta-analysis. Public Health Nutr 23(10):1778–1790, 2020 32174292

Power M, Uphoff E, Kelly B, et al: Food insecurity and mental health: an analysis of routine primary care data of pregnant women in the Born in Bradford cohort. J Epidemiol Community Health 71(4):324–328, 2017 28275045

Pryor L, Lioret S, van der Waerden J, et al: Food insecurity and mental health problems among a community sample of young adults. Soc Psychiatry Psychiatr Epidemiol 51(8):1073–1081, 2016 27294729

Pryor L, Melchior M, Avendano M, et al: Childhood food insecurity, mental distress in young adulthood and the supplemental nutrition assistance program. Prev Med 168:107409, 2023 36592677

Pulgar CA, Trejo G, Suerken C, et al: Economic hardship and depression among women in Latino farmworker families. J Immigr Minor Health 18(3):497–504, 2016 26022147

Rabbitt MP, Reed-Jones M, Hales LJ, et al: Household food security in the United States in 2023 (rep. no. ERR-337). September 4, 2024. U.S. Department of Agriculture, Economic Research Service. Available at: https://www.ers.usda.gov/publications/pub-details?pubid=109895. Accessed March 29, 2025.

Rani D, Singh JK, Acharya D, et al: Household food insecurity and mental health among teenage girls living in urban slums in Varanasi, India: a cross-sectional study. Int J Environ Res Public Health 15(8):1585, 2018 30049971

Reed-Jones M: Prevalence of food insecurity differs by disability status in 2023. November 12, 2024. Available at https://www.ers.usda.gov/data-products/charts-of-note/chart-detail?chartId=110370#:~:text=In%202023%2C%20the%20prevalence%20of,with%203.4%20percent%20of%20households). Accessed March 29, 2025.

Reeder N, Tapanee P, Persell A, et al: Food insecurity, depression, and race: correlations observed among college students at a university in the southeastern United States. Int J Environ Res Public Health 17(21):8268, 2020 33182386

Reesor-Oyer L, Cepni AB, Lee CY, et al: Disentangling food insecurity and maternal depression: which comes first? Public Health Nutr 24(16):5506–5513, 2021 33517950

Richards M, Weigel M, Li M, et al: Household food insecurity and antepartum depression in the national children's study. Ann Epidemiol 44:38–44.e1, 2020 32220512

Romo ML, Abril-Ulloa V, Kelvin EA: The relationship between hunger and mental health outcomes among school-going Ecuadorian adolescents. Soc Psychiatry Psychiatr Epidemiol 51(6):827–837, 2016 27083901

Rose-Jacobs R, Black MM, Casey PH, et al: Household food insecurity: associations with at-risk infant and toddler development. Pediatrics 121(1):65–72, 2008 18166558

Ross JM, Sanchez A, Epps JB, et al: The impact of a food recovery-meal delivery program on homebound seniors' food security, nutrition, and well-being. J Nutr Gerontol Geriatr 41(2):175–189, 2022 35179450

Royer MF, Ojinnaka CO, Bruening M: Food insecurity is related to disordered eating behaviors among college students. J Nutr Educ Behav 53(11):951–956, 2021 34561153

Sampaio J, Henriques A, Ramos E, et al: Influence of social adversity on perceived health status and depressive symptoms among Portuguese older people. Int J Environ Res Public Health 19(11):6355, 2022 35681940

Seligman HK, Jacobs EA, López A, et al: Food insecurity and glycemic control among low-income patients with type 2 diabetes. Diabetes Care 35(2):233–238, 2012 22210570

Selvamani Y, Elgar F: Food insecurity and its association with health and well-being in middle-aged and older adults in India. J Epidemiol Community Health 77(4):252–257, 2023 36754599

Shafiee M, Vatanparast H, Janzen B, et al: Household food insecurity is associated with depressive symptoms in the Canadian adult population. J Affect Disord 279:563–571, 2021 33152560

Sharkey JR, Johnson CM, Dean WR: Relationship of household food insecurity to health-related quality of life in a large sample of rural and urban women. Women Health 51(5):442–460, 2011 21797678

Shim RS, Compton MT: The social determinants of mental health: psychiatrists' roles in addressing discrimination and food insecurity. Focus 18(1):25–30, 2020 32047394

Siefert K, Heflin CM, Corcoran ME, et al: Food insufficiency and the physical and mental health of low-income women. Women Health 32(1–2):159–177, 2001 11459368

Siefert K, Heflin CM, Corcoran ME, et al: Food insufficiency and physical and mental health in a longitudinal survey of welfare recipients. J Health Soc Behav 45(2):171–186, 2004 15305758

Silverman J, Krieger J, Kiefer M, et al: The relationship between food insecurity and depression, diabetes distress and medication adherence among low-income patients with poorly-controlled diabetes. J Gen Intern Med 30(10):1476–1480, 2015 25917659

Slopen N, Fitzmaurice G, Williams DR, et al: Poverty, food insecurity, and the behavior for childhood internalizing and externalizing disorders. J Am Acad Child Adolesc Psychiatry 49(5):444–452, 2010 20431464

Smith L, Il Shin J, McDermott D, et al: Association between food insecurity and depression among older adults from low- and middle-income countries. Depress Anxiety 38(4):439–446, 2021 33687122

Spencer AE, Baul TD, Sikov J, et al: The relationship between social risks and the mental health of school-age children in primary care. Acad Pediatr 20(2):208–215, 2020 31751774

Srivastava S, Muhammad T: Rural-urban differences in food insecurity and associated cognitive impairment among older adults: findings from a nationally representative survey. BMC Geriatr 22(1):287, 2022 35387591

Stang J, Taft Bayerl C, Flatt MM: Position of the American Dietetic Association: child and adolescent food and nutrition programs. J Am Diet Assoc 106(9):1467–1475, 2006 16986233

Stickley A, Leinsalu M: Childhood hunger and depressive symptoms in adulthood: findings from a population-based study. J Affect Disord 226:332–338, 2018 29031183

Stickley A, Koyanagi A, Inoue Y, et al: Childhood hunger and thoughts of death or suicide in older adults. Am J Geriatr Psychiatry 26(10):1070–1078, 2018 30076079

Strike C, Rudzinski K, Patterson J, et al: Frequent food insecurity among injection drug users: correlates and concerns. BMC Public Health 12(1):1058, 2012 23216869

Stuff JE, Casey PH, Szeto KL, et al: Household food insecurity is associated with adult health status. J Nutr 134(9):2330–2335, 2004 15333724

Tani Y, Suzuki N, Fujiwara T, et al: Neighborhood food environment and dementia incidence: the Japan gerontological evaluation study cohort survey. Am J Prev Med 56(3):383–392, 2019 30777158

Tarasuk V, Gundersen C, Wang X, et al: Maternal food insecurity is positively associated with postpartum mental disorders in Ontario, Canada. J Nutr 150(11):3033–3040, 2020 32856046

Teasdale SB, Morell R, Lappin JM, et al: Prevalence and correlates of food insecurity in community-based individuals with severe mental illness receiving long-acting injectable antipsychotic treatment. Br J Nutr 124(4):470–477, 2020 32234106

Tetteh J, Ekem-Ferguson G, Quarshie ENB, et al: Food insecurity and its impact on substance use and suicidal behaviours among school-going adolescents in Africa: evidence from the global school-based student health survey. Eur Child Adolesc Psychiatry 33(2):467–480, 2024 36859592

Tirfessa K, Lund C, Medhin G, et al: Food insecurity among people with severe mental disorder in a rural Ethiopian setting: a comparative, population-based study. Epidemiol Psychiatr Sci 28(4):397–407, 2019 29143723

Tirfessa K, Lund C, Medhin G, et al: Impact of integrated mental health care on food insecurity of households of people with severe mental illness in a rural African district: a community-based, controlled before-after study. Trop Med Int Health 25(4):414–423, 2020 31925844

Tomita A, Ramlall S, Naidu T, et al: Major depression and household food insecurity among individuals with multidrug-resistant tuberculosis (MDR-TB) in South Africa. Soc Psychiatry Psychiatr Epidemiol 54(3):387–393, 2019 30758540

Tomita A, Cuadros DF, Mabhaudhi T, et al: Spatial clustering of food insecurity and its association with depression: a geospatial analysis of nationally representative South African data, 2008–2015. Sci Rep 10(1):13771, 2020 32792498

Tripodi E, Jarman R, Morell R, et al: Prevalence of food insecurity in community-dwelling people living with severe mental illness. Nutr Diet 79(3):374–379, 2022 34608729

Tsai AC, Tomlinson M, Comulada WS, et al: Food insufficiency, depression, and the modifying role of social support: evidence from a population-based, prospective cohort of pregnant women in peri-urban South Africa. Soc Sci Med 151:69–77, 2016 26773296

Tseng KK, Park SH, Shearston JA, et al: Parental psychological distress and family food insecurity: sad dads in hungry homes. J Dev Behav Pediatr 38(8):611–618, 2017 28742541

Turner VE, Demissie Z, Sliwa SA, et al: Food insecurity and its association with alcohol and other substance use among high school students in the United States. J Sch Health 92(2):177–184, 2022 34841533

Umeda M, Ullevig SL, Chung E, et al: Depression mediates the relationship between food insecurity and pain interference in college students. Int J Environ Res Public Health 18(1):78, 2020 33374231

U.S. Department of Agriculture, U.S. Department of Health and Human Services: Dietary Guidelines for Americans, 2010, 7th Edition. Washington, DC, U.S. Government Printing Office, December 2010

Vilar-Compte M, Martínez-Martínez O, Orta-Alemán D, et al: Functional limitations, depression, and cash assistance are associated with food insecurity among older urban adults in Mexico City. J Health Care Poor Underserved 27(3):1537–1554, 2016 27524783

Walker RE, Keane CR, Burke JG: Disparities and access to healthy food in the United States: a review of food deserts literature. Health Place 16(5):876–884, 2010 20462784

Walker RJ, Garacci E, Ozieh M, et al: Food insecurity and glycemic control in individuals with diagnosed and undiagnosed diabetes in the United States. Prim Care Diabetes 15(5):813–818, 2021 34006474

Wang DD, Li Y, Afshin A, et al: Global improvement in dietary quality could lead to substantial reduction in premature death. J Nutr 149(6):1065–1074, 2019 31049577

Wang EA, McGinnis KA, Goulet J, et al: Food insecurity and health: data from the veterans aging cohort study. Public Health Rep 130(3):261–268, 2015 25931630

Ward WL, Swindle TM, Kyzer AL, et al: Maternal depression: relationship to food insecurity and preschooler fruit/vegetable consumption. Int J Environ Res Public Health 17(1):123, 2019 31877981

Weigel MM, Armijos RX, Racines M, et al: Association of household food insecurity with the mental and physical health of low-income urban Ecuadorian women with children. J Environ Public Health 2016:5256084

Weinreb L, Wehler C, Perloff J, et al: Hunger: its impact on children's health and mental health. Pediatrics 110(4):e41, 2002 12359814

Whitaker RC, Phillips SM, Orzol SM: Food insecurity and the risks of depression and anxiety in mothers and behavior problems in their preschool-aged children. Pediatrics 118(3):e859–e868, 2006 16950971

Wilkinson R, Pickett K: The Spirit Level: Why Greater Equality Makes Societies Stronger. New York, Bloomsbury Press, 2009

Willis SK, Simonsen SE, Hemmert RB, et al: Food insecurity and the risk of obesity, depression, and self-rated health in women. Womens Health Rep (New Rochelle) 1(1):308–317, 2020 33786494

Woldetensay YK, Belachew T, Biesalski HK, et al: The role of nutrition, intimate partner violence and social support in prenatal depressive symptoms in rural Ethiopia: community based birth cohort study. BMC Pregnancy Childbirth 18(1):374, 2018 30219050

Wolfe WS, Olson CM, Kendall A, et al: Hunger and food insecurity in the elderly: its nature and measurement. J Aging Health 10(3):327–350, 1998 10342935

Wong JC, Scott T, Wilde P, et al: Food insecurity is associated with subsequent cognitive decline in the Boston Puerto Rican health study. J Nutr 146(9):1740–1745, 2016 27466603

The World Bank. World Bank Country and Lending Groups, 2024. https://datahelpdesk.worldbank.org/knowledgebase/articles/906519-world-bank-country-and-lending-groups. Accessed April 1, 2025.

Wright L, Vance L, Sudduth C, et al: The impact of a home-delivered meal program on nutritional risk, dietary intake, food security, loneliness, and social well-being. J Nutr Gerontol Geriatr 34(2):218–227, 2015 26106989

Wu Q, Harwood RL, Feng X: Family socioeconomic status and maternal depressive symptoms: mediation through household food insecurity across five years. Soc Sci Med 215:1–6, 2018 30195125

Yang F, Shen Y, Nehring D: Maltreatment and depression among left-behind adolescents in rural China: the moderating roles of food security and depression literacy. Child Abuse Negl 114:104976, 2021 33548688

Zheng S, Ngo AL, Forman MR, et al: Associations of household food insufficiency with childhood depression and anxiety: a nationwide cross-sectional study in the USA. BMJ Open 11(9):e054263, 2021 34493526

Zlotorzynska M, Sanchez T: Food insecurity as a social determinant of sexual health and substance use independent of poverty status among men who have sex with men in the United States. Ann Epidemiol 74:97–103, 2022 35788033

6

Food- and Nutrition-Related Rating Scales and Assessment in the Clinical Setting

Mariam Motunrayo Sulaimon, M.A.
Michael T. Compton, M.D., M.P.H.

"Your body is the direct result of what you eat as well as what you don't eat."

—Gloria Swanson (1899–1983), American actor

In mental health care, we increasingly recognize the importance of food and nutrition to well-being. For clinicians, understanding the influence of dietary factors on mental health outcomes is essential for providing comprehensive care. Food- and nutrition-related assessments, such as those examining food security, nutrition security, and diet quality, offer valuable insights into a patient's overall health status and well-being. These assessments not only consider what patients eat but also explore their access to nutritious food and their motivation for dietary change. In this chapter, we delve into the practical tools available for clinicians to assess these factors. By incorporating food- and nutrition-related rating scales and assessment into mental health care, practitioners can better support patients in improving their overall health. The focus here is on measures that are short and simple enough to be integrated into mental health care visits, in which practitioners often face time constraints.

Food Security/Insecurity Measures

Food insecurity can occur at the family or individual level when the availability of nutritionally adequate and safe foods is limited or uncertain, and it disproportionately affects ethnic minorities and socioeconomically disadvantaged populations (National Institute on Minority Health and Health Disparities 2023). Being economically disadvantaged results in reduced intake of fruits, vegetables, and other micronutrient-rich foods that are essential for good health (Shim and Compton 2020). Food insecurity is associated with increased risk for multiple chronic health conditions and mental health disorders, and about 12% of U.S. households are food insecure (National Institute on Minority Health and Health Disparities 2023). Assessing food insecurity in clinical settings is crucial to identify patients who may be at risk of poor nutritional outcomes and associated health problems, including worsening of mental health. Food security assessments play a crucial role in identifying individuals or households that may be at risk of not having reliable access to enough food. These tools—briefly described here and also summarized in Table 6.1—vary in length (we discuss them in order from longer to shorter) and complexity but are designed to provide insight into the extent of food insecurity within a given population such as a clinic, or among individuals.

The Radimer/Cornell Hunger and Food Insecurity Scale (Radimer et al. 1992) measures hunger and food insecurity at both individual and household levels. This scale assesses food anxiety, food quality, and food intake to identify individuals or families at risk. Its focus on the psychological and emotional aspects of food insecurity, such as anxiety about food, makes it valuable for understanding the mental health impacts of food insecurity. The scale consists of 10 items, although the number may vary depending on the respondent's knowledge of their family situation or their children's food insecurity, if applicable (Radimer et al. 1992). By identifying individuals or families at risk of food insecurity, clinicians can better understand and address the mental health impacts of food insecurity.

Table 6.1 Overview of clinically useful food security/insecurity measures and rating scales

Measure	Key/original reference	Number of items	Description/notes
Radimer/Cornell Hunger and Food Insecurity Scale	Radimer et al. 1992	Varies	Measures hunger and food insecurity at the individual and household levels, focusing on food anxiety, food quality, and food intake; used to identify at-risk individuals
The Child Food Security Survey Module	Connell et al. 2004	9	Specifically designed to measure food security among children in a household; assesses children's access to adequate food and experiences of hunger
Household Food Insecurity Access Scale (HFIAS)	Coates et al. 2007	9	Assesses household food insecurity by measuring access to food over the past 4 weeks; evaluates the severity of food insecurity based on anxiety about food supply, insufficient food quality, and insufficient food intake
Food Insecurity Experience Scale (FIES)	Ballard et al. 2013	8	Suitable for global use and can be adapted to different cultural contexts; measures the severity of food insecurity at the household or individual level over the past 12 months
Community Childhood Hunger Identification Project (CCHIP)	Wehler et al. 1992	8	Measures whether adults or children are affected in the household by food insecurity, food shortages, perceived food insufficiency, or altered food intake due to constraints on resources; constructed as a measure of hunger appropriate for the socioeconomic conditions of the U.S.; part of a survey instrument developed to document the prevalence of hunger among low-income families (≤185% of the federal poverty level) having at least one child under age 12

Table 6.1 Overview of clinically useful food security/insecurity measures and rating scales (*continued*)

Measure	Key/original reference	Number of items	Description/notes
Six-Item Short Form of the Food Security Survey Module	Blumberg et al. 1999	6	Shorter version of the 18-item Household Food Security Survey Module, designed for quick screening; reliable for identifying households or individuals with low or very low food security
Household Hunger Scale (HHS)	Ballard et al. 2011	6	Derived directly from the HFIAS, assesses only the most severe experiences of food insecurity; consists of three "occurrence" and three "frequency-of-occurrence" questions that should be answered according to household food security experience in the previous 30 days; suitable for clinical and research settings, including low-resource environments
Hunger Vital Sign	Hager et al. 2010	2	Identifies household food insecurity in clinical settings; quick screening tool consisting of two simple questions derived from the Household Food Security Survey Module that address concerns about food running out and the ability to afford balanced meals; easy to administer and interpret; ideal for use in busy clinical environments
A single-question screening tool	Kleinman et al. 2007	1	Brief screening item to identify food insecurity in primary care: "In the past month, was there any day when you or anyone in your family went hungry because you did not have enough money for food?"; developed after a review of existing hunger surveys and consultation with several experts in the field

The Child Food Security Survey Module specifically measures food security among children in a household. This tool focuses on children's direct experiences with hunger and their access to adequate food. It consists of nine items and has been validated and found to be reliable for assessing food security among children (Connell et al. 2004). It is valuable in identifying children who may be at risk for food insecurity, and it is important in clinical settings, as childhood food insecurity has been linked to various negative outcomes, including depressive symptoms, anxiety, and behavioral problems (Thomas et al. 2019).

The Household Food Insecurity Access Scale (HFIAS) (Coates et al. 2007) also consists of nine items. It measures the severity of food insecurity by assessing household anxiety regarding food supply, the quality of food available, and the quantity of food consumed. It covers a 4-week recall period, making it suitable for short-term monitoring. The HFIAS has demonstrated good internal consistency and reliability across different cultural contexts (Coates et al. 2007).

The Food Insecurity Experience Scale (FIES) is a globally applicable tool designed to measure food insecurity at either the household or individual level. This eight-item scale is unique in that it is culturally adaptable and relies on people's direct yes/no responses to eight brief questions regarding their access to adequate food (Ballard et al. 2013). It is used across a variety of populations and settings. It has been validated in both high-income and low-income countries, providing a valuable resource for both clinical and research activities aiming to assess food insecurity. It has good reliability and internal consistency (Grimaccia and Naccarato 2020). The FIES has undergone extensive methodological development and validation, demonstrating its reliability and accuracy in more than 140 countries (Nord et al. 2016). It is an essential tool for global food security monitoring and for guiding actions aimed at achieving food security targets outlined in the 2030 Sustainable Development Agenda (Nord et al. 2016).

The Community Childhood Hunger Identification Project (CCHIP) (Wehler et al. 1992) measures food insecurity and hunger, specifically among low-income families with children. This eight-item tool is designed to assess whether children and adults within a household are affected by food shortages, food insufficiency, or altered food intake due to resource constraints (Wehler et al. 1992). It was originally developed to capture hunger experiences in the U.S. socioeconomic context and is widely used to document food insecurity prevalence among vulnerable families.

The Six-Item Short Form of the Food Security Survey Module (Economic Research Service 2024) is a reasonable substitute for settings that cannot implement the more comprehensive version that the U.S. Department of Agriculture (USDA) uses for nationally representative, population-based surveys. Its primary advantage is that it provides quick yet reliable screening for households that may be experiencing low food security. Although the six-item form sacrifices some detail for efficiency and does not measure the most severe level of food insecurity, it is highly suitable for busy clinical settings in which time constraints may limit the feasibility of longer assessments. Despite its brevity, it maintains strong validity and reliability in identifying food-insecure households with high specificity and sensitivity (Blumberg et al. 1999). Additionally, the USDA Economic Research Service has conducted assessments showing that the six-item module performs well with minimal bias compared to the 18-item measure. This makes it a trusted tool for identifying patients who may need intervention.

Another important tool is the Household Hunger Scale (HHS) developed by Ballard et al. (2011), which is derived from the HFIAS. It is different from the other tools in that it focuses solely on the most severe instances of food insecurity. Its six items assess whether households have experienced hunger due to food insecurity over the past 30 days (Ballard et al. 2011). The simplicity of this measure, combined with its ability to capture severe food insecurity, makes it particularly useful in low-resource environments and clinical settings dealing with highly vulnerable populations. The HHS has been validated for cross-cultural use, ensuring that it produces valid and comparable results across different settings (Ballard et al. 2011).

The Hunger Vital Sign (Hager et al. 2010) is another highly efficient screening tool. Comprising just two questions, it was designed specifically for use in pediatric clinical settings to identify food insecurity among children. The two items are derived from the Household Food Security Survey Module, focusing on concerns about food running out and the household's ability to afford balanced meals. This measure is quick to administer, easy to interpret, and ideal for clinical settings in which time and resource limitations are common, especially in settings that serve low-income populations. This two-item screener has been validated in clinical settings, demonstrating strong reliability and validity in identifying food-insecure households with high specificity and sensitivity among low-income families with young children (Hager et al. 2010). The two items are: "Within the past 12 months, we worried whether our food would run out before we got money to buy more," and "Within the past 12 months, the food we bought just didn't last and we didn't have money to get more," with response options being "Often true," "Sometimes true," or "Never true." The tool provides a quick indication of potential food insecurity and allows clinicians to refer patients for further assessment or services if needed.

The Single-Question Screening Tool (Kleinman et al. 2007) is a brief tool designed to identify hunger in clinical settings, particularly in low-income urban populations. It consists of one question that assesses whether any family member has gone hungry in the past month owing to a lack of money for food: "In the past month, was there any day when you or anyone in your family went hungry because you did not have enough money for food?" Response options are "Yes" or "No." This simple tool was developed for use in primary care and serves as a quick way to identify families at risk of hunger, leading to timely interventions. This single-question tool has been evaluated for its reliability and validity in identifying hunger among low-income urban populations. Studies have shown that this tool is both reliable and valid for quickly screening families at risk of hunger in clinical settings.

Nutrition Security/ Insecurity Measures

Food insecurity and nutrition insecurity are often used interchangeably, but they address distinct concepts. Nutrition security means "consistent and equitable access to healthy, safe, affordable foods essential to optimal health and well-being" (USDA). The USDA has shifted its focus to include nutrition security to promote health equity and address structural inequities. Whereas food insecurity focuses on the availability and affordability of food (regardless of how healthy or unhealthy the food might be), the concept of nutrition security/insecurity emphasizes whether that food is nutritious and balanced and supports overall well-being.

Ensuring nutrition security in clinical settings is essential for promoting optimal health outcomes and preventing disease. This concept is important in addressing health disparities among racial/ethnic minority populations, low-income groups, and rural communities, which often face barriers to accessing nutritious foods (Mozaffarian et al. 2011). By focusing on the quality of food and its impact on health, clini-

Table 6.2 Overview of clinically useful nutrition security/insecurity measures and rating scales

Measure	Key/original reference	Number of items	Description/notes
Household Nutrition Security Measure	Calloway et al. 2022	4	Assesses a household's perceived ability to acquire healthful foods without resource limitations or worry
Household Dietary Choice	Calloway et al. 2022	3	Assesses the degree of control a household perceives they have in acquiring foods that meet their food preferences
Household Healthfulness Choice	Calloway et al. 2022	3	Assesses the degree of control a household perceives they have in acquiring foods that meet their healthfulness needs
Brief Nutrition Security Screener (BNSS)	Calloway et al. 2024	1	A one-item screener used in health-related social needs screening in clinical and community settings

cians can better support patients in achieving a balanced and healthful diet, thereby reducing the risk of chronic diseases and improving overall health. Measures of nutrition security/insecurity—briefly described here and also summarized in Table 6.2—vary in length but provide insight into the extent of nutrition insecurity in the clinical setting. Again, we describe them here in order based on the number of items, from longer instruments to shorter ones.

The Household Nutrition Security Measure identifies households that may have access to sufficient food but still face nutritional deficiencies. The four items cover aspects such as eating foods that are not good for health because other types of foods could not be obtained, concerns about the food being eaten hurting health, and eating the same food several days in a row due to a shortage of funds (Calloway et al. 2022).

Clinicians can use this measure to understand the broader context of a patient's dietary environment, focusing on the household's control over food choices and the nutritional quality of food. Calloway et al. (2022) found that the measure has reliability and construct validity, effectively captures the nuances of nutrition security, and correlates well with other indicators of food security and health outcomes.

The Household Dietary Choice (Calloway et al. 2022) is a three-item tool that assesses the degree of control that households perceive they have over their food choices, focusing on how external factors such as income or food availability affect diet quality. This measure is particularly useful for evaluating nutrition security, as it considers the extent to which households can acquire foods that meet their health needs and preferences. Calloway et al. (2022) found this measure to be both reliable and valid.

The Household Healthfulness Choice measure, also developed by Calloway et al. (2022), is a three-item tool that assesses a household's perceived control over acquiring foods that meet their healthfulness needs. This measure is useful for understanding how households navigate their food environments and the extent to which they can access and choose healthy foods. Calloway et al. (2022) also highlighted the reliability and validity of this measure and its usefulness for assessing risk for poor diet and related adverse health outcomes even after controlling for household food security status and sample characteristics.

The Brief Nutrition Security Screener (BNSS) is a concise tool designed for rapid assessment of nutrition security in clinical and community settings. This one-item screener is part of the broader Health-Related Social Needs (HRSN) screening toolkit, which aims to identify a number of social determinants of health. Its primary advantage is its brevity, making it especially suitable for busy healthcare environments with time constraints. The one-item question is, "In the last 12 months, we worried that the food we were able to eat would hurt our health and well-being." Responses of "Sometimes," "Often," or "Always" (as opposed to the response of "Never") constitute a positive screen for nutrition insecurity (Calloway et al. 2024). Despite its simplicity, the screener has strong validity and reliability in identifying households experiencing nutrition insecurity with high specificity (78%) and sensitivity (93%), meaning it correctly identifies as many households in need (or true positives) as possible, while limiting false positives (Calloway et al. 2024). As such, the BNSS screener offers a single, critical question that assesses the household's ability to consistently access nutritious food.

Measures of Nutritional Status/Malnutrition

Measures of nutritional status and malnutrition—described here and in Table 6.3, from more to less complex—are critical in understanding the adequacy of dietary intake and its implications for health. These assessments, along with the other measures of diet quality described, can help to measure the quality of food and whether it meets the nutritional needs necessary for health. Poor nutrition can exacerbate or contribute to a wide range of physical and mental health issues, including obesity, depression, and anxiety. For instance, malnutrition in older adults is especially concerning, as it can lead to increased frailty and a higher risk of adverse health outcomes, including mortality (Wei et al. 2018). Nutritional status assesses actual intake and its adequacy in preventing malnutrition. This is especially relevant for vulnerable populations, such as older adults, who may have limited access to or knowledge about healthy food choices. By using effective measures of nutritional status, health care providers can identify individuals at risk of malnutrition and implement targeted interventions to improve dietary intake and overall health outcomes.

The Subjective Global Assessment (SGA) is a comprehensive clinical tool used to evaluate a patient's nutritional status through a combination of medical history and physical examination. It involves assessing factors such as recent weight loss, changes in dietary intake, gastrointestinal symptoms, and functional capacity. SGA categorizes patients into three nutritional status groups: well-nourished, moderately malnourished, or severely malnourished. This tool is valuable in clinical settings because of its ability to provide a holistic view of a patient's nutritional health, making it suitable for various populations, including mental health settings in which nutritional status can significantly impact treatment outcomes. SGA has been widely validated and is considered the gold standard for diagnosing malnutrition. It correlates well with objective measures of nutritional status and has good interrater reliability and accuracy in identifying patients who would benefit from nutritional interventions (Detsky et al. 1987).

The Nutrition Screening Initiative (NSI) Checklist was developed to address malnutrition, particularly in older adults. This tool consists of 10 items that assess dietary intake, weight loss, and overall health status. It is simple to administer and is designed for quick identification of individuals who may be at risk for malnutrition. In clinical settings,

Table 6.3 Overview of clinically useful measures of nutritional status/malnutrition

Measure name	Key/original reference	Number of items	Description/notes
Subjective Global Assessment (SGA)	Detsky et al. 1987	7	Uses a patient's medical history and physical examination to assess nutritional status; highly effective in identifying malnutrition; original version uses seven items from a medical history and four items from a physical exam to screen for malnutrition
Nutrition Screening Initiative (NSI) Checklist	ADA, NCA, and AAFP 1991	10	Developed to address the prevalence of malnutrition among older adults and to identify individuals at risk of malnutrition; easy to administer; includes questions on dietary intake, weight loss, and health status
Malnutrition Universal Screening Tool (MUST)	Elia 2003	5	Designed to identify adults who are malnourished or at risk of malnutrition; includes BMI, weight loss, and acute disease effect scores
Nutrition Risk Screening 2002 (NRS-2002)	Kondrup et al. 2003	4	Designed to identify patients at risk of malnutrition; includes items on BMI, recent weight loss, appetite, and disease severity; commonly used in hospitals for quick assessment
Mini Nutritional Assessment–Short Form (MNA-SF)	Rubenstein et al. 2001	6	Used to assess nutritional status in older adults; evaluates factors such as weight loss, mobility, psychological stress, and BMI; quick to administer and effective in identifying malnutrition or the risk of malnutrition in clinical settings

Table 6.3 Overview of clinically useful measures of nutritional status/malnutrition (*continued*)

Measure name	Key/original reference	Number of items	Description/notes
Simplified Nutritional Appetite Questionnaire (SNAQ)	Wilson et al. 2005	4	Assesses appetite, satiety, taste of food, and number of meals per day in older adults
Short Nutritional Assessment Questionnaire (SNAQ)	Kruizenga et al. 2005	3	Consists of the three most highly predictive questions related to presence and degree of unintentional weight loss, changes in appetite, and use of supplemental drinks or tube feeding
Malnutrition Screening Tool (MST)	Ferguson et al. 1999	2	Used to identify patients at risk of malnutrition; includes questions on recent weight loss and appetite; used in various clinical settings

AAFP = American Academy of Family Physicians; ADA = American Dietetic Association; BMI = body mass index; NCA = National Council on Aging.

the NSI Checklist is often used in primary care or geriatric assessments to ensure early detection of nutritional risks among older adult patients. The NSI Checklist includes the DETERMINE Your Nutritional Health Checklist, including disease, eating poorly, tooth loss/mouth pain, economic hardship, reduced social contact, multiple medicines, involuntary weight loss or gain, needs assistance in self-care, or elder years (age ≥80) (American Dietetic Association et al. 1991). These factors are often interconnected with mental health issues, making the NSI Checklist a useful tool in identifying patients who may be at risk of both nutritional and mental health problems. The tool's focus on factors such as social isolation, malnutrition, poor dietary habits, and economic hardship is especially relevant in mental health settings, in which these issues are common among patients (American Dietetic Association et al. 1991; Posner et al. 1993). The NSI Checklist has been validated in various studies and has shown good reliability and validity. For example, a study conducted by Posner et al. (1993) found that the NSI Checklist was effective in identifying older adults at risk of malnutrition with a high degree of sensitivity and specificity. The tool's reliability has also been supported by its consistent use in clinical and community settings over the years, demonstrating its robustness in different populations and environments (Posner et al. 1993).

The Malnutrition Universal Screening Tool (MUST) was developed by the Malnutrition Advisory Group, a standing committee of the British Association for Parenteral and Enteral Nutrition. This tool identifies adults who are malnourished, at risk of malnutrition (undernutrition), or obese. It is a five-step screening tool that includes management guidelines to help develop a care plan. The steps involve measuring height and weight to calculate body mass index (BMI), noting the percentage of unplanned weight loss, considering the effect of acute disease, adding the scores to determine overall risk, and using management guidelines to develop a care plan (Elia 2003). MUST has been validated in a number of studies and has shown good reliability and validity in identifying malnutrition risk. It is widely used in hospitals, community-based clinical settings, and other care environments. Neelemaat et al. (2011) documented specificity and sensitivity among inpatient samples.

The Nutrition Risk Screening 2002 (NRS-2002), developed by Kondrup et al. (2003), is another tool designed to identify hospitalized patients who are malnourished or at risk of malnutrition. This four-item screening tool assesses BMI, recent weight loss, appetite, and disease severity. It is commonly used in hospital settings to identify malnutrition risk, making it an essential part of patient care. The tool's focus on both nutritional status and disease severity makes it highly relevant in acute-care settings, in which patients often experience rapid changes in their health status (Kondrup et al. 2003). The validity and reliability of NRS-2002 have been confirmed, and its sensitivity and specificity have been evaluated. Neelemaat et al. (2011) showed greater than 70% sensitivity and specificity to effectively identify patients at risk or severe risk of malnutrition. The tool's reliability is supported by its ability to distinguish between patients who will benefit from nutritional support and those who will not (Kondrup et al. 2003).

The Mini Nutritional Assessment–Short Form (MNA-SF) is a widely used screening tool designed to identify older adults who are malnourished or at risk of malnutrition. It provides a quick and simple method for assessing nutritional status in different settings, including hospitals, long-term-care facilities, and community environments (Rubenstein et al. 2001). This tool is valuable because it takes only 5 minutes to complete, making it practical for routine use in many clinical settings. MNA-SF consists of six questions that cover food intake, weight loss, mobility, psychological stress or acute disease, neuropsychological problems, and BMI. The tool has been validated in international studies and has been shown to correlate with morbidity and mortality (Rubenstein et al. 2001). It has also been found to have excellent sensitivity among older adults (Neelemaat et al. 2011).

The Simplified Nutritional Appetite Questionnaire (SNAQ) was developed by Wilson et al. (2005) as a brief and practical tool to assess appetite and predict weight loss primarily in older adults. It consists of four questions that evaluate appetite, satiety, taste of food, and frequency of meals. Each question is scored, and the total score helps identify individuals at risk of malnutrition due to poor appetite. SNAQ is useful in clinical settings, including mental health environments, where appetite can be significantly affected by psychological conditions. Its simplicity and ease of use make it an efficient screening tool for health care providers. SNAQ has demonstrated good reliability, as well as sensitivity and specificity, making it a useful predictor of malnutrition in both specialized and nonspecialized older adult populations. For instance, a study conducted in Singapore validated SNAQ among community-dwelling older adults, confirming its effectiveness in identifying those at risk of malnutrition (Lau et al. 2020).

The Short Nutritional Assessment Questionnaire is also referred to as "SNAQ." It is a concise tool consisting of three questions designed to quickly identify individuals at risk of malnutrition. Developed to be user-friendly and efficient, SNAQ consists of a few key questions that assess weight loss, appetite, and dietary intake. Its simplicity makes it suitable for various clinical settings, including mental health, where time and resources may be limited. It has demonstrated good validity and reliability in different populations, ensuring consistent and accurate identification of nutritional risk. Its development involved rigorous testing and validation to ensure it effectively screens for malnutrition, making it an asset in both general and specialized health care environments, where it has been proven to have excellent criterion validity and high sensitivity and specificity (Kruizenga et al. 2005; Neelemaat et al. 2011).

The Malnutrition Screening Tool (MST), developed by Ferguson et al. (1999), is a two-item screening tool designed for quick identification of malnutrition risk. It is a straightforward and efficient instrument to identify adults at risk of malnutrition. The two questions are, "Have you lost weight recently (in the last 6 months) without trying?" and "Have you been eating poorly because of a decreased appetite?" Each question is scored as a "yes" (1 point) or "no" (0 points), with a combined score used to determine malnutrition risk. The MST is useful in clinical settings due to its simplicity and quick administration, making it suitable for a number of different patient populations, including those in mental health settings, where nutritional status can significantly impact overall well-being. The tool has demonstrated good reliability and validity across different studies, including those involving older adults and hospital patients (Ferguson et al. 1999). The MST showed sensitivity and specificity of at least 70% in an inpatient sample (Neelemaat at al. 2011). Its effectiveness in early detection and intervention helps improve patient outcomes by addressing malnutrition promptly.

Measures of Food Intake and Diet Quality

Food intake refers to the total amount of food and beverages consumed by an individual, encompassing both the quantity and quality of nutrients ingested. It plays a crucial role in maintaining energy balance, supporting bodily functions, and promoting overall health. Healthy food intake involves a balanced diet in terms of macronutrients (carbohydrates, proteins, and fats) and being rich in micronutrients (vitamins and minerals) and fiber. Poor dietary intake, particularly low consumption of fruits and vegetables, is associated with increased risk for chronic diseases such as type 2 diabetes, cardiovascular disease, and cancer, as well as premature mortality (Głąbska et al. 2020). Better diet quality also promotes positive emotions and improved mental health (Głąbska et al. 2020).

Assessing food intake is essential in clinical practice, as dietary habits are closely linked to both physical and mental health outcomes. Monitoring and adjusting food intake can help prevent nutritional deficiencies, manage weight, and reduce the risk of chronic diseases (World Health Organization 2008). Food intake assessments are important in understanding how patients' food choices impact their physical and mental health. The following tools—also summarized in Table 6.4—focus on assessing specific aspects of food intake, such as overall dietary patterns or the consumption of specific food groups such as fruits and vegetables.

The Household Dietary Diversity Score (HDDS) is a tool whose number of items varies by administration. Developed by Swindale and Bilinsky (2006), it measures food security by evaluating the diversity of food groups consumed by a household. It is a qualitative tool with the number of food groups varying depending on the household's dietary intake. The questionnaire typically takes about 10–15 minutes to complete, depending on the respondent's familiarity with their household's dietary habits (Swindale and Bilinsky 2006). The tool provides a snapshot of diet quality and helps clinicians understand whether households have access to a variety of foods, which is crucial for maintaining nutritional health.

The Mini-EAT (Eating Assessment Tool) is a brief, nine-item dietary screener designed to assess an individual's dietary patterns and food intake (Lara-Breitinger et al. 2023). It is useful in clinical settings because of its simplicity and quick administration time, making it feasible for routine use by health care professionals. Mini-EAT has demonstrated good test-retest reliability, as well as validity, correlating well with comprehensive food frequency questionnaires and the Healthy Eating Index 2015 (Vadiveloo et al. 2023). Its brevity and ease of use make it relevant in mental health settings. It is suitable for integration into clinical decision support systems, enhancing the overall care provided to patients (Vadiveloo et al. 2023).

The Starting the Conversation (STC) screener is an eight-item simplified food frequency instrument designed for use in primary care and health-promotion settings (Paxton et al. 2011). It is relevant in clinical settings for assessing patients' dietary patterns and guiding nutri-

Table 6.4 Overview of clinically useful measures of food intake and diet quality

Measure	Key/original reference	Number of items	Description/notes
Household Dietary Diversity Score (HDDS)	Swindale and Bilinsky 2006	Qualitative (Varies)	Assesses food security by evaluating the diversity of food groups consumed by a household; quick to administer and provides a snapshot of diet quality related to food security
Mini-EAT (Eating Assessment Tool)	Lara-Breitinger et al. 2023	9	Validated brief dietary screener that correlates well with a comprehensive food frequency questionnaire; assesses dietary patterns and food intake; designed for quick and simple use in clinical settings
Starting the Conversation (STC)	Paxton et al. 2011	8	Brief dietary screener focusing on diet quality, including questions on fruits, vegetables, sugar-sweetened beverages, and fat intake; designed to be used in clinical settings
Fruit & Vegetable Intake Screeners (EATS)	Thompson et al. 2000	7	Brief dietary assessment tool designed to estimate the frequency of fruit and vegetable intake over the past month; includes questions on the consumption of different types of fruits and vegetables, excluding potatoes; provides a quick and practical way to assess dietary intake in large-scale surveys or clinical settings; has been validated against more comprehensive dietary assessments and is particularly useful for evaluating adherence to dietary guidelines related to fruit and vegetable consumption

tional counseling, which can help in the prevention and management of chronic diseases (Paxton et al. 2011). The STC has demonstrated good reliability and validity, with moderate intercorrelations among items ($r = 0.39–0.59$; $P < 0.05$) and significant correlations with the National Cancer Institute fat screener ($r = 0.39$; $P < 0.05$) (Paxton et al. 2011). Additionally, STC is sensitive to changes in dietary behavior, making it a useful tool for monitoring progress in dietary interventions (Paxton et al. 2011).

Another widely used tool is the Fruit & Vegetable Intake Screener. Developed as part of Eating at America's Table Study (EATS), it is a short, seven-item assessment tool designed to measure the intake of fruits and vegetables in specific population groups (Thompson and Byers 1994). It has been widely used to track changes in fruit and vegetable consumption and has shown good reliability and validity compared to 24-hour dietary recalls (Thompson et al. 2000). In clinical mental health settings, these screeners can be especially relevant, as adequate fruit and vegetable intake is associated with better mental health outcomes in part by promoting higher levels of optimism and self-efficacy, as well as reducing the level of psychological distress and depressive symptoms (Głąbska et al. 2020). EATS screeners are practical for use in clinical settings owing to their brevity and ease of administration, allowing health care providers to quickly assess dietary habits and implement necessary nutritional interventions.

Measures of Other Food- and Nutrition-Related Constructs

In addition to food security/insecurity, nutrition security/insecurity, nutritional status/malnutrition, and food intake and diet quality, several related constructs contribute to a comprehensive understanding of a patient's food- and nutrition-related behaviors. Some of these constructs include food satisfaction, emotional eating, meal preparation skills, obesity risk, and readiness for nutritional counseling. Assessing these areas, when necessary, helps clinicians better understand how a patient's relationship with food might be affecting their physical and mental health, which will guide a tailored approach to intervention. Measures assessing these constructs are briefly described here and summarized in Table 6.5.

These assessments can reveal underlying patterns and behaviors that contribute to physical and mental health challenges, which will

Table 6.5 Overview of other clinically useful food- and nutrition-related measures and rating scales

Measure	Key/original reference	Number of items	Description/notes
Food satisfaction measures			
Mealtime Satisfaction Questionnaire (MSQ)	Keller and Martos 2013	14	Assesses satisfaction with meals, especially in retirement and long-term care settings, focusing on the overall mealtime experience rather than individual meals
Salzburg Emotional Eating Scale (SEES)	Meule et al. 2018	20	Assesses emotional eating by distinguishing between emotional overeating and undereating, with subscales for happiness, sadness, anger, and anxiety
NutriMental Screener	Teasdale et al. 2021	Varies (about 10–20)	Identifies at-risk populations with mental illnesses who may have dietary and nutritional concerns, facilitating referrals to specialized clinical care
Positive Eating Scale (PES)	Sproesser et al. 2018	8	Focuses on general satisfaction with one's eating behavior, including the pleasure experienced while eating; emphasizes eating as a general act in a normal, nonpathological context, moving away from dieting and restrictive eating patterns
Food Enjoyment Scale for Older Adults	Vailas and Nitzke 1998	6	Assesses aspects of food enjoyment among older adults, including sensory enjoyment, the impact of dietary restrictions, and limitations related to oral, financial, social, and functional factors

Table 6.5 Overview of other clinically useful food- and nutrition-related measures and rating scales (*continued*)

Measure	Key/original reference	Number of items	Description/notes
Meal preparation skills			
Cooking Skills Confidence Measure	Lavelle et al. 2017	14	Assesses confidence in cooking skills including food preparation techniques and cooking methods
Staff-Administered Meal Independence Rating Scale	Ehntholt et al. 2024	20	Designed for use among patients with serious mental illness to assess their independence in meal preparation
Lawton Instrumental Activities of Daily Living (IADL) Scale	Lawton and Brody 1969	8	Evaluates the ability to perform daily tasks, including food preparation, shopping, and housekeeping
Overweight/obesity			
Body mass index (BMI)	Keys et al. 1972	1	A simple measure of body fat based on height and weight; widely used in clinical settings to assess for overweight/obesity; often combined with waist circumference for a more comprehensive assessment
Waist circumference	World Health Organization 2008	1	Assesses central obesity, which is a risk factor for metabolic syndrome; quick and easy to measure; useful alongside BMI

help clinicians develop interventions that address specific needs. For example, identifying emotional eating patterns can prompt clinicians to implement strategies that improve emotional regulation, and understanding a patient's mealtime satisfaction or cooking confidence can guide targeted nutritional counseling and skill-building. Moreover, tracking obesity risk through measures such as BMI and waist circumference allows clinicians to monitor patients' progress and intervene early in cases where dietary adjustments or lifestyle changes are warranted. By using these tools in an integrated way, clinicians can create comprehensive, personalized care plans that support both the mental and physical aspects of well-being.

The Mealtime Satisfaction Questionnaire (MSQ) is a 14-item tool designed to assess the overall satisfaction of older adults with their mealtime experiences in retirement and long-term-care settings. Unlike tools that focus on food intake, MSQ captures the patient's general satisfaction with mealtime; it covers aspects such as the timing of meals, food variety, taste, temperature, portion size, dining atmosphere, and interactions with dining staff (Keller and Martos 2013). It is useful for identifying issues such as dissatisfaction with meal routines, which may contribute to poor food choices or disordered eating behaviors. Clinicians working with patients who struggle with meal planning or eating in structured environments may find this tool helpful in developing interventions that improve the mealtime experience. MSQ has demonstrated good internal consistency, test-retest reliability, and construct validity (Pizzola et al. 2013).

The Salzburg Emotional Eating Scale (SEES) is a 20-item self-report questionnaire designed to assess emotional eating by differentiating between specific emotional states and the increase or decrease of food intake in response to these emotions (Meule et al. 2018). SEES includes four subscales: happiness, sadness, anger, and anxiety, each with five items (Meule et al. 2018). It has demonstrated good reliability, with acceptable internal consistency for each subscale, and its validity has been supported through significant correlations with BMI and eating pathology (Meule et al. 2018). This tool could be useful in clinical settings for patients with mood disorders or those who use food as a coping mechanism for emotional distress. It helps clinicians identify patterns of emotional eating, which can be a target for behavioral interventions aimed at improving both emotional regulation and eating habits.

The NutriMental Screener is a nutrition and eating-behavior risk screening tool specifically developed for use in mental health settings to identify individuals at risk for nutrition-related issues, including both overnutrition and undernutrition (Teasdale et al. 2021). The number of items varies depending on the specific version used. It can be adapted to include more or fewer items based on the population being assessed or the specific focus of the screening. This tool is relevant in mental health settings, where it helps clinicians identify patients who may need further nutritional assessment and intervention (Teasdale et al. 2021). The development of the NutriMental Screener involved multiple phases, including literature reviews, service-user interviews, and international workshops to ensure its comprehensiveness and relevance (Teasdale et al. 2021). Preliminary validation studies have shown promising results regarding its feasibility and validity, making it a valuable tool for improving the nutritional care of individuals with serious mental illness (Teasdale et al. 2021), among others.

The Positive Eating Scale (PES) is a self-report questionnaire designed to assess positive eating behaviors by focusing on general satisfaction with one's eating habits. Unlike scales that focus on restrictive or disordered eating patterns, PES emphasizes the pleasure and satisfaction derived from eating, which can promote a healthy relationship with food. It has been validated in various populations, including samples from Germany, the United States, and India (Sproesser et al. 2018). The scale has demonstrated good reliability, with internal consistency and test-retest reliability over 6 months (Sproesser et al. 2018). Its validity is supported by significant associations with health risk factors, and it has been shown to be a useful tool for promoting physical and psychological health by encouraging a positive relationship with eating (Sproesser et al. 2018). Encouraging positive eating experiences can lead to better mental and physical health outcomes.

The Food Enjoyment Scale for Older Adults is a six-item instrument designed to measure the sensory enjoyment of food among older adults, considering factors such as dietary restrictions, oral health, financial limitations, social interactions, and functional abilities (Vailas and Nitzke 1998). The scale uses a five-point response format ranging from "very true" to "not at all true" (Vailas and Nitzke 1998). It has demonstrated good reliability and validity, making it a valuable tool for assessing food enjoyment in older adults and understanding the impact of several factors on their eating experiences (Vailas and Nitzke 1998). This scale can be useful in both clinical and research settings aiming to improve the quality of life and nutritional status of older adults (Vailas and Nitzke 1998).

There are also tools that assess meal preparation skills, as exemplified by the Cooking Skills Confidence Measure. It is a validated tool designed to assess an individual's confidence in their cooking abilities. Developed by Lavelle and colleagues in 2017, this measure evaluates cooking skills such as chopping, boiling, and baking, using a self-report format (Lavelle et al. 2017). The tool has demonstrated good reliability, with internal consistency and reliability across different cohorts, and has shown significant temporal stability (Lavelle et al. 2017). The measure is useful in both clinical and community settings for identifying areas where individuals may need additional support or training to improve their cooking skills and confidence (Lavelle et al. 2017). By assessing cooking skills, clinicians can provide targeted support or referrals to programs that teach cooking techniques, helping patients improve their diet quality through home cooking.

The Staff-Administered Meal Independence Rating Scale (SAMIRS) is a tool designed to assess meal preparation skills and independence among individuals with serious mental illness (Ehntholt et al. 2024). This scale was developed to address the lack of tailored rating scales for this population, which often faces challenges in meal preparation that can hinder their ability to live independently. SAMIRS includes items that evaluate aspects of meal preparation, such as planning, cooking, and cleaning up, and it is completed by staff in inpatient and residential settings who know the client well (Ehntholt et al. 2024). The scale has demonstrated high internal consistency, reliability, and strong validity, with significant correlations with Specific Levels of Functioning (SLOF) scale items (Ehntholt et al. 2024). This makes SAMIRS a valuable tool in clinical settings for identifying functional needs and guiding interventions to improve meal independence among individuals with serious mental illness.

The Lawton Instrumental Activities of Daily Living (IADL) scale, developed by Lawton and Brody (1969), evaluates complex activities necessary for functioning in community settings, such as telephone use, shopping, food preparation, housekeeping, laundry, transportation, medication management, and handling finances. The IADL scale is particularly relevant in clinical settings for identifying functional decline and planning appropriate interventions to support independent living (Lawton and Brody 1969). It has demonstrated good reliability, with inter-rater reliability and 6-month test-retest reliability (Lawton and Brody 1969). The scale's validity is supported by significant correlations with other measures of functional status.

Body mass index (BMI) is a widely used measure to assess body fat based on an individual's weight and height. It is calculated by dividing a person's weight in kilograms by the square of their height in meters. In clinical settings, BMI is often used to screen for weight categories that may lead to health problems, such as underweight, overweight, and obesity. Additionally, BMI has been found to have significant associations with mental health outcomes. For instance, He et al. (2022) found a positive correlation between BMI and increased risk of depression. The reliability and validity of BMI as a measure have been thoroughly documented, with many studies demonstrating its consistent association with a number of health outcomes across different populations (He et al. 2022). It is important to note, however, that BMI does not account for muscle mass, bone density, and other factors that may influence body composition, which can limit its accuracy in certain situations.

Waist circumference is a simple and effective measure of abdominal obesity, which is crucial for assessing health risks associated with excess visceral fat. In clinical settings, waist circumference is used to predict the risk of cardiovascular disease, type 2 diabetes, and overall mortality (World Health Organization 2008). The measurement is taken at the midpoint between the lower margin of the last palpable rib and the top of the iliac crest, ensuring consistency and accuracy (World Health Organization 2008). Waist circumference is relevant in mental health settings, as obesity is linked to several mental health disorders, including depression (He et al. 2022). The reliability and validity of waist circumference as a measure are well documented. However, it is important to ensure proper measurement techniques to maintain accuracy and consistency.

Food- and Nutrition-Related Measures Used Primarily in Research Settings

Although many tools exist for assessing food- and nutrition-related measures, some are too long or complex for use in routine clinical settings. These measures are frequently used in research environments, where detailed and comprehensive data collection is required to assess long-term dietary patterns, nutritional status, or food security. Below are some key research-based tools and their descriptions.

Several types of 24-Hour Dietary Recall are widely used in nutrition research. They require a detailed interview or a detailed self-report measure designed to capture an individual's full food and beverage intake over the past 24 hours. Such measures provide a comprehensive snapshot of daily consumption, including portion sizes and meal timing, which allows for accurate nutrient intake analysis. One of these is the Automated Self-Administered 24-Hour Dietary Assessment Tool (ASA24), a web-based dietary recall system developed by the National Cancer Institute. This innovative tool allows participants to self-report their food and beverage intake over the previous 24 hours without the need for an interviewer, thereby streamlining the data collection process. Research has demonstrated that the ASA24 can provide high-quality dietary intake data comparable to data gathered by more conventional methods, making it a valuable resource for both epidemiological and clinical research (Kirkpatrick et al. 2014).

The Food Frequency Questionnaires (FFQs) are widely used tools in nutritional epidemiology for assessing dietary intake over extended periods. Developed to capture habitual food consumption patterns, an FFQ typically consists of a structured list of food items, with respondents indicating how often they consume them. The design of FFQs allows for the estimation of nutrient intake and dietary patterns, making them useful in studies examining the relationship between diet and chronic diseases. The validity of FFQs can vary, however, based on the population and context in which they are used. Some studies have reported systematic overestimations of dietary intake when using FFQs compared with multiple 24-hour recalls, highlighting the importance of careful validation against more accurate dietary assessment methods (Cade et al. 2002).

The Block Dietary Fat Screener is a brief, computerized tool with 17 questions designed to rate individuals on their fat intake. This screener is commonly used in research to investigate dietary fat consumption trends in populations. Although it is relatively quick to administer compared with more detailed tools, it is primarily used to assess dietary fat intake, and that specific focus makes it less suitable for a comprehensive assessment of the overall diet. Nevertheless, it remains highly valuable for targeted research. Studies have shown that dietary fat intake is closely linked to health issues including cardiovascular disease and obesity (Block et al. 2000).

The Five-A-Day Community Evaluation Tool (FACET) (Ashfield-Watt et al. 2007) assesses fruit and vegetable intake with a specific focus on the "5-a-day" recommendation for daily consumption. Comprising 14 items, it is frequently used in community-based research to evaluate adherence to dietary guidelines, particularly in studies targeting dietary interventions or public health campaigns. It is relatively short, and its specialized focus on fruits and vegetables makes it more appropriate for research assessing specific dietary interventions than general clinical practice.

The Household Food Security Survey Module (HFSSM), developed and used by the USDA, is a well-established tool used in both clinical and research settings to measure food security. The full 18-item version provides a comprehensive assessment of food access, affordability, and experiences of hunger. The tool is widely used in research exploring food insecurity trends. Researchers use the HFSSM to examine the relationship between food insecurity and health outcomes such as mental health disorders, malnutrition, and chronic disease. The six-item short form is feasible in clinical settings, but the full version remains a preferred option in research for its depth and reliability.

The Eating Behavior Patterns Questionnaire (EBPQ) (Schlundt et al. 2003) is a 51-item tool designed to evaluate multiple dimensions of eating behaviors, including emotional eating, eating control, and dietary restraint. This comprehensive measure is often used in research to identify unhealthy eating patterns, especially in studies focused on obesity, disordered eating, and eating behaviors related to mental health. EBPQ is valuable in understanding how psychological factors influence eating habits, making it a frequent choice in behavioral nutrition and public health research. Although it is insightful, its length makes it more suitable for research than for clinical use. EBPQ has been shown to effectively capture the complexities of eating behaviors, providing valuable insights for interventions aimed at improving dietary habits and addressing issues related to obesity and mental health.

The Three-Factor Eating Questionnaire (TFEQ) (Stunkard and Messick 1985) is a well-known research tool that assesses cognitive restraint, uncontrolled eating, and emotional eating. The original version includes 51 items, although shortened versions of 16–20 items exist. Despite these shorter adaptations, TFEQ remains a relatively detailed tool, making it best suited for research studies examining the psychological aspects of eating behaviors. It is commonly used in studies of obesity, eating disorders, and diet-related mental health conditions, helping researchers draw links between eating behaviors and long-term health outcomes (Stunkard and Messick 1985).

The Eating Attitudes Test (EAT-26) (Garner et al. 1982) is a widely used tool in research focused on eating disorders, such as anorexia nervosa and bulimia. With 26 items, it assesses attitudes and behaviors associated with disordered eating. Given its relevance to mental health, this tool is frequently used in studies exploring the prevalence and risk factors for eating disorders, especially among adolescents and young adults. Its length and focus on mental health make it most suitable for research environments or specialized clinical settings.

Biomarkers, such as hemoglobin measurements and serum vitamin D levels, are also commonly used in research settings to assess micronutrient deficiencies. These measures provide objective data on nutrient status, making them valuable in studies exploring the effects of diet on health outcomes. For example, hemoglobin measurements are often used to assess anemia in studies of undernutrition, whereas serum vitamin D levels are critical in research on bone health and chronic diseases such as osteoporosis. These tests, while routine in clinical settings, are especially important in research for understanding the broader population-level impacts of nutrient deficiencies (Alonso et al. 2023).

Future Research Directions

Several areas within the field of nutrition assessment require further exploration. Research on food and nutrition insecurity remains vital, particularly in underserved populations where these issues significantly affect diet quality and health outcomes. Longitudinal studies are needed to understand the long-term effects of food insecurity on both physical and mental health and determine how interventions can best address these issues. The role of dietary interventions in mental health care is another area that warrants deeper investigation. Although emerging evidence suggests that diet plays a role in mental health, more research is needed to determine the effectiveness of specific dietary changes in managing conditions such as depression, anxiety, and psychosis. Finally, more research is needed on optimal ways to incorporate select rating scales and assessments into varying mental health practice settings.

Clinical Pearls

- Given the burden of comorbidity, chronic diseases, and early mortality faced by many individuals with mental illnesses, clinicians should assess food- and nutrition-related constructs in mental health settings.
- Clinicians should be aware that food insecurity may be highly prevalent in some mental health settings, and straightforward

screening tools and rating scales—which may be as brief as one or two items—can be incorporated to determine which clients warrant further assessment and intervention.

- Beyond food security (or availability and access to sufficient amounts of food), both nutrition security, which focuses on sufficient healthy food, and diet quality, or an eating pattern that reduces risk of chronic diseases and improves overall health, can also be easily assessed in routine clinical practice.
- Measures of nutritional status and malnutrition may be warranted in some clinical settings, especially those serving older adults facing social adversities, living with chronic health conditions, or living with social isolation.
- For clinicians to assess food- and nutrition-related issues in mental health practice settings is consistent with a whole-person, holistic care approach to both physical and mental health.

Key Chapter Points

- By incorporating food- and nutrition-related rating scales and assessment into their practice, mental health professionals can better support their clients' overall health.
- In addition to measures of food security, nutrition security, diet quality, nutritional status and malnutrition, and overweight/obesity status, measures of other food- and nutrition-related constructs may be tailored to individual clients' needs. These might include measures of satisfaction with mealtime experiences, emotional eating, eating-behavior risks, food enjoyment, and cooking skills confidence and meal independence.
- Both body mass index (BMI) and waist circumference are important measures of overweight/obesity status that should be used in nearly all clinical settings.
- Beyond the clinical setting, a number of more complex and comprehensive food- and nutrition-related measures—such as 24-hour dietary recalls—are used primarily in research settings.
- Once food- and nutrition-related screening is accomplished in the mental health practice setting, more thorough assessment can be conducted using culturally informed and motivation-enhancing discussion with clients, as detailed in the next chapter.

References

Alonso N, Zelzer S, Eibinger G, et al: Vitamin D metabolites: analytical challenges and clinical relevance. Calcif Tissue Int 112(2):158–177, 2023 35238975

American Dietetic Association, National Council on Aging, American Academy of Family Physicians: Nutrition Screening Initiative: Determine Your Nutritional Health Checklist. 1991. Available at: https://acl.gov/sites/default/files/nutrition/NSI_checklist_508%20with%20citation.pdf. Accessed on November 20, 2024.

Ashfield-Watt PA, Welch AA, Godward S, et al: Effect of a pilot community intervention on fruit and vegetable intakes: use of FACET (Five-a-Day Community Evaluation Tool). Public Health Nutr 10(7):671–680, 2007 17381948

Ballard T, Coates J, Swindale A, et al: Household Hunger Scale: Indicator Definition and Measurement Guide. Food and Nutrition Technical Assistance III project (FANTA-2), USAID, 2011. Available at: https://www.fantaproject.org/sites/default/files/resources/HHS-Indicator-Guide-Aug2011.pdf. Accessed November 18, 2024.

Ballard T, Kepple A, Cafiero C: The Food Insecurity Experience Scale: development of a global standard for monitoring hunger worldwide. Food and Agriculture Organization of the United Nations (FAO), 2013. Available at: https://openknowledge.fao.org/server/api/core/bitstreams/29506589-c91c-44aa-b628-b032ea38f691/content. Accessed November 18, 2024.

Block G, Gillespie C, Rosenbaum EH, et al: A rapid food screener to assess fat and fruit and vegetable intake. Am J Prev Med 18(4):284–288, 2000 10788730

Blumberg SJ, Bialostosky K, Hamilton WL, et al: The effectiveness of a short form of the household food security scale. Am J Public Health 89(8):1231–1234, 1999 10432912

Cade J, Thompson R, Burley V, et al: Development, validation and utilisation of food-frequency questionnaires: a review. Public Health Nutr 5(4):567–587, 2002 12186666

Calloway EE, Carpenter LR, Gargano T, et al: Development of new measures to assess household nutrition security, and choice in dietary characteristics. Appetite 179:106288, 2022 36049571

Calloway EE, Coakley KE, Carpenter LR, et al: Benefits of using both the hunger vital sign and brief nutrition security screener in health-related social needs screening. Transl Behav Med 14(8):445–451, 2024 38954835

Coates J, Swindale A, Bilinsky P: Household Food Insecurity Access Scale (HFIAS) for Measurement of Food Access: Indicator Guide (v.3). Food and Nutrition Technical Assistance Project (FANTA), 2007

Connell CL, Nord M, Lofton KL, et al: Food security of older children can be assessed using a standardized survey instrument. J Nutr 134(10):2566–2572, 2004 15465749

Detsky AS, McLaughlin JR, Baker JP, et al: What is subjective global assessment of nutritional status? JPEN J Parenter Enteral Nutr 11(1):8–13, 1987 3820522

Economic Research Service. Food Security in the U.S. – Survey Tools: Six-Item Short Form of the Food Security Survey Module. U.S. Department of Agriculture, Economic Research Service, 2024. Available at: https://www.ers.usda.gov/topics/food-nutrition-assistance/food-security-in-the-u-s/survey-tools/#six. Accessed November 6, 2024.

Ehntholt A, Fu E, Pope LG, et al: Introducing the Staff-Administered Meal Independence Rating Scale for use among patients with serious mental illnesses. J Nerv Ment Dis 212(2):71–75, 2024 37788339

Elia M: The 'MUST' Report: Nutritional screening of adults: a multidisciplinary responsibility. BAPEN, 2003. Available at: https://www.bapen.org.uk/pdfs/must/must-report.pdf. Accessed December 3, 2024.

Ferguson M, Capra S, Bauer J, et al: Development of a valid and reliable malnutrition screening tool for adult acute hospital patients. Nutrition 15(6):458–464, 1999 10378201

Garner DM, Olmsted MP, Bohr Y, et al: The Eating Attitudes Test: psychometric features and clinical correlates. Psychol Med 12(4):871–878, 1982 6961471

Głąbska D, Guzek D, Groele B, et al: Fruit and vegetable intake and mental health in adults: a systematic review. Nutrients 12(1):115, 2020 31906271

Grimaccia E, Naccarato A: Confirmatory factor analysis to validate a new measure of food insecurity: perceived and actual constructs. Qual Quant 54:1211–1232, 2020

Hager ER, Quigg AM, Black MM, et al: Development and validity of a 2-item screen to identify families at risk for food insecurity. Pediatrics 126(1):e26–e32, 2010 20595453

He K, Pang T, Huang H: The relationship between depressive symptoms and BMI: 2005–2018 NHANES data. J Affect Disord 313:151–157, 2022 35753497

Keller H, Martos T: Mealtime Satisfaction Questionnaire (MSQ). 2013. Available at: https://the-ria.ca/wp-content/uploads/2018/08/Final-MSQ-web-version.pdf. Accessed November 18, 2024.

Keys A, Fidanza F, Karvonen MJ, et al: Indices of relative weight and obesity. J Chronic Dis 25(6–7):329–343, 1972

Kirkpatrick SI, Subar AF, Douglass D, et al: Performance of the automated self-administered 24-hour recall relative to a measure of true intakes and to an interviewer-administered 24-h recall. Am J Clin Nutr 100(1):233–240, 2014 24787491

Kleinman RE, Murphy JM, Little M, et al: Hunger in children in the United States: potential behavioral and emotional correlates. Pediatrics 101(1):E3, 1998 9417167

Kleinman RE, Murphy JM, Wieneke KM, et al: Use of a single-question screening tool to detect hunger in families attending a neighborhood health center. Ambul Pediatr 7(4):278–284, 2007 17660098

Kondrup J, Allison SP, Elia M, et al: Educational and Clinical Practice Committee, European Society of Parenteral and Enteral Nutrition (ESPEN): ESPEN guidelines for nutrition screening 2002. Clin Nutr 22(4):415–421, 2003 12880610

Kruizenga HM, Seidell JC, de Vet HC, et al: Development and validation of a hospital screening tool for malnutrition: the Short Nutritional Assessment Questionnaire (SNAQ). Clin Nutr 24(1):75–82, 2005 15681104

Lara-Breitinger KM, Medina Inojosa JR, Li Z, et al: Validation of a brief dietary questionnaire for use in clinical practice: Mini EAT (Eating Assessment Tool). J Am Heart Assoc 12(1):e025064, 2023 36583423

Lau S, Pek K, Chew J, et al: The Simplified Nutritional Appetite Questionnaire (SNAQ) as a screening tool for risk of malnutrition: optimal cutoff, factor structure, and validation in healthy community-dwelling older adults. Nutrients 12(9):2885, 2020 32967354

Lavelle F, McGowan L, Hollywood L, et al: The development and validation of measures to assess cooking skills and food skills. Int J Behav Nutr Phys Act 14(1):118, 2017 28865452

Lawton MP, Brody EM: Assessment of older people: self-maintaining and instrumental activities of daily living. Gerontologist 9(3):179–186, 1969 5349366

Meule A, Reichenberger J, Blechert J: Development and preliminary validation of the Salzburg Emotional Eating Scale. Front Psychol 9:88, 2018 29467700

Mozaffarian D, Hao T, Rimm EB, et al: Changes in diet and lifestyle and long-term weight gain in women and men. N Engl J Med 364(25):2392–2404, 2011 21696306

National Institute on Minority Health and Health Disparities (NIMHD): Food accessibility, insecurity and health outcomes. NIMHD, 2023. Available at: https://www.nimhd.nih.gov/resources/understanding-health-disparities/food-accessibility-insecurity-and-health-outcomes.html. Accessed December 3, 2024.

Neelemaat F, Meijers J, Kruizenga H, et al: Comparison of five malnutrition screening tools in one hospital inpatient sample. J Clin Nurs 20(15–16):2144–2152, 2011 21535274

Nord M, Cafiero C, Viviani S: Methods for estimating comparable prevalence rates of food insecurity experienced by adults in 147 countries and areas. J. Phys Conf. Ser 772:012060, 2016

Paxton AE, Strycker LA, Toobert DJ, et al: Starting the conversation performance of a brief dietary assessment and intervention tool for health professionals. Am J Prev Med 40(1):67–71, 2011 21146770

Pizzola L, Martos Z, Pfisterer K, et al: Construct validation and test-retest reliability of a mealtime satisfaction questionnaire for retirement home residents. J Nutr Gerontol Geriatr 32(4):343–359, 2013 24224941

Posner BM, Jette AM, Smith KW, et al: Nutrition and health risks in the elderly: the nutrition screening initiative. Am J Public Health 83(7):972–978, 1993 8328619

Radimer KL, Olson CM, Greene JC, et al: Understanding hunger and developing indicators to assess it in women and children. J Nutr Educ 24(1):36S–44S, 1992

Rubenstein LZ, Harker JO, Salvà A, et al: Screening for undernutrition in geriatric practice: developing the Short-Form Mini-Nutritional Assessment (MNA-SF). J Gerontol A Biol Sci Med Sci 56(6):M366–M372, 2001 11382797

Schlundt DG, Hargreaves MK, Buchowski MS: The eating behavior patterns questionnaire predicts dietary fat intake in African American women. J Am Diet Assoc 103(3):338–345, 2003 12616256

Shim RS, Compton MT: The social determinants of mental health: psychiatrists' roles in addressing discrimination and food insecurity. Focus 18(1):25–30, 2020 32047394

Sproesser G, Klusmann V, Ruby MB, et al: The positive eating scale: relationship with objective health parameters and validity in Germany, the USA and India. Psychol Health 33(3):313–339, 2018 28641449

Stunkard AJ, Messick S: The three-factor eating questionnaire to measure dietary restraint, disinhibition and hunger. J Psychosom Res 29(1):71–83, 1985 3981480

Swindale A, Bilinsky P: Household Dietary Diversity Score (HDDS) for Measurement of Household Food Access: Indicator Guide (v.2). Food and Nutrition Technical Assistance Project (FANTA), 2006. Available at: https://www.fantaproject.org/sites/default/files/resources/HDDS_v2_Sep06_0.pdf. Accessed December 3, 2024.

Teasdale SB, Moerkl S, Moetteli S, et al: The development of a nutrition screening tool for mental health settings prone to obesity and cardiometabolic complications: study protocol for the NutriMental Screener. Int J Environ Res Public Health 18(21):11269, 2021 34769787

Thomas MMC, Miller DP, Morrissey TW: Food insecurity and child health. Pediatrics 144(4):e20190397, 2019 31501236

Thompson FE, Byers T: Dietary assessment resource manual. J Nutr 124(11)(Suppl):2245S–2317S, 1994 7965210

Thompson FE, Kipnis V, Subar AF, et al: Evaluation of 2 brief instruments and a food-frequency questionnaire to estimate daily number of servings of fruit and vegetables. Am J Clin Nutr 71(6):1503–1510, 2000 10837291

Vadiveloo MK, Thorndike AN, Lichtenstein AH: Integrating diet screening into routine clinical care: the time is now. J Am Heart Assoc 12(1):e028583, 2023 36583426

Vailas RL, Nitzke SA: Food enjoyment scale for older adults: development and application in a Wisconsin population. J Nutr Elder 17(3):59–64, 1998

Wehler CA, Scott RI, Anderson JJ: The Community Childhood Hunger Identification Project: a model of domestic hunger: demonstration project in Seattle, Washington. J Nutr Educ 24(1):29S–35S, 1992

Wei K, Nyunt MS, Gao Q, et al: Association of frailty and malnutrition with long-term functional and mortality outcomes among community-dwelling older adults: results from the Singapore Longitudinal Aging Study 1. JAMA Netw Open 6;1(3):e180650, 2018

Wilson MM, Thomas DR, Rubenstein LZ, et al: Appetite assessment: simple appetite questionnaire predicts weight loss in community-dwelling adults and nursing home residents. Am J Clin Nutr 82(5):1074–1081, 2005 16280441

World Health Organization (WHO): Waist circumference and waist-hip ratio: report of a WHO expert consultation. Geneva, World Health Organization, 2008. Available at: https://www.who.int/publications/i/item/9789241501491. Accessed December 3, 2024.

7

Assessing and Addressing Food- and Nutrition-Related Issues in the Clinical Setting

B. Lynette Staplefoote-Boynton, M.D., M.P.H.

Listening to patients is the cornerstone of patient-centered care.

—Don Berwick, former Administrator of the Centers for Medicare and Medicaid Services

Although the evidence is convincing for healthy nutrition as a high-yield tool for chronic disease prevention and management, incorporating nutrition and dietary counseling into regular practice is a new and emerging skill for most physicians and advanced practice providers. Given that most providers have had limited education or guidance during their training programs on nutrition and dietary counseling, they often find it challenging to incorporate this type of counseling into their practice. In a 2020 study, many resident physicians felt that they needed to be more adequately trained in nutrition and dietary counseling (Jain et al. 2020). The same study showed that residents trained with nutrition education curricula felt more confident in their knowledge of nutrition interventions to address chronic diseases after receiving instruction. Even so, this confidence may not always translate into clinical practice because of the lack of a framework and approach for addressing behavioral changes around food consumption and nutrition. This chapter provides a practical clinical framework for how a provider can help improve patients' nutrition.

Overview of Public Health and Medical Societies' Guidelines on Nutrition

Poor nutrition, or malnutrition, is one of the leading causes of morbidity and mortality in the United States. The World Health Organization (WHO) defines malnutrition as an imbalance in nutritional intake, including deficiencies and excesses in energy intake, in macronutrients, and in micronutrients (Kesari and Noel 2024). In the United States, the most significant disease burden comes from an excess of calories. This excess or imbalance has been implicated in the increased risk for diseases such as hypertension, type 2 diabetes, and atherosclerotic disease, which increase an individual's risk for coronary artery disease, peripheral artery disease, and stroke. Cardiovascular disease is the leading cause of death in the United States. Individuals with serious mental illness carry a heavier burden. The rate of cardiovascular disease in this population is more than twice that of the general population. This population also has a life expectancy that is 15–20 years shorter than the general population, largely due to the heavy disease burden of cardiovascular disease and other chronic physical health conditions (Hjorthøj et al. 2017; Lambert et al. 2022; Saha et al. 2007).

Data are accumulating that support the interdependent relationship between cardiometabolic diseases and serious mental illness (Goldfarb et al. 2022). Although most psychiatrists will not be actively managing chronic medical conditions, many patients will have cardiovascular or metabolic comorbidities, which may further complicate the treatment of a patient's mental illness. Given that nutrition serves a foundational role in achieving outcomes for cardiovascular and metabolic conditions, mental health professionals can play an active role in chronic disease management by promoting healthy nutrition. This possibility highlights the importance of being aware of medical society guidelines pertaining to nutrition. Society guidelines recommend lifestyle modification as the first line for prevention and as the primary intervention in a comprehensive treatment plan for cardiovascular disease and type 2 diabetes (ElSayed 2023; Grundy et al. 2019).

The American Diabetes Association recommends that providers evaluate the need for medical nutrition therapy (MNT), which will be discussed later, in four key phases in a patient's care: 1) at diagnosis; 2) annually or when the patient is not meeting diabetes treatment targets (e.g., an A1C goal); 3) when physical, medical, or psychosocial stressors develop; and 4) when transitions in life or care occur (ElSayed et al. 2023).

Although this guideline is expert opinion, it highlights the need to consider ongoing nutrition counseling throughout a patient's treatment course.

The most recent guidelines from the American College of Cardiology (ACC) and the American Heart Association (AHA) for adults with elevated blood pressure or hypertension recommend four diet-related nonpharmacological interventions, all of which have a high level of evidence (Whelton et al. 2018): 1) the DASH (Dietary Approaches to Stop Hypertension) diet; 2) a reduction of approximately 1,000 mg per day of sodium; 3) increasing dietary potassium, primarily through at least four to five servings of fruits and vegetables (although it may be contraindicated in those with chronic kidney disease or potassium-sparing medications contributing to hyperkalemia); and 4) for individuals who drink, reducing alcohol consumption to ≤2 drinks daily for men and ≤1 drink daily for women. These interventions can decrease systolic blood pressure 4–11 mmHg for patients with hypertension. Encouraging these changes in diet can be a cost-conscious and effective way to address a patient's blood pressure without contributing to drug-drug interactions or adverse medication reactions.

The ACC's and AHA's most recent guidelines on the management of blood cholesterol also have general recommendations surrounding diet (Grundy et al. 2019): 1) review dietary habits, endorse a healthy lifestyle, and provide relevant advice, material, or referrals when engaging in clinician-patient shared decision-making for initiating statin therapy; and 2) give lifestyle counseling using principles of the Mediterranean and DASH diets that are consistent with the patient's racial/ethnic preferences to avoid weight gain and address blood pressure and lipids.

An estimated 32.8% of adult males and 36.2% of adult females have a total cholesterol of ≥200 mg/dL, and about 25% of adults have a low-density lipoprotein (LDL) cholesterol of ≥130 mg/dL (Tsao et al. 2023). Patients with serious mental illness are particularly at risk for elevated

LDL. Although many mental health professionals may not decide to prescribe statins (instead referring to and collaborating with primary care), by incorporating dietary counseling into routine mental health practice, they can contribute to the overall efforts to reduce cardiovascular risks in their patients.

The Clinical Approach

The argument for the importance of dietary counseling in clinical practice has been made clear by many medical society guidelines. Even so, the logistics of how to do this is not always obvious. A provider with basic nutrition knowledge can contribute to healthy behavioral change in a patient by following a simple approach to addressing nutrition. As detailed below, providers should strive to 1) assess, 2) discuss, 3) refer and collaborate, and 4) follow up throughout the treatment course.

Assess

Although nutrition assessments are not usually included in most psychiatric evaluations, they should be considered during initial assessment or throughout the course of treatment with a patient. This is especially important for patients with difficult-to-treat or refractory illness, who may be experiencing cardiovascular or metabolic side effects such as weight gain or elevated blood pressure contributed to by the use of psychotropic medications, or who have existing comorbidities that complicate treatment.

Screen for and Assess Food Insecurity and Nutrition Insecurity

When assessing a patient's nutrition and dietary habits, it is important to have a baseline and ongoing understanding of their food and nutrition security status. Food and nutrition insecurity are too often barriers to dietary changes and serve as an unmet health-related social need that affects many patients. Health care payers and accrediting agencies, such as the Centers for Medicare and Medicaid Services, the Joint Commission, and the National Commission for Quality Assurance, require health care organizations to screen for and address health disparities. Given these requirements, most large health care systems are incorporating food insecurity screening into patient clinic flow and storing it in the electronic health record. This can vary from setting to setting, even within the same health system or organization. It is important for the clinician to understand how patients are screened and to know where to access this screening information. Even if a patient has been screened by another member of the health care team, the treating provider should round out the assessment of food insecurity by discussing screening findings directly with the patient to confirm and gain a richer understanding of a patient's unmet health-related social needs. In general, every patient should be screened for food insecurity. Recent research suggests that screening using an iPad or on paper yields more positive screens for food insecurity than screening done verbally, which may be due to the stigma associated with food insecurity (Palakshappa et al. 2019).

Assessing Dietary Behaviors Based on the Framework of Thomas Campbell, M.D.

Dr. Thomas Campbell provided a practical approach for assessing patients' dietary habits (Campbell 2022). As detailed in Table 7.1, providers should ask about food choice, eating structure, and food volume. Assessing at least one of these three aspects of eating habits during a visit is part of a 5-minute dietary counseling approach that is explained in further detail in this section. Assessment of food choice encompasses understanding what a person chooses to eat. Ask questions about food choices by doing a simple 24-hour food recall or reviewing a diet diary. Diet diaries covering a short period (e.g., one weekday and one weekend day) are the most likely to be completed. However, diaries that cover a longer stretch of time can give a more realistic view of what a patient typically eats based on different life circumstances. Assessing eating structure encompasses understanding the when, where, and how often of people's eating habits throughout the day. Ask questions about eating structure to understand what time of day meals are eaten, if meals are often skipped, how many meals a day a person eats with others, and whether snacking is done during the day. Assessment of food volume includes understanding the typical amount of food eaten during meals and snacks and screening for restrictive or binge eating behaviors. This approach can include short-term calorie monitoring using smartphone apps such as MyFitnessPal. In addition to monitoring calories, assessing food volume should focus on helping patients identify episodes of high-volume eating and gain self-awareness of comfortable satiety rather than being overly full.

Table 7.1 Assessing and targeting dietary behaviors based on the framework of Thomas Campbell, M.D.

Behavior	How to assess	Behavioral change targets
Food choice	Help patient to do a 24-hour diet recall. Example questions include: What did you eat for dinner, lunch, breakfast, and snacks yesterday? Review a diet diary written on paper or in an app.	Address misinformation about foods to avoid vs. foods to enjoy. Help patients identify a concrete change with the message, "Eat less of _ and replace it with _." For instance: Drink less sugar-sweetened soda or tea and replace it with water flavored with fruit. Eat less white bread or pasta and replace it with whole-grain bread or pasta. Help establish a SMART goal and follow up during visits.
Eating structure	Understand how the time of day, social networks, and other factors (e.g., emotions, work schedule) influence food choices and volume. Example questions include, Did you eat any food after dinner? How does skipping meals affect how much you eat the following meal? Do you eat with others?	Promote consistent eating patterns to reduce impulse snacking. Explore ways to minimize snacking on unhealthy foods. Encourage involvement of social supports in dietary change goals.

Table 7.1 Assessing and targeting dietary behaviors based on the framework of Thomas Campbell, M.D. (*continued*)

Behavior	How to assess	Behavioral change targets
Food volume	Perform a short-term trial of calorie-counting using smart phone apps. Example questions include: Have you ever eaten what most people would consider an excessive amount in a brief period of time? Have you eaten an excessive amount and immediately felt guilty about it? Do you eat past fullness? Do you ever eat when you are not hungry?	Encourage tools that promote awareness around food portions, such as calorie tracking or portion control dinnerware. If binge or emotional eating is a factor, consider pharmacologic or psychotherapy treatment. Promote mindful eating. Help patients explore their fullness cues and identify how they experience "comfortable fullness."

SMART = specific, measurable, attainable, realistic, and time-bound.

Discuss

Food Insecurity

Every patient should be screened for food insecurity. Even if a person has a negative screen for food insecurity, it is a good practice to confirm that and discuss it briefly during a visit. Once someone screens positive for food insecurity, it is essential to continue the conversation in a sensitive manner that minimizes stigma and embarrassment. When discussing food insecurity, remain curious and open-minded. Financial issues may not be the only barrier to food security—others include limited transportation, insufficient local availability (e.g., living in a food desert), and psychiatric symptoms (e.g., depression, anxiety, negative symptoms of schizophrenia) (Compton and Shim 2015). Continue the conversation with the 3 A's: acknowledge, affirm, and ask. *Acknowledge* that discussing food insecurity may come with stigma. Help patients offload self-blame for food insecurity by recognizing societal factors (e.g., competing costs of housing, health care, and medications; the role of food deserts and food swamps). Display gratitude that the patient has entrusted that information to you. *Affirm* how important it is to you, as the clinician, that food insecurity is addressed. Mention that the use of available community resources is a proactive step in reaching health goals. Let patients know that food insecurity is quite common and that they are not alone. *Ask* if the patient is interested in being connected to services. Do not assume that a patient wants to be connected or is ready to receive services.

Nutrition Education: Approaches Based on Time Available in a Visit

Although physicians and other clinicians have a role in health promotion, it is important to recognize that most providers have limited training and significant time barriers in the context of the current health care environment. Depending on the allotted time, be prepared with a 5-minute, 2-minute, or 1-minute approach to promoting healthy eating habits. With any approach, delivering it with cultural humility and mindfulness of social context is critical.

5-Minute Approach to Dietary Counseling

Allot at least 5 minutes during a visit to target one domain of Dr. Campbell's framework for dietary counseling. After assessing a patient's food choice, eating structure, or food volume, use motivational interviewing to gauge readiness to make dietary changes by fostering the patient's own curiosity and awareness about their diet and their eating behaviors and how they impact health. Then use motivational interviewing techniques to support the patient's efforts to improve their nutrition. Focus on one of the three domains at a time to facilitate achievable small changes and promote the patient's self-efficacy for making dietary changes. Table 7.1 provides specific examples of behavioral change targets for each domain.

2-Minute Approach to Dietary Counseling

A 2-minute approach for dietary counseling can be used to provide concrete information about healthy nutrition based on the current research. This approach focuses on choosing one evidence-based diet and communicating the principles and benefits of the diet based on the current evidence. This can be helpful for patients who are in the *contemplation* stage of behavioral change. Providing general information about an evidence-based diet and communicating the benefits based on data provides information that could lead a patient to move into the *preparation* stage of change. The three diets that have the most data are the Mediterranean diet, the DASH diet (Dietary Approaches to Stop Hypertension), and the MIND diet (Mediterranean–DASH Intervention for Neurodegenerative Delay).

The Mediterranean diet encourages consumption of plenty of fruits, vegetables, whole grains, and legumes; olive oil as the primary fat source; and moderate amounts of fish, poultry, and dairy. This diet is typically a good approach for most people, but it has compelling evidence for patients with or at an elevated risk for atherosclerotic cardiovascular disease to reduce the risk of future major adverse cardiovascular events (Grundy et al. 2019). The DASH diet encourages the consumption of fruits, vegetables, whole grains, lean proteins, and low-fat dairy while reducing saturated fat, cholesterol, and sodium. This evidence-based diet is for patients with elevated blood pressure or hypertension who want to add to their pharmacologic treatment. This diet has the most evidence for decreasing blood pressure; studies suggest that following the DASH diet can decrease systolic blood pressure by 11 mmHg for individuals with hypertension (Whelton et al. 2018). The MIND diet is based on both diets and focuses on foods that improve brain health, such as green leafy vegetables, nuts, berries, and whole grains. This diet is known best for promoting healthy aging

Table 7.2 Examples of websites with handouts that can provide useful information for clients

Name	Organization	URL
CardioSmart	American College of Cardiology	https://www.cardiosmart.org/
Healthy Eating	American Heart Association	https://www.heart.org/en/healthy-living/healthy-eating
Heart Healthy Toolbox	Preventive Cardiovascular Nurses Association	https://pcna.net/clinical-resources/patient-handouts/heart-healthy-toolbox/
Diabetes Plate	American Diabetes Association	https://www.diabetesfoodhub.org/articles/what-is-the-diabetes-plate-method.html

and overall heart and brain health. Studies suggest that following the MIND diet can reduce one's risk of dementia (Arjmand et al. 2022).

1-Minute Approach to Dietary Counseling

When time is short, use a 1-minute approach to print out or secure-message a resource for the patient to refer to after the visit. Be prepared to have a handout ready for a patient to review after the appointment. This can be helpful when a patient is in the *preparation* or *action* stage of change. Handouts vetted and created by health organizations to be patient-friendly and easily understood, including the ones discussed in Table 7.2, can provide important information as patients prepare to make changes and need reliable information.

Cultural Considerations and Mindfulness of Social Context

Cultural humility in efforts to improve the nutrition of patients is often underappreciated, but it is a critical component of dietary counseling. Incorporating cultural humility involves self-evaluation and critical awareness of biases while maintaining openness for learning, communicating, offering help, and making clinical decisions with patients (National Association of Social Workers n.d.; Tervalon and Murray-García 1998). No matter the background of a patient, it is vital to consider and discuss how the principles of the diets mentioned earlier can be adapted to their own culture or family. Research suggests that culturally tailored nutrition counseling can improve diet quality (Hammons et al. 2019). A central start to this approach is not making assumptions, being curious, and encouraging the patient to be curious about their background and the significant foods in their culture/subculture. Have discussions about how cultural beliefs and practices influence their diet. In addition to encouraging open dialogue, offer culturally appropriate nutrition information resources that they can explore. Furthermore, beyond integrating cultural considerations into nutrition education, it is imperative to be attentive to patients' social contexts, such as their health-related social needs profile and interpersonal and community networks. Ways to promote cultural humility and to include social context into the conversations are shown in Table 7.3.

Refer and Collaborate

Becoming an expert on local community resources is not feasible for most providers, thus highlighting the importance of interprofessional collaboration. Each community varies in the resources available to address food insecurity, and it is important to become aware of the resources available to the patients you serve. Although you may not directly refer patients to services, you will likely work with a case manager, social worker, or community health worker to do so. Understanding the basic community-based infrastructure available helps you guide and collaborate with your interprofessional colleagues. Presented briefly here are some common community resources, and more information is given in Chapter 9 ("Food- and Nutrition-Related Policies and Programs"). Familiarity with these resources can help you work with your patients and other health care team members to address food insecurity.

Overview of Clinical and Community Resources Related to Addressing Food Insecurity

Food pantries are distribution centers where families can receive food. Often, food pantries offer mainly shelf-stable foods distributed to them by the regional food bank. Some food pantries also provide fresh produce and meats based on availability. Food pantries are often located in community locations such as schools or faith-based organizations.

Table 7.3 **Ways to promote cultural humility and to include social context into conversations**

Action	Notes
Promote cultural humility	Don't make assumptions; be curious about the patient's background and culture/subculture. Encourage the patient to be curious about foods important to their culture/subculture that may align with the diets being recommended. Focus on strengths and not weaknesses. Discuss how cultural beliefs influence nutritional choices. Be mindful of language barriers; use an interpreter if necessary. Also, try to have text and printouts translated into the patient's preferred language. Highlight that dietary changes can help prevent or even treat disease without the use of medications. This tends to be a value important to many cultures/subcultures. Offer culturally appropriate resources for patients to explore.
Include social context into conversations	Screen and discuss food insecurity. Be aware of community resources to help address food insecurity and refer patients to someone who can connect them to the right resources. Gain a basic understanding of the patient's relationship with food. The patient may have a history of food-related trauma or emotional distress (e.g., food insecurity in childhood or in country of origin). Therapy may be needed to address this. Gain a basic understanding of the patient's attitudes, self-efficacy, and skills around food preparation. Based on the patient's response, interventions and referrals can be tailored to the patient's needs. Be mindful of any medical, psychiatric, or cognitive comorbidities that can serve as barriers to food selection and preparation. Include the patient's family and loved ones in the conversation. Food choices are significantly influenced by family and friends.

Mobile food pantries are also available in some communities. *Senior congregate meal* programs provide nutritionally balanced meals in group settings. They are often served in community or senior centers, schools, or faith-based locations. This service aims to address both the food insecurity and social needs of seniors. *Delivered meals to seniors* (e.g., Meals on Wheels) provide nutritionally balanced meals to homebound seniors, which also allows for a quick safety check and a friendly visit. This service aims to address food insecurity and social needs of seniors.

A number of federally funded programs are available, as given in Table 7.4; some of these are described further in Chapter 9.

Food Is Medicine

Food Is Medicine (FIM) efforts are a proposed solution for decreasing food and nutrition insecurity while addressing chronic diseases. FIM interventions offered by health care organizations or insurance plans include medically tailored meals, medically tailored groceries, and produce prescription programs that provide benefits for participants to purchase fruits and vegetables (Bleich et al. 2023). These programs are described in detail in Chapter 8.

Working With Registered Dietitians

Physicians have limited training and little time during routine visits to address nutrition and dietary habits. Although taking a few minutes at each visit to discuss healthy eating habits is invaluable, it is important to recognize when patients need more time and expertise. Incorporate interprofessional collaboration with a registered dietitian into your practice. Nutrition services, also known as Medical Nutrition Therapy (MNT), may be reimbursed by Medicaid, Medicare, and some private insurance plans. Other nutrition-related community resources are also available to help patients make dietary changes. Consider a nutrition referral for any patient with 1) pre-diabetes, new-onset diabetes, or uncontrolled diabetes; 2) Stage I hypertension, new-onset hypertension, and uncontrolled Stage II hypertension; 3) an intermediate-risk profile for atherosclerotic cardiovascular disease; 4) weight gain or metabolic syndrome while taking antipsychotics; and 5) unintended weight loss after medical causes have been ruled out.

You may be in a health system that already incorporates qualified professionals to provide MNT. When referring patients to nutrition services, provide them with information about dietitians' qualifica-

Table 7.4 Federally funded programs related to food and nutrition

Program	Description	Website
Supplemental Nutrition Assistance Program (SNAP)	Available in all 50 states, the District of Columbia, Puerto Rico, the Virgin Islands, and Guam; provides money to purchase food; formerly known as "food stamps"	www.fns.usda.gov/snap
SNAP-Ed	Provides nutrition education and recipes; policy, system, and environmental change approaches; and social marketing tools	https://snaped.fns.usda.gov
Special Supplemental Nutrition Program for Women, Infants, and Children (WIC) Program	Provides money to purchase prespecified foods based on nutrition standards for pregnant or postpartum women, infants, and children	www.fns.usda.gov/wic
WIC Farmers Market Nutrition Program (FMNP)	Associated with WIC; eligible WIC participants are issued FMNP coupons in addition to their regular WIC benefits; coupons can be used to buy eligible foods from farmers, farmers markets, or roadside stands that have been approved by the state agency to accept FMNP coupons	https://www.fns.usda.gov/fmnp/wic-farmers-market-nutrition-program
School Breakfast Program	Provides free or reduced-price breakfast for income-eligible students of all ages	www.fns.usda.gov/sbp/school-breakfast-program
National School Lunch Program	Provides free or reduced-price lunch for income-eligible students of all ages	https://www.fns.usda.gov/nslp
SUN Meals (Summer Food Service Program)	Offers free healthy meals for students age ≤18 during the summer months when school is not in session	www.fns.usda.gov/sfsp/summer-food-service-program

Table 7.4 Federally funded programs related to food and nutrition (*continued*)

Child and Adult Care Food Program	Provides reimbursements for nutritious meals and snacks to eligible children and adults who are enrolled for care at participating child care centers, day care homes, and adult day care centers	https://www.fns.usda.gov/cacfp
Seniors Farmers Market Nutrition Program	Like the WIC FMNP, offers vouchers for low-income seniors for farmers markets, farm stands, and community-supported agriculture programs	https://www.fns.usda.gov/sfmnp/senior-farmers-market-nutrition-program
Commodity Supplemental Food Program	Serves eligible low-income seniors with a monthly food package	https://www.fns.usda.gov/csfp/commodity-supplemental-food-program
Food Distribution Program on Indian Reservations	Provides USDA foods to income-eligible households living on Indian reservations and to Native American households residing in designated areas near reservations or in Oklahoma	https://www.fns.usda.gov/fdpir/food-distribution-program-indian-reservations
The Emergency Food Assistance Program	Helps supplement the diets of people with low income by providing them with emergency food assistance at no cost; USDA provides 100% American-grown USDA foods and administrative funds to states to operate the program	https://www.fns.usda.gov/tefap/emergency-food-assistance-program

Table 7.4 Federally funded programs related to food and nutrition (*continued*)

Expanded Food and Nutrition Education Program	The nation's first nutrition education program for low-income populations and remains at the forefront of nutrition education efforts to reduce nutrition insecurity of low-income families and youth; a federal extension (community outreach) program that operates through land-grant universities in every state, the District of Columbia, and the six U.S. territories: American Samoa, Guam, Micronesia, Northern Marianas, Puerto Rico, and the Virgin Islands	https://www.nifa.usda.gov/grants/programs/capacity-grants/efnep/expanded-food-nutrition-education-program
Eldercare (Administration for Community Living) and Area Agencies on Aging	Local agencies may not directly provide food or nutrition assistance but often are able to connect seniors to food and local nutrition services and can serve as a vital resource to seniors	https://eldercare.acl.gov/
Veterans Service Organizations	The Veteran's Administration implements this program and offers a range of services, including assistance with benefit claims and emergency food assistance	www.va.gov/vso
USDA National Hunger Hotline	Hotline available to providers or other members of the healthcare team; can assist with referrals for food banks and other social services	1-866-348-6479 (TTY: 711), 7 a.m.–10 p.m., Eastern time; text the automated service at 914-342-7744
Feeding America	National organization that maintains a registry of local resources for feeding programs, including information about food banks and their respective local food distribution sites (e.g., food pantries)	www.feedingamerica.org/find-your-local-foodbank

tions and help them understand the differences between dietitians and nutritionists, as detailed in Table 7.5.

The *Find a Nutrition Expert* database lists credentialed nutrition and dietetics practitioners by specialty, language, or insurance/payment type: https://www.eatright.org/find-a-nutrition-expert.

Follow Up Throughout the Treatment Course

Ongoing follow-up and repeat assessments of nutrition—including food security, food choice, eating structure, and food volume—are critical for encouraging ongoing nutrition improvement with a patient. This consistency signals to the patient that nutrition is an essential part of their medical management, and it gives the provider opportunities to help patients troubleshoot any issues or stumbling blocks. With these discussions about nutrition, it is vital to maintain cultural humility and mindfulness of social context, as conversations about a patient's food and nutrition can often come with stigma, making conversations counterproductive.

Continuing the discussion about nutrition and the resources available to achieve goals can be instrumental in keeping patients in the *maintenance* stage of change. These discussions should include learning more about the role that interdisciplinary colleagues and community organizations play in nutrition improvement efforts. Once you refer patients to community resources, do not think this is where your involvement ends. Following up on your patients' experience with a particular community resource and how the resource may have affected their efforts for behavioral change serves many purposes:

1. It shows the patient that you care about their food insecurity and nutritional status. Even if you cannot directly change their food insecurity status, discussing their ongoing journey shows them that it is important to you.
2. Continuing the conversation reduces the stigma of seeking help for food insecurity. Reducing this stigma can reinforce that receiving help to improve their diet and their health is the right thing to do.
3. Following up helps improve your understanding of how community resources can affect your patients' diet habits. Much like we check in on how medications or therapies such as physical

Table 7.5 Differences between dietitians and nutritionists, based on Campbell (Cleveland Clinic 2023)

Characteristic	Dietitian	Nutritionist
Professional title	Registered dietitian (RD) or registered dietitian nutritionist (RDN)	No official professional title; some may call themselves nutrition coach
Educational requirements	Bachelor's degree from an accredited dietetics program; as of January 2024, master's degree from an accredited dietetics program	Online certification courses, some as brief as 8 weeks
Supervision prior to independent practice	1,000 supervised hours of clinical practice	No requirement
Competency exam	Must pass a national exam called the Registration Examination for Registered Dietitians	Some programs may have an exam to receive certification
Continuing education	Every 5 years: 75 continuing professional education units must be completed	No requirement
Specialty certifications	Yes; examples include: sports dietetics (CSSD); gerontological nutrition (CSG); pediatric nutrition (CSP); obesity and weight management (CSOWM); and diabetes care and education (CDCES)	Yes; some are available to non-RDs or RD/RDNs
Insurance reimbursement	Certain services are reimbursed by Medicaid, Medicare, and some private insurance plans	Services are not covered by any major insurance

therapy or psychotherapy affect our patients, we should follow up on how community resources affect them.

4. Following up can bring to your attention any barriers to services your patient may experience. Sometimes, patients do not get the needed services and may require assistance with troubleshooting.

Following up on your patients' experience with resources can be as simple as asking how things went during their next visit. It does not need to be too time-consuming. Occasionally, issues arise during the conversation that go beyond your scope as the physician or clinician, presenting a great opportunity to reengage your interprofessional colleagues.

Clinical Pearls

- Clinicians should be aware of and recommend the Dietary Approaches to Stop Hypertension (DASH) diet for adults with elevated blood pressure or hypertension.
- Clinicians with basic nutrition knowledge can contribute to healthy behavioral change by following a simple approach to addressing nutrition: 1) assess, 2) discuss, 3) refer and collaborate, and 4) follow up throughout the treatment course.
- Clinicians should be familiar with recommendations around dietary counseling, including the 5-minute approach, the 2-minute approach, and the 1-minute approach.
- Clinicians providing dietary counseling should discuss with patients how recommendations can be adapted to their own culture or family. Culturally tailored nutrition counseling can improve diet quality.
- Clinicians should be familiar with community resources related to addressing food insecurity, including local food pantries, Food Is Medicine programs, and working with registered dietitians.

Key Chapter Points

- Several medical societies recommend nutrition assessment, dietary counseling, and lifestyle change as key aspects of disease treatment and prevention.
- Dietary counseling to improve nutrition is often a new skill for providers but can be incorporated into patient visits even

within the time constraints of visits primarily for medication management.

- All patients should be screened for food insecurity as a part of the effort to improve their food security, nutritional status, and diet quality.
- Nutritionists, registered dietitians, case managers, social workers, and community health workers are important partners in improving patients' nutrition.
- Follow-up with patients after dietary counseling and referrals to interprofessional colleagues and community organizations is vital in supporting patients' nutrition improvement in the long term.

References

Arjmand G, Abbas-Zadeh M, Eftekhari MH: Effect of MIND diet intervention on cognitive performance and brain structure in healthy obese women: a randomized controlled trial. Sci Rep 12(1):2871, 2022 35190536

Bleich SN, Dupuis R, Seligman HK: Food is medicine movement: key actions inside and outside the government. JAMA Health Forum 4(8):e233149, 2023 37561480

Campbell T: An approach to nutritional counseling for family physicians: focusing on food choice, eating structure, and food volume. J Fam Pract 71(Suppl 1 Lifestyle):eS117–eS123, 2022

Cleveland Clinic: Dietitians vs. Nutritionists: What's the Difference? June 5, 2023. Available at: https://health.clevelandclinic.org/dietitian-vs-nutritionist. Accessed February 19, 2025.

Compton MT, Shim R: The Social Determinants of Mental Health. Washington, DC, American Psychiatric Association Publishing, 2015

ElSayed NA, Aleppo G, Aroda VR, et al: 5. Facilitating positive health behaviors and well-being to improve health outcomes: standards of care in diabetes. Diabetes Care 46(Suppl 1):S68–S96, 2023 36507648

Goldfarb M, De Hert M, Detraux J, et al: Severe mental illness and cardiovascular disease. J Am Coll Cardiol 80(9):918–933, 2022 36007991

Grundy SM, Stone NJ, Bailey AL, et al: 2018 AHA/ACC/AACVPR/AAPA/ABC/ACPM/ADA/AGS/APhA/ASPC/NLA/PCNA Guideline on the management of blood cholesterol: executive summary: a report of the American College of Cardiology/American Heart Association task force on clinical practice guidelines. J Am Coll Cardiol 73(24):3168–3209, 2019 30423391

Hammons AJ, Hannon BA, Teran-Garcia M, et al: Effects of culturally tailored nutrition education on dietary quality of Hispanic mothers:

a randomized control trial. J Nutr Educ Behav 51(10):1168–1176, 2019 31375361
Hjorthøj C, Stürup AE, McGrath JJ, et al: Years of potential life lost and life expectancy in schizophrenia: a systematic review and meta-analysis. Lancet Psychiatry 4(4):295–301, 2017 28237639
Jain S, Feldman R, Althouse AD, et al: A nutrition counseling curriculum to address cardiovascular risk reduction for internal medicine residents. MedEdPORTAL 16:11027, 2020 33204843
Kesari A, Noel JY: Nutritional Assessment, in StatPearls. Treasure Island, FL, StatPearls Publishing, 2024
Lambert AM, Parretti HM, Pearce E, et al: Temporal trends in associations between severe mental illness and risk of cardiovascular disease: a systematic review and meta-analysis. PLoS Med 19(4):e1003960, 2022 35439243
National Association of Social Workers. Standards and Indicators for Cultural Competence in Social Work Practice. NASW, n.d. Available at: https://www.socialworkers.org/Practice/NASW-Practice-Standards-Guidelines/Standards-and-Indicators-for-Cultural-Competence-in-Social-Work-Practice. Accessed February 19, 2025.
Palakshappa D, Goodpasture M, Albertini L, et al: Written versus verbal food insecurity screening in one primary care clinic. Acad Pediatr 20(2):203–207, 2019 31629943
Saha S, Chant D, McGrath J: A systematic review of mortality in schizophrenia: is the differential mortality gap worsening over time? Arch Gen Psychiatry 64(10):1123–1131, 2007 17909124
Tervalon M, Murray-García J: Cultural humility versus cultural competence: a critical distinction in defining physician training outcomes in multicultural education. J Health Care Poor Underserved 9(2):117–125, 1998 10073197
Tsao CW, Aday AW, Almarzooq ZI, et al: Heart disease and stroke statistics—2023 update: a report from the American Heart Association. Circulation 147(8):e93–e621, 2023 36695182
Whelton PK, Carey RM, Aronow WS, et al: 2017 ACC/AHA/AAPA/ABC/ACPM/AGS/APhA/ASH/ASPC/NMA/PCNA Guideline for the prevention, detection, evaluation, and management of high blood pressure in adults: a report of the American College of Cardiology/American Heart Association task force on clinical practice guidelines. Circulation 138(17):e426–e483, 2018 30354655

8

Food Is Medicine

Amy Ehntholt, Sc.D.

Let food be thy medicine and medicine be thy food.

—Hippocrates

Hippocrates, the ancient Greece physician and philosopher, is often cited as the author of the words above. While the attribution is likely apocryphal, the millennia-old recognition of the connection between diet and health is undisputed. Whether or not the father of medicine penned (on his papyrus!) those particular words, surviving texts indicate that Hippocrates was indeed thinking and writing about the influence of food on the human body during the classical era. The idea that diet and health are intertwined is documented in even earlier civilizations (e.g., Egypt, China, and India) where food and nutrition were fundamental features of medical and healing traditions.

Food Is Medicine

Today, "Food Is Medicine" is not just a pithy phrase. Food Is Medicine (FIM)—sometimes referred to as Food As Medicine—is a movement driven by the recognition of the vital importance of nutritious food in achieving and maintaining good health.

Nutrition has not traditionally been a focus of the U.S. health care system, despite evidence of its impact on health outcomes and the associated financial and societal burdens. Access to and delivery of nutritious food, according to the FIM philosophy, is as important to health as prescription drugs and should therefore be incorporated into, or at least coordinated with, health care systems. FIM initiatives aim to do just that: integrate food-based interventions into health care systems, often accompanied by an element of nutrition counseling or education. FIM treats an individual's interactions with the health care system as an opportunity to offer evidence-based interventions to reduce food and nutrition insecurity, improve diet, and manage diverse diet-related illnesses. Although certain components of FIM approaches are not new—as described in this chapter, in the United States it has firm roots in community-based initiatives that include meal delivery at the peak of the HIV/AIDS epidemic, as well as in the early work of a pioneer of social medicine in 1960s Mississippi—FIM has gained great momentum in the past decade. FIM initiatives address both medical conditions and food security—or more accurately, *nutrition security,* which the U.S. Department of Agriculture (USDA) defines as "consistent and equitable access to healthy, safe, affordable foods essential to optimal health and well-being" (U.S. Department of Agriculture 2024). FIM initiatives have the potential not only to improve health and well-being, but also to significantly advance health equity. They could also help reduce the United States's outsized health care costs (e.g., the Rockefeller Foundation estimates that diet-related medical conditions cost the U.S. $1.1 trillion a year in excess health care spending and lost productivity; Rockefeller Foundation 2021).

The modern-day rise of diet-related chronic conditions such as obesity, cardiovascular disease, and type 2 diabetes profoundly demonstrates the powerful role that the food we eat plays in our health and well-being. Less than 7% of U.S. adults have optimal cardiometabolic health (O'Hearn et al. 2022), in part because of unhealthy dietary choices. It is estimated that poor diets directly contribute to more than 300,000 cardiovascular disease deaths (Micha et al. 2017) and 80,000 new cases of cancer in the United States each year (Zhang et al. 2019). Diet-related medical conditions result in more than a million deaths every year, more than those caused by smoking.

It is critical to note that the incidence of these diet-related chronic diseases and the consequent mortality is not evenly distributed across the U.S. population; nor is the prevalence of food insecurity, which is estimated to affect 13.5% of U.S. households (Rabbitt et al. 2024).

Indeed, food insecurity and diet-related medical conditions are closely connected. Healthier food, after all, is more expensive than highly processed, calorie-dense, nutrient-weak food. Those of lower income, with less educational and employment opportunities, and the historically marginalized are more likely to be food-insecure and also to have cardiometabolic disease. These health disparities continue to widen. Among those who suffer disproportionately from diet-related, preventable physical illnesses are individuals with serious mental illness (SMI).

Clinicians treating individuals with SMI are working with a population that, on average, has a far higher prevalence of obesity, hypertension, diabetes, cardiovascular disease, and other diet-related medical conditions. For those with SMI, some of these conditions (e.g., obesity) are brought on or exacerbated by side effects of medications or by the disease itself, as well as by illness-related social and contextual challenges to maintaining an active lifestyle and healthy diet (Muralidharan et al. 2020). These conditions contribute greatly to the lower life expectancy (15–20 years lower than peers; Brown et al. 2010) seen among this population. The syndemic nature of SMI and food insecurity has been understudied, but a recent systematic review suggests that 4 in 10 individuals with SMI experience food insecurity—a prevalence three times that found among peers without SMI (Teasdale et al. 2023). Recent informal research revealed that some individuals with SMI have expressed the desire to extend their stays in psychiatric hospitals solely for "access to hot meals" and that "although it is a sensitive subject, patients would welcome an opportunity to talk to mental health practitioners about food insecurity if this would result in some support to access services" (Smith et al. 2022).

Among mental health clinicians, FIM interventions represent largely overlooked yet promising resources, as research has abundantly demonstrated that improving diet can improve client outcomes (Bleich et al. 2023). Mental health clinicians are uniquely positioned to identify clients who may be most in need and to connect them with FIM programs. Clinicians treating individuals with SMI often see them living with the very diseases—and food and nutrition insecurity—that FIM programs are specifically designed to address. But because of complex barriers (e.g., not going to a primary care physician, the nature of illness symptoms), individuals with SMI are less likely to get involved in FIM programs. And it is not only individuals with SMI that FIM interventions could greatly benefit; these initiatives also hold great potential for those in recovery for substance or alcohol use disorders (Jeynes and Gibson 2017) and for individuals with less severe forms of mental illness.

Core Food Is Medicine Programs and Interventions

The Food Is Medicine movement encompasses a range of programs and policies integrated into the health care system to promote health and reduce disease burden through the provision of nutritious food. FIM programs tend to operate under the direction of a clinician. Funded by health care, government, or philanthropy, they are offered at low or no cost to the client. The FIM framework—and the initiatives falling under its umbrella—can be visualized as adjacent circles of increasing size (Figure 8.1), with interventions and programs for individuals with the greatest need positioned in the smallest circle at the left, and progressively less intensive approaches toward the right in larger circles. Examples of the populations targeted by programs within each of the first three circles—the core FIM programs—are presented in Table 8.1. Those eligible for the programs in the smallest circles are very specific subgroups; the target of the policies and programs falling within the largest circle are far wider (i.e., at the population level). The policies appearing in that largest circle include federal programs such as the Supplemental Nutrition Assistance Program (SNAP), which is discussed in Chapter 9 ("Food- and Nutrition-Related Policies and Programs"). These population-level initiatives have historically been geared more toward addressing *food* insecurity rather than *nutrition* insecurity and are more preventive in nature. FIM services described below typically focus on treatment and management of an existing condition and the nutrition needs connected to that condition.

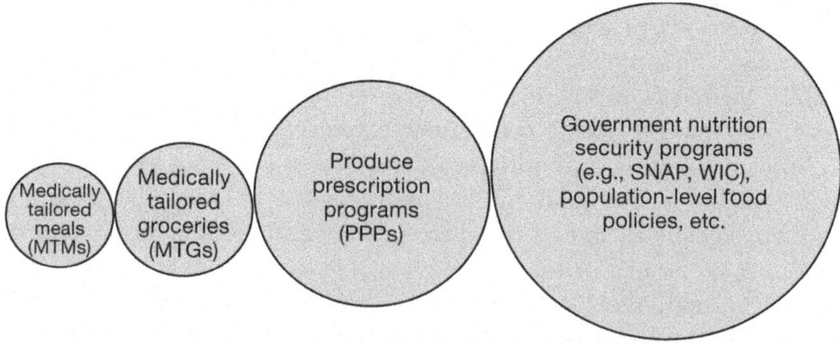

Figure 8.1 **Food Is Medicine programs**

SNAP = Supplemental Nutrition Assistance Program; WIC = Special Supplemental Nutrition Program for Women, Infants, and Children.

Table 8.1 Summary of core Food Is Medicine (FIM) programs

Program	Population served	Intervention	Evidence for effectiveness
Medically tailored meals (MTMs)	Individuals with serious medical conditions that are complex and often nutrition-sensitive, who are limited in their ability to shop and prepare food	Referral from a medical professional or health care plan; meals tailored by a registered dietitian nutritionist, prepared, and delivered to the recipient—generally 10–21 per week, with a nutrition education component	Healthier eating scores, greater food security, improved medication adherence, reduced hospitalizations, cost savings
Medically tailored groceries (MTGs)	Individuals with one or more major diet-related conditions able to make their own meals; prioritization is often given to people of low income or those with food insecurity	Healthy food items are chosen by a registered dietitian nutritionist or other qualified professional and provided to eligible individuals, with a nutrition/culinary education component	Increased food security; mixed evidence (associations) with health outcomes
Produce prescription programs (PPPs)	Individuals of low income or with food insecurity, or with at least one diet-sensitive health condition (e.g., diabetes, hypertension, obesity, heart disease)	Free or subsidized produce (fruits and vegetables; sometimes nuts, seeds, beans, whole grains, dairy, and eggs) given via voucher or electronic benefit transfer card, to be filled at grocery stores, farmers markets, health care settings, or home delivered, with a nutrition/culinary education component	Increased food security, improved blood pressure, lower hemoglobin A1C (among those with type 2 diabetes), and decreased BMI

Source. Adapted from Mozaffarian et al. 2024.
BMI = body mass index.

Medically Tailored Meals

Medically tailored meals (MTMs; sometimes called "therapeutic meals") are home-delivered, fully prepared, ready-to-eat meals, which (as the name suggests) have been designed specifically to meet the nutritional needs of individuals living with certain chronic or complex medical conditions. These programs are appropriate for the most high-needs health care clients, who are often unable to shop and prepare food for themselves and whose medical conditions are complex and nutrition-sensitive. The nonprofit Food Is Medicine Coalition (FIMC; fimcoalition .org)—an organization that convenes MTM providers, establishes best practices, trains nonprofits on how to implement MTMs, and provides technical assistance—emphasizes that MTMs go beyond simply placing a client on a diet and providing food; the complexities of these individuals' lives require a more specialized intervention, as this population often includes individuals who also have pressing social needs. An organization (e.g., Meals on Wheels) can contract with a managed care plan in its county to deliver to health care plan members. Along with provision of the meals themselves, MTM providers often offer some level of nutrition education.

Agencies preparing MTMs are required to use only fresh ingredients, with no added preservatives. They also must pass local food safety standards checks (Sharma and Sharma 2024). Hospitals offering MTMs must have a provider (e.g., physician, social worker, registered dietitian) on hand to coordinate meal delivery by a partnered delivery service. Typically, a health care provider or plan refers an individual to an agency providing MTMs. Intake and eligibility assessment are done by the agency. Eligibility is generally based on the presence of at least one diet-sensitive condition (usually cardiometabolic) and one social need (e.g., food insecurity, homelessness, financial strain). Upon confirmation of eligibility, a registered dietitian nutritionist designs an MTM and care plan based on the nutrition needs for management or treatment of a specific condition. For example, an MTM for an individual living with high blood pressure would limit or avoid sodium and would include foods known to be heart-healthy. Common conditions of recipients of MTMs are diabetes, heart disease, cancer, and HIV/AIDS. Meals are usually home-delivered, although shipment or pick-up by recipients are sometimes available. MTMs typically deliver 10 to 21 meals per week; a reassessment is usually done after 6 months.

MTMs are not a new phenomenon. The concept first emerged in the early days of the HIV/AIDS epidemic in the United States. Long before the virus was well understood or any treatment was available, volunteers at grassroots organizations such as Project Open Hand in San Francisco and God's Love We Deliver in New York City prepared and delivered meals to the sick, the isolated, and the dying in their homes. These interventions soon relied on registered dietitians to design meals tailored to individuals' specific nutrition and medical needs in recognition of the importance of keeping people as healthy as possible for as long as possible. Services were largely covered by the Ryan White CARE Act (U.S. Government Information 1990), which includes "medical nutrition therapy" in its core medical services. In 2023, according to the Food Is Medicine Coalition, more than 15 million MTMs were delivered to nearly 60,000 people in the United States through the coalition's growing network of certified nonprofit organizations serving as MTM providers.

Medically Tailored Groceries

Medically tailored groceries (MTGs, sometimes called "food boxes," "food packages," "food pharmacies," or "food farmacies") are the next-largest circle of FIM programs. MTG interventions are similar to MTMs but provide raw ingredients—rather than fully prepared meals—tailored to an individual's specific diet-related medical condition, whether it be acute or chronic. This approach serves a larger subgroup of individuals than MTM programs, as it is not limited to the smaller subpopulation of those unable to shop for and prepare their own meals. As with MTMs, MTGs are selected by a registered dietitian nutritionist or other qualified nutrition professional based on the recipient's particular medical condition and nutrition needs. MTGs are often given in conjunction with some form of nutrition or culinary education. The groceries made possible by the Special Supplemental Nutrition Program for Women, Infants, and Children (WIC) to pregnant and breastfeeding people, and children up to 5 years of age, are related to MTG programs, although groceries are sourced directly by the WIC recipient and paid for using electronic benefit transfer (EBT). Although MTGs demand more from the recipient than what MTMs require, they tend to be less expensive to implement, and by their very nature they allow more flexibility in meeting individuals' tastes in food and meal preparation, which may vary by culture.

Produce Prescription Programs

The third level of FIM interventions are produce prescription programs (PPP), a service through which eligible individuals are referred by a health care provider or health insurance plan and provided a prescription for fresh, healthy foods (e.g., fruits and vegetables; nuts, seeds, beans, dairy, eggs, and whole grains are sometimes available). The recipient can then redeem the prescription—subsidized at low cost or free—for healthful foods at participating grocery stores, farmers markets, or community food pantries.

Although these programs are seen as innovative, they too are not entirely new. During the United States Civil Rights Era, public health leader and social medicine pioneer Dr. H. Jack Geiger recognized the importance of addressing social factors in medical practice. At his first community health center in the Mississippi delta region in the 1960s, he famously prescribed food to the poor and malnourished. His retort when the governor of the state expressed displeasure at his prescribing food to be reimbursed by the health center's pharmacy was, "Yeah, well, the last time I looked in my medical textbooks, they said the specific therapy for malnutrition was food" (Lubinger 2016). This effort provided a model for similar activities in the 1980s and 1990s, with state health departments and nonprofits assisting families of low income with produce purchased at farmers markets. It became part of nutrition-assistance programs in the 1990s and 2000s and was codified in the 2014 Farm Bill (Food Insecurity Nutrition Incentive [FINI]; later the Gus Schumacher Nutrition Incentive Program [GusNIP]). More recently, PPPs have broadened to include programs such as the one in Flint, Michigan, where a pediatrician offers vouchers for every child seen, to be used in a farmers market housed in the same building as the doctor's office (McKenna 2024). Among FIM initiatives, as described here, PPPs are the most heterogeneous. A review of PPPs in the United States found that most PPPs have a nutrition education component and include a health care visit, and that the most common criterion for eligibility is diabetes, followed by food insecurity or economic risk (Newman et al. 2022).

Government and Private-Sector Involvement

Federal Funding

Evidence of the growing interest in FIM initiatives can be seen in recent increases in federal funding of the USDA's GusNIP, which was expanded to $250 million in 2018, with up to 10% of those funds to support PPPs from 2019 through 2023. GusNIP data from 2023 show that the extent of participation in FIM programs has ballooned, along with the number of FIM sites and providers. The escalating enthusiasm and support for FIM culminated in the 2022 White House Conference on Hunger, Nutrition, and Health and the Biden administration's pledge of $8 billion for funding (public and private) for work in this realm. A major focus of that conference was the integration of nutrition and health; one outcome was the U.S. Department of Health and Human Services (HHS) Food Is Medicine initiative, launched in 2023. Congress has directed funding to HHS, in collaboration with other federal agencies (e.g., Departments of Veterans Affairs [VA], Housing and Urban Development, USDA), to develop a national strategy to address diet-related chronic disease and food insecurity, and to improve health and racial equity. Efforts to widen access to FIM initiatives and increase research also include a toolkit, released online in September 2024 (www.health.gov/foodismedicine), in which a collection of resources are housed to help organizations develop and implement FIM. It presents case studies, state and federal policies supporting FIM initiatives, and information on measurement and research.

State Medicaid Section 1115 Demonstration Waivers

Another big win for the FIM movement came with the integration of FIM programs into Medicaid through Section 1115 of the Social Security Act. Since the 2010s, U.S. State Medicaid Section 1115 demonstration waivers have given states the opportunity to pilot innovative approaches to health care, including for nontraditional services for health-related social needs (HRSNs). This has offered a way for states to have nutrition interventions covered through Medicaid (under federal law, food provision is not allowed to be covered directly by Medicaid outside of the demonstration waivers). Any state Medicaid agency can submit a Section 1115 proposal to the Centers for Medicare and Medicaid Services (CMS), as long as the proposed pilot will further the Medicaid program's objectives and its impact will be "budget neutral." Massachusetts was the first state to receive an FIM-related waiver providing direct food-related intervention in 2016 (extended in 2022) for a broad range of programs including MTMs, MTGs, and PPPs. Other states with early FIM waivers were Oregon and California. In November 2023, CMS published guidance to help states specifically interested in including FIM in their HRSN 1115 demonstration waivers. A survey of states' applications and approvals for Medicaid Section 1115 waivers showed a sharp increase in such waivers since 2021 (Hanson et al. 2024). States newly approved for food-related 1115 demonstrations in more recent years include New Jersey, Washington, New York, New Mexico, Delaware, and Illinois.

In addition to the integration of FIM pilot programs into Medicaid through 1115 demonstration waivers, Medicare Advantage plans may offer nutritional benefits if they choose, although this option has yet to reach many Medicare recipients. The VA and the U.S. Indian Health Service are also experimenting with pilot programs of similar initiatives.

Health Plans/Insurance Companies

Health plans and insurance companies have shown a marked interest in the FIM movement through large investments in recent years. Perhaps the biggest provider to do so is Kaiser Permanente, which in 2022 pledged $50 million to work to incorporate FIM into its model of care, including through the creation of a Food Is Medicine Center of Excellence, launched in April 2024. Kaiser's vision for the center is a clinical, research, and collaborative hub that also offers services in the FIM realm, such as MTMs and PPPs. Kaiser's announcement of the center's launch described ambitions to expand member screening and clinical nutrition training; create novel and scalable approaches for providing evidence-based FIM programs; serve as a research hub; and expand partnerships. One example of many of Kaiser's ongoing partnerships is the provider's work with Instacart, through which Kaiser is examining the impact of offering more options to members of California's Medicaid program, Medi-Cal, using grocery stipends for the purchase of fresh produce and other food via a virtual storefront.

The for-profit Elevance Health (formerly Anthem, Inc.) has also created an FIM program. At the time of writing, Elevance had invested nearly $30 million in programs addressing food insecurity over 3 years. This money is funding programs such as a FIM Coalition pilot to expand access to MTMs and other nutrition services in Colorado and California.

Geisinger Health and other health care systems have also been investing in efforts to study and scale up FIM initiatives such as MTMs and PPPs, while also engaging in efforts to build the technological infrastructure to ensure that clients in need of nutrition services can easily enroll and benefit from them (Mozaffarian et al. 2022).

Public-Private and Other Partnerships

In addition to health plans and insurance companies, companies in the private sector have shown increasing interest in this rapidly evolving area. Partnerships abound, only a small sampling of which are mentioned here.

Three public-private partnerships were first announced by HHS at its inaugural Food Is Medicine Summit in early 2024 (U.S. Department of Health and Human Services 2024). In collaboration with the online grocery delivery and pickup service Instacart, the not-for-profit Rockefeller Foundation, and the 501(c)3 nonprofit organization Feeding America, HHS plans to leverage the technology, the research capabilities, and the nationwide network of food banks, pantries, and community-based organizations each of these entities brings to further the FIM movement. Instacart Health had already been offering to systems including Boston Children's Hospital a suite of technology products through which providers are able to set up FIM programs, including the prescribing of healthy foods. Instacart has also been a partner with health systems and academic institutions in ongoing evaluation of FIM initiatives provided to clients. Instacart's competitor Uber has more recently joined the Food Is Medicine realm and is helping with FIM scale-up. Planned efforts include a partnership between Uber and one of the largest grocery companies in the United States, Albertsons Companies, to enable community-based organizations and health providers to deliver FIM groceries through Uber Health-Uber Eats, allowing payment by clients' benefits, including through their health insurance.

The Rockefeller Foundation, the American Heart Association, and Kroger have committed $250 million to improve the existing evidence base for FIM initiatives. This collaboration first entails funding of 20 randomized, controlled trials, which will then expand to cohort studies of 2,000–5,000 people. Kroger had also begun a pilot launched in 2019 in Ohio in which a doctor could refer individuals with diabetes to a Kroger supermarket to meet with and receive guidance from a Kroger Health registered dietitian, and to fill a written food prescription at the local Kroger.

The Milken Institute recently released a report (Freishtat et al. 2024) on the role that National Association of Chain Drug Stores (NACDS) pharmacists can play in providing FIM services: by identifying clients eligible for FIM interventions, connecting them to the right resources, and providing follow-up on health outcomes of interest. The institute convened stakeholders from private and public sectors—pharmacies, food retailers, government, and others—in Washington, DC, to discuss possible payment pathways, needed technology infrastructure, and workflow.

Effectiveness of Food Is Medicine: A Look at the Evidence

Efforts to assess the efficacy of FIM interventions have increased considerably in recent years. A 2024 systematic review of 72 papers on federal programs offering food assistance in the United States evaluated the different subprograms falling under the FIM umbrella, including MTMs, MTGs, and PPPs (Sharma and Sharma 2024). The reviewers found evidence that FIM programs improve food security and can strengthen individuals' management of their health. They also reported on evidence that some FIM initiatives have improved multiple health outcomes and have, as a consequence, lowered health care costs.

Among FIM programs, MTMs have the strongest evidence base. One randomized cross-over trial of 44 adults with type 2 diabetes and food insecurity providing 12 weeks of MTMs (vs. usual care for controls) found not only improved Healthy Eating Index (HEI) scores among participants receiving MTMs (71.3 vs. 39.9 for controls), but also lower reported food insecurity (42% vs. 62% for controls) (Berkowitz et al. 2019). Another MTM study described in the 2024 review was a 6-month pre- and post-study of 52 adults diagnosed with HIV/AIDS and/or type 2 diabetes and living at income levels ~300% lower than the federal poverty line (Palar et al. 2017). The MTMs contained the full daily energy requirements and met guidelines for a healthy diet. From baseline to 6-month follow-up, prevalence of very low food insecurity fell from 59.6% to 11.5% ($P < 0.0001$); consumption frequency of fats fell, and that of fruits and vegetables increased. Improvements among those with diabetes included a decrease in sugar consumption, depressive symptoms, and binge drinking, as well as an increase in positive measures of diabetes self-management. Among those with HIV/AIDS, high (95%) adherence to retroviral therapy rose from 47% to 70% ($P = 0.046$). A separate assessment running a population-level cohort policy simulation model estimated that, if MTMs were expanded nationally to all those with diet-sensitive medical conditions and activity limitations, roughly 1.6 million hospitalizations could be avoided, and approximately $13.6 billion might be saved every year (Hager et al. 2022).

Studies examining programs providing MTGs and PPPs have also shown a positive association with food security measures, and in some cases an indication of improvements in health outcomes (Sharma and Sharma 2024). For example, results of a 6-month randomized, controlled trial for individuals with type 2 diabetes ($n = 568$) who received food designed to improve glycemic control showed no significant differences between treatment and control in indicators for self-management (depressive symptoms, diabetes distress, self-care, hypoglycemia, self-efficacy) or in hemoglobin A1C, although food security and intake of fruits and vegetables increased (Seligman et al. 2018). A 2022 systematic scoping review reported that individual studies have shown positive associations between PPPs and some health outcomes, for instance, in blood pressure (though results have been mixed); in weight loss (also mixed); and, importantly, in qualitative studies noting participants' perceived improvements in their health (Little et al. 2022). The review concluded, however, that although PPPs are a promising intervention, the evidence on their efficacy for improving food security and fruit and vegetable intake is not completely robust—and for diet-related health outcomes, it is limited and mixed.

That conclusion is similar to that of a 2021 systematic review and meta-analysis of food prescription programs' impact on dietary behavior and cardiometabolic risk factors (Bhat et al. 2021). Although pooled estimates showed decreased BMI and increased fruit and vegetable consumption, the authors stressed that the findings "should be interpreted with caution in light of considerable heterogeneity, methodological limitations of the included studies, and moderate to very low certainty of evidence." And while a 2023 systematic review of PPPs found that 21 of 22 programs suggested improvements in intake of fruits and vegetables, that review's authors also cautioned that overall study quality was weak (Veldheer et al. 2020). Mozaffarian and colleagues (2024) have acknowledged limitations of much of the current assessments of FIM interventions but have pointed to the more rigorous studies now underway, including several randomized trials to test the effectiveness of FIM programs for such varied health outcomes as cancer, diabetes, and high-risk pregnancy.

Future Directions for Food Is Medicine

A necessary next step for the FIM movement is reflected in that common theme running through most of the recent papers reviewing the evidence on FIM's efficacy: more rigorous studies and more data. Existing FIM research has relied heavily on pre/post studies and quasi-experimental designs rather than randomized, controlled trials, and the studies are exceptionally heterogeneous. The consensus of leaders in the FIM field is that the quality of studies must improve—larger sample sizes, longer study periods, inclusion of control groups, and consistent use of validated measures of food security, dietary intake, and other health outcomes—to achieve a successful, scaled-up integration of FIM into health care systems. It is necessary to determine the optimal dose (e.g., how many meals per week, how much nutrition education should be delivered), the right duration, and the ideal target population. One effort at the federal level is the HHS's convening of leaders to develop metrics for measuring success of FIM programs. As Mozaffarian and colleagues (2024) have noted, FIM's success relies on "multiparty partnerships to assess, optimize, and scale these promising treatments to advance health and health equity."

Other obstacles to overcome include "low levels of clinician nutrition knowledge and awareness of interventions, and narrow access to appropriate services and programmes" (Downer et al. 2020). Efforts to improve clinician knowledge of nutrition, as well as practitioners' awareness of existing interventions, must continue to be made, beginning with—but not limited to—nutrition education in medical school. This extends to the education of mental health clinicians on each level of FIM programs. Finally, while FIM holds much promise, equally important is advocating for the well-established population-level food policies and programs with a long-established and very strong evidence base (particularly early-life interventions, e.g., SNAP, WIC, the School Breakfast Program, the National School Lunch Program; to be discussed in the next chapter) (Barnidge et al. 2020; Moran and Roberto 2023).

Clinical Pearls

- Clinicians can familiarize themselves with existing local Food Is Medicine services for food-insecure individuals and for those managing complex health conditions, and work to establish strong links with these organizations.
- Clinicians can screen for food insecurity and other social and clinical needs, taking advantage of their unique position treating individuals who may be most in need, and for whom FIM programs could be particularly appropriate.
- Clinicians can share information and connect clients to FIM programs for which clients may not know they are eligible.

- Clinicians can further educate themselves and their clients about the connection between diet and health, emphasizing the importance of nutrient-dense foods such as fruits, vegetables, legumes, nuts, seeds, whole grains, and lean meats.
- Clinicians can also advocate for challenging and changing the upstream factors (e.g., social and economic policies, food industry behavior) responsible for food insecurity and disparities in health—and not lose sight of the fact that these are, at their core, *social* problems, rather than *medical* problems.

Key Chapter Points

- The Food Is Medicine movement in the United States has deep roots in the past but has gained great momentum in recent years, as evidenced by a number of significant public and private investments and partnerships.
- Food Is Medicine programs target both food insecurity and chronic disease through nutrition-related initiatives such as medically tailored meals, medically tailored groceries, and produce prescription programs—interventions that could be of particular value to individuals with serious mental illness, a population disproportionately affected by the very conditions Food Is Medicine is designed to address.
- Food Is Medicine programs have been shown to improve food security and some dietary outcomes. As the evidence base continues to grow, more rigorous studies will allow for clearer assessment of the impact of Food Is Medicine on other outcomes and should guide future directions for implementation.
- Some individuals with mental illness may be eligible for Food Is Medicine programs (e.g., if it is covered in their state by Medicaid), although they might not be aware of the potential opportunity.
- A good starting point for clinicians and others seeking resources on various Food Is Medicine initiatives—including local services available—is the Food Is Medicine Coalition's website: fimcoalition.org.

References

Barnidge EK, Stenmark SH, DeBor M, et al: The right to food: building upon "Food Is Medicine." Am J Prev Med 59(4):611–614, 2020 32800425

Berkowitz SA, Delahanty LM, Terranova J, et al: Medically tailored meal delivery for diabetes patients with food insecurity: a randomized crossover trial. J Gen Intern Med 34(3):396–404, 2019 30421335

Bhat S, Coyle DH, Trieu K, et al: Healthy food prescription programs and their impact on dietary behavior and cardiometabolic risk factors: a systematic review and meta-analysis. Adv Nutr 12(5):1944–1956, 2021 33999108

Bleich SN, Dupuis R, Seligman HK: Food is medicine movement—key actions inside and outside the government. JAMA Health Forum 4(8):e233149, 2023 37561480

Brown S, Kim M, Mitchell C, et al: Twenty-five year mortality of a community cohort with schizophrenia. Br J Psychiatry 196(2):116–121, 2010 20118455

Downer S, Berkowitz SA, Harlan TS, et al: Food is medicine: actions to integrate food and nutrition into healthcare. BMJ 369:m2482, 2020 32601089

Freishtat H, Roesler AR, Lin-Schweitzer A, et al: Catalyzing action for pharmacist-provided food is medicine care. Milken Institute, June 2024. Available at: https://nppc.health/catalyzing-action-for-pharmacist-provided-food-is-medicine-care/. Accessed December 16, 2024.

Hager K, Cudhea FP, Wong JB, et al: Association of national expansion of insurance coverage of medically tailored meals with estimated hospitalizations and health care expenditures in the US. JAMA Netw Open 5(10):e2236898, 2022 36251292

Hanson E, Albert-Rozenberg D, Garfield KM, et al: The evolution and scope of Medicaid Section 1115 demonstrations to address nutrition: a US survey. Health Aff Sch 2(2):qxae013, 2024 38577164

Jeynes KD, Gibson EL: The importance of nutrition in aiding recovery from substance use disorders: a review. Drug Alcohol Depend 179:229–239, 2017 28806640

Little M, Rosa E, Heasley C, et al: Promoting healthy food access and nutrition in primary care: a systematic scoping review of food prescription programs. Am J Health Promot 36(3):518–536, 2022 34889656

Lubinger B: A Public Health Pioneer. Think Magazine. Spring 2016. Case Western Reserve University. Archived from the original on December 5, 2016. Available at: https://case.edu/think/spring2016/public-health-pioneer.html. Accessed November 27, 2024.

McKenna M: Produce prescriptions sound good, but data to support them are lacking—that could soon change. JAMA 331(17):1433–1436, 2024 38607621

Micha R, Peñalvo JL, Cudhea F, et al: Association between dietary factors and mortality from heart disease, stroke, and type 2 diabetes in the United States. JAMA 317(9):912–924, 2017 28267855

Moran AJ, Roberto CA: A "Food Is Medicine" approach to disease prevention: limitations and alternatives. JAMA 330(23):2243–2244, 2023 38032668

Mozaffarian D, Blanck HM, Garfield KM, et al: A Food Is Medicine approach to achieve nutrition security and improve health. Nat Med 28(11):2238–2240, 2022 36202998

Mozaffarian D, Aspry KE, Garfield K, et al: "Food Is Medicine" strategies for nutrition security and cardiometabolic health equity: JACC State-of-the-Art Review. J Am Coll Cardiol 83(8):843–864, 2024 38383100

Muralidharan A, Brown CH, Zhang Y, et al: Quality of life outcomes of web-based and in-person weight management for adults with serious mental illness. J Behav Med 43(5):865–872, 2020 31741204

Newman T, Lee JS, Thompson JJ, et al: Current landscape of produce prescription programs in the US. J Nutr Educ Behav 54(6):575–581, 2022 35618406

O'Hearn M, Lauren BN, Wong JB, et al: Trends and disparities in cardiometabolic health among U.S. adults, 1999–2018. J Am Coll Cardiol 80(2):138–151, 2022 35798448

Palar K, Napoles T, Hufstedler LL, et al: Comprehensive and medically appropriate food support is associated with improved HIV and diabetes health. J Urban Health 94(1):87–99, 2017 28097614

Rabbitt MP, Reed-Jones M, Hales LJ, et al: Household food security in the United States in 2023 (rep. no. ERR-337). U.S. Department of Agriculture, Economic Research Service, 2024

Rockefeller Foundation: True Cost of Food: Measuring What Matters to Transform the U.S. Food System. Targeted News Service, 2021. Available at: https://www.rockefellerfoundation.org/report/true-cost-of-food-measuring-what-matters-to-transform-the-u-s-food-system/. Accessed January 8, 2025.

Seligman HK, Smith M, Rosenmoss S, et al: Comprehensive diabetes self-management support from food banks: a randomized controlled trial. Am J Public Health 108(9):1227–1234, 2018 30024798

Sharma V, Sharma R: Food Is Medicine initiative for mitigating food insecurity in the United States. J Prev Med Public Health 57(2):96–107, 2024 38487843

Smith J, Ker S, Archer D, et al: Food insecurity and severe mental illness: understanding the hidden problem and how to ask about food access during routine healthcare. BJPsych Adv 29(3):204–212, 2022

Teasdale SB, Müller-Stierlin AS, Ruusunen A, et al: Prevalence of food insecurity in people with major depression, bipolar disorder, and schizophrenia and related psychoses: a systematic review and meta-analysis. Crit Rev Food Sci Nutr 63(20):4485–4502, 2023 34783286

U.S. Department of Agriculture. USDA Delivers on Promise to Expand Access to Nutrition Resources in Underserved Communities by Funding Three New Nutrition Hubs. USDA, 2024. Available at: https://www.usda.gov/about-usda/news/press-releases/2024/12/19/usda-delivers-promise

-expand-access-nutrition-resources-underserved-communities-funding -three-new. Accessed July 15, 2025.

U.S. Department of Health and Human Services: HHS Hosts First-Ever 'Food Is Medicine' Summit, Launches Three Public-Private Partnerships. HHS Press Office, 2024. Available at: https://www.hhs.gov/about/news/2024/02/02/hhs-hosts-first-ever-food-medicine-summit-launches-three-public-private-partnerships.html. Accessed December 10, 2024.

U.S. Government Information: Ryan White CARE Act: Ryan White Comprehensive AIDS Resources Emergency Act (Ryan White CARE Act), Pub. L. No. 101-38, 104 Stat. 576 1990. Available at: https://www.govinfo.gov/content/pkg/STATUTE-104/pdf/STATUTE-104-Pg576.pdf. Accessed January 8, 2025.

Veldheer S, Scartozzi C, Knehans A, et al: A systematic scoping review of how healthcare organizations are facilitating access to fruits and vegetables in their patient populations. J Nutr 150(11):2859–2873, 2020 32856074

Zhang FF, Cudhea F, Shan Z, et al: Preventable cancer burden associated with poor diet in the United States. JNCI Cancer Spectr 3(2):pkz034, 2019 31360907

9

Food- and Nutrition-Related Policies and Programs

Julie C. Suarez, M.A.

Malnourishment is a national concern because we are a nation that cares about its people, how they feel, how they live.... We have an agricultural abundance that ranks as a miracle of the modern world. This Nation cannot long continue to live with its conscience if millions of its own people are unable to get an adequate diet.

—President Richard Nixon,
Remarks at the 1969 White House
Conference on Food, Nutrition, and Health

President Richard Nixon opened the first White House Conference on Food, Nutrition, and Health in 1969 with a focus on the moral imperative of ending hunger for all (Nixon 1969). Using terminology about income inequality, President Nixon cited the negative impacts of poverty on children and families, and called for a significant expansion of federal governmental actions to alleviate want. The President reflected on the experiences of many with hunger during the Great Depression and World War II and portrayed a unity of purpose and a belief in government's role to solve problems that is not always seen in politics today. Genuine hunger today is not as common as it was during the Depression because the United States has a wider array of hunger safety nets in federal policy and emergency feeding programs, although access to those programs may change in 2025–2026. Hunger and food insecurity are still significant problems, however: 13.5% of United States households reported food insecurity in 2023—well after the COVID-19 pandemic (Economic Research Service 2024b). Food insecurity has lifelong affects on childhood development, sets the stage for learning and behavioral problems, and is linked to suicidal ideation in teenage years; it is also highly detrimental to the mental and physical health of adults (Hoefer and Curry 2012).

Federal Nutrition Policy and Programs

The term *food insecurity,* rather than the more one-dimensional term *hunger,* was adopted by the U.S. Department of Agriculture (USDA) in 2006 to holistically assess and measure economic considerations surrounding a household's food availability. Hunger is experienced on an individual, physical basis and can be a direct result of food insecurity. Food security means that an individual has enough access to food to sustain an active, healthy lifestyle. Food security, or the lack of it by household, is now measured by the USDA in annual surveys in four tiers—high food security, marginal food security, low food security, and very low food security (Wunderlich and Norwood 2006). Although changing terminology from *hunger* to *food insecurity* allows clinicians to more accurately measure household status, some academics have credibly argued that dropping the term *hunger* lessens, in the minds of the general public, the very real experience of living with hunger (Himmelgreen and Romero-Daza 2010). To the extent that public views on the perception of *hunger*—versus *food insecurity*—as a serious policy issue affect decision-making of elected officials, this change in terminology may be more significant to funding levels for programs that truly work to end hunger.

Clinicians, particularly those using social determinants of health as a framework in their practice, may wish to pay attention to the unique role of food and nutrition security in determining health outcomes for greater client well-being. In the aftermath of the COVID-19 pandemic, clinicians should also be aware of the significant inequities linked to food and nutrition access and health outcomes. In the United States, Indigenous people died from COVID-19 at a 7.19% greater rate than White people; the Latina and Latino death rate was 3.85% higher and the Black death rate was 2.59% higher than the death rate of White people (Freeman 2022). Many factors affected death rates during the pandemic, but clinicians should be particularly aware that Indigenous, Black, and Latina/Latino and Hispanic populations have a documented higher prevalence of food insecurity rates that may play a greater role in overall client well-being and health (Hales and Coleman-Jensen 2024). This chapter provides clinicians with a broad understanding of U.S. policies and programs designed to alleviate hunger and food insecurity, which may assist in client referrals, when appropriate.

Historical Framing

The historical origins of the nation's first foray into providing nutrition education and guidance to a burgeoning population began in 1894, when the USDA's Wilbur Atwater, an agricultural chemist, first published dietary guidance in the form of food tables recommending consumption levels of nutrients from five key food groups: fruits and vegetables, meats and other proteins, cereals and starchy foods, sweets, and foods that were considered fatty (Jahns et al. 2018). At that time, the federal government's concern was primarily alleviating hunger and malnutrition, while encouraging a balance to ensure good health during a time when food was less widely available and food perishability limited variety.

The nation's first federal policy aimed at alleviating actual hunger, as opposed to providing dietary guidance, through federal food programs occurred in the 1933 Agricultural Adjustment Act also known as the first "Farm Bill" (Compton and Suarez 2023). Faced with the Great Depression and a surfeit of agricultural commodities (e.g., wheat, corn, cotton), Congress adopted the first food relief programs distributing surplus farm goods directly to people in need and piloted school meal programs for children (Himmelgreen and Romero-Daza 2010). During World War II, federal hunger programs waned as attention shifted to feeding soldiers overseas, but the nation's broad social upheavals during the 1960s catalyzed and demanded action—action to solve, once and for all, the serious problem of hunger among the nation's citizens (Woteki et al. 2020).

Although that ambition to solve hunger in the United States has not been realized, federal policies have evolved along three broad program areas: income-based approaches to alleviating hunger, programs addressing childhood hunger and nutrition, and approaches that support family farms while concomitantly improving access to fresh fruits and vegetables. Many of these programs have their origins in or were made permanent because of recommendations of the 1969 White House Conference on Food, Nutrition, and Health.

Organized by Dr. Jean Mayer, a hunger researcher and nutritionist, the first conference was a 3-day affair with more than 5,000 engaged participants. President Nixon's charge to Dr. Mayer was to answer five key questions primarily focused on improving nutritional outcomes through consistent measurement, focus on vulnerable populations, food production and technology, and a Presidential concern about improving nutrition education in the nation's populace. Twenty-six subcommittees framed and reported on more than 1,800 recommendations developed in a consensus-based approach with academics, policymakers, and influential public citizens active in hunger and nutrition. A subsequent nutrition summit 2 years later, led by Dr. Mayer at President Nixon's request, found significant progress on an incredible 1,650 recommendations (Woteki et al. 2020).

The nation's overall nutrition policy framework was influenced significantly by Congressional adoption in 1990 of the National Nutrition Monitoring and Related Research Act (NNMRR). Designed to provide some consistency into how the United States conducts, compiles, and identifies nutritional issues in the population, it is administered jointly by the USDA and the Department of Health and Human Services (HHS) (Moshfegh 1994). In the absence of actual data, it is challenging for policymakers to tweak or design innovative programs or nutrition experts to make recommendations to improve dietary choices. NNMRR helps fill in the data gaps by encouraging collaboration between the 22 different federal entities tasked with food- and nutrition-related activities, including data collection and use of nutrition information. NNMRR created a National Nutrition Monitoring Advisory Council, which serves as a scientific guidance committee. NNMRR also established the requirement that dietary guidelines be published every 5 years to provide citizens and nutrition educators with up-to-date and relevant nutritional information and guidance. It is important to note that the USDA dietary guidelines, discussed later in this chapter, are the basis for nutrition program implementation.

Income-Based Approaches to Alleviating Hunger

Hunger and nutrition program use spiked during the pandemic, and it may be helpful for clinicians to understand the overall participation rates in income-based programs designed to alleviate food insecurity. According to the USDA, 12.6% of U.S. residents received Supplemental Nutrition Assistance Program (SNAP) benefits in 2023. A comparison shows that SNAP participation is higher after the pandemic, but other income-based programs have leveled off to the more usual participation rates (see Figure 9.1).

Originally piloted to ameliorate the twin problems of high hunger levels and a surplus of agricultural commodities during the Great Depression, what we now know as SNAP was signed into law as part of President Johnson's "War on Poverty" in 1964. The Food Stamp Act created a systemic approach to addressing poverty as a root cause of hunger by adopting an income-based threshold. Eligible individuals and households could purchase food stamps with their normal food budget and receive in return enough stamps to provide a nutrition-

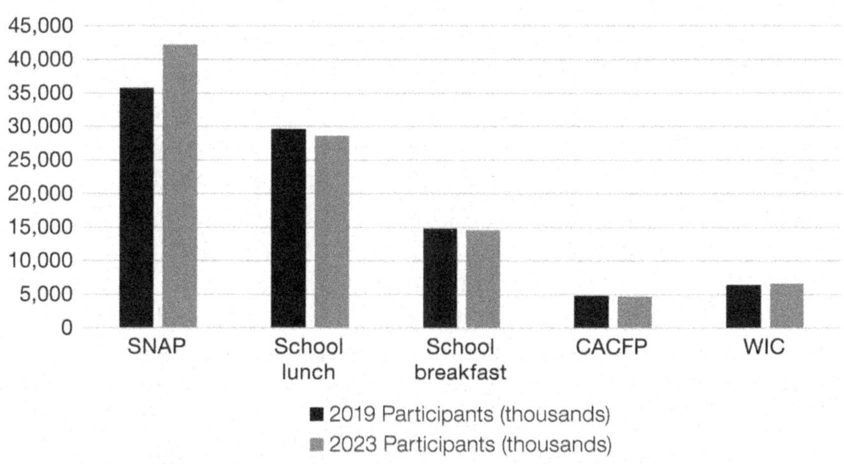

Figure 9.1 Nutrition program participants, 2019–2023

Source. U.S. Department of Agriculture, Food and Nutrition Service, Program Summary Data 2019–2023. Supplemental Nutrition Assistance Program (SNAP), School Lunch Program, School Breakfast Program, Child and Adult Care Feeding Program (CACFP), and Special Supplemental Nutrition Program for Women, Infants, and Children (WIC).

ally adequate diet. The Food Stamp Act of 1964 set the framework for income thresholds in nutrition programs, created a critical role for state administrative and eligibility control, and importantly, prohibited states from discriminating against issuance of benefits on the basis of race or religion (Food and Nutrition Service 2024a).

As one can imagine, the Food Stamp Act was a subject of a considerable number of recommendations for improvement during the 1969 White House Conference, and during the early to mid-1970s, several key changes occurred. Uniform standards of national eligibility were adopted, work requirements were instituted, and the benefit level was set at an amount thought to provide adequate nutrition. Notably, funding for the program was included in subsequent iterations of the 5-year Farm Bills, providing an inextricable policy linking farmers and nutrition advocates for decades to come. In the 2008 Farm Bill, the program was renamed the Food and Nutrition Act, and states were encouraged to reduce stigma in using food stamps by transitioning to the terminology *SNAP benefits* (Food and Nutrition Service 2024b).

Clinicians should know that the general qualification for SNAP is 130% of the poverty level for gross income; eligibility or ease of access varies across the states. Recent data released by the USDA analyzing SNAP participation rates from 2020 to 2022 found that 88% of SNAP-eligible participants were receiving benefits, which was the highest level in 50 years. SNAP participation was highest among populations reporting no to minimal income and lowest among older adults (Alma and Rahimi 2024). Clinicians should also be aware that signing up for SNAP benefits is not necessarily an easy process, and that different states have different rules for access. Clinicians should also be aware that changes adopted by Congress in the One Big Beautiful Bill Act (2025) may restrict eligibility for SNAP in 2028, as work requirements and state cost-share requirements phase in, unless amended by subsequent Congressional action. Research has shown that more restrictive administrative procedures at a state level can discourage participation, and that states with a unified, longer-term Democratic majority political structure have greater participation rates (Newby and Chen 2022).

A survey of SNAP participants on their own perspectives of the program found that a majority would support expansion of the monthly benefits and policies to promote more healthful eating and ease of access (Leung and Wolfson 2019). Forty-four states and U.S. territories have applied for Broad-Based Categorical Eligibility, which ensures that participants do not have to complete a SNAP application and asset test if they qualify for other basic income protection programs such as Temporary Assistance for Needy Families (TANF), a federal relief program that provides block grants to individual states, ensures a certain level of income protection for families with children, and offers work placement assistance and worker retraining. TANF is administered by each state, so clinicians who have clients with families can get information on eligibility criteria by searching their state's TANF-administering agency.

Applicants not automatically qualifying for income-based nutrition support need to file a regular application for SNAP, which often includes an asset or means test that can be challenging for those experiencing stress. Research on SNAP participation rates over the years has found that some participants are troubled by the stigma of being perceived as needing "food stamps," although the switch to an electronic benefits transfer (EBT) similar to a debit card and program renaming to SNAP has alleviated some but not all of that concern (Ivancic and Dooling 2023). Research has also shown real learning costs in how people cycle in and out of SNAP, and that changes to make feeding programs easier to access during times of high economic insecurity (for instance, during the pandemic) were not uniformly understood by participants, nor were they communicated clearly enough to realize the full benefit of ensuring access to food relief. Challenges in understanding changing rules and access barriers are particularly acute for already underserved and marginalized populations, as well as individuals experiencing psychological distress (Barnes and Riel 2022).

Another income-based nutrition assistance program is specifically geared toward providing food assistance to income-eligible Indigenous and tribal community members, primarily in the form of surplus commodities. Surplus commodities are shelf-stable food products—such as canned vegetables and fruit juices, grains, canned meats, and dairy products—purchased by the USDA from authorized food processors to distribute in both domestic and foreign hunger relief programs and emergency disaster relief responses. Known as the Food Distribution Program on Indian Reservations (FDPIR), the program is designed to assist participants living on reservation lands, where SNAP sign-up offices and grocery stores may be in short supply. Under this program, participants directly receive USDA surplus commodities, through an authorized tribal partner or a state agency operating on the reservation land.

Adding to the complexity of programs that are not always readily understood, USDA also operates the Emergency Feeding Assistance Program, which functions as an income-based program that provides USDA commodities directly to states based on unemployment levels and the proportion of people living in poverty. Modeled on a not-for-profit-public sector partnership, states provide the commodities through a network of state-selected food banks, pantries, and community-based hunger relief agencies. Clinicians should be aware that accessing this program is easy for participants, who simply need to show up at a local food bank or pantry, but accessibility barriers exist based on distribution locations, transportation availability, and the types of food provided.

Childhood Hunger and Nutrition Programs

Childhood hunger has weighed heavily on the minds of Americans since the early 1900s, with a variety of ad hoc, temporary, and pilot programs created at the federal and state levels designed to alleviate nutritional deficits. The first solid attempt to systematically address childhood hunger was the 1946 adoption of the National School Lunch Program, followed by the School Breakfast Program (authorized in 1966 as the Child Nutrition Act), which also continued the National School Lunch Program. After the 1969 White House Conference on Food, Nutrition, and Health, Congress made these two programs permanent and adopted the Summer Food Service Assistance program to meet childhood hunger needs during the summer (Hopkins and Gunther 2015). Policymakers and nutritionists have long been concerned about the nutritional standards of these popular childhood programs, which are governed nationally but implemented locally. Over the years, standards have changed from a simple requirement of serving food to children in three broad categories toward assuring that children's meals for both breakfast and lunch follow the USDA Dietary Guidelines for Americans.

Increasing concern over childhood nutrition and rising levels of childhood obesity in the 2000s led to the adoption of the Healthy, Hunger-Free Kids Act of 2010. Initially, childhood feeding programs were far more concerned with addressing overall caloric needs for children who were unable to receive enough food at home for healthy development (Hirschman and Chriqui 2013). Over time, the scientific community has debated whether childhood food programs were contributing to the rise in childhood obesity, with high-refined-carbohydrate meals and less of an emphasis on fresh fruits and vegetables. The Healthy, Hunger-Free Kids Act led to the exclusion of candy, full-calorie sodas, and certain high-sugar snacks being sold in vending machines in schools while improving the quality of school meals by imposing new restrictions on trans fats and sodium, adding whole-grain requirements, and serving more fruits and vegetables (Hopkins and Gunther 2015).

The Child and Adult Care Feeding Program began as a pilot program prior to the 1969 White House Conference, when Congress recognized that children in day care programs (both at-home and center-based) facing food insecurity needed access to healthy foods. Making this program permanent was one of the plethora of recommendations from the 1969 White House Conference, and that was achieved in 1975. The addition of nutrition support for older adults came about in 1985, making the Child and Adult Care Feeding Program a key provider of healthy meals for society's most vulnerable youth and senior citizens. Although this is a federal program, states serve as administrators and provide reimbursement to eligible care providers for meals. Program eligibility is on an areawide basis, using both census data and school data, with qualifying programs being those that are located in areas where school populations have 50% or more of students eligible for free or reduced-cost meals (Chriqui and Asada 2023).

The Special Supplemental Nutrition Program for Women, Infants, and Children (WIC) is focused on pregnant and postpartum women and children up to 5 years of age. Designed to ensure nutritional outcomes specific to these groups, WIC provides benefits to eligible participants—like SNAP, through EBT cards. Participants can receive both WIC and SNAP benefits simultaneously. WIC packages are designed for the stage of pregnancy or child development of the program participant and include products such as infant formula as well as food types meeting specific protein and nutrient needs like peanut butter and canned tuna. Eligibility is set at 185% of the federal poverty level, and sign-up is at the state level (Hoynes and Schanzenbach 2015).

WIC participants also receive an added benefit of having in-person meetings with WIC program staff. This personal touch makes the WIC program more accessible to participants and reduces barriers to understanding program usage (Barnes et al. 2023).

Farmer-Friendly Programs Incentivizing Fresh Fruits and Vegetables

Added into the 1973 Farm Bill, the Nutrition Title provides mandatory funding in the approximately every 5-year authorization process for the next Farm Bill, which ensures that the annual agricultural appropriations process will include funding for critical programs to alleviate hunger. In the most recent Farm Bill, nutrition programs accounted for slightly more than 75% of the total monies projected to be expended in the 2018 Farm Bill (Economic Research Service 2018). This inclusion in the Farm Bill has meant that farmers and their trade associations have a vested interest in supporting the Nutrition Title, while nutrition and antihunger advocates have a similar vested interest in supporting the Commodities and Risk Management Titles of the Farm Bill, which are important to farmers. The 2018 Farm Bill has been extended in a variety of congressional supplemental appropriations authorization bills; a new 5-year Farm Bill has not been successfully passed and signed into law despite being well over 2 years late.

This alliance between farming advocates and nutrition and antihunger advocates has led to an increasing number of connected programs seeking to incentivize access to local and regional fresh fruits and vegetables for low-income, food-insecure consumers. These reciprocal benefit programs have their genesis in the 2008 Farm Bill, with the first Food Insecurity Nutrition Incentive Program (FINI). FINI piloted community-based grants designed to increase access of SNAP participants to local or regionally sourced fresh fruits and vegetables. Providing a $0.30 incentive to "match," SNAP participants purchasing at farmers markets were able to find fresher products and stretch the food dollar further. In the 2014 Farm Bill, the program was renamed the Gus Schumacher Nutrition Incentive Program (GusNIP), and the 2018 Farm Bill expanded program funding to $56 million annually (National Institute of Food and Agriculture 2024).

Benefiting both local farmers and low-income consumers, GusNIP grants have led to exciting program innovations. Double Up Food Bucks, administered by a national not-for-profit, Fair Field Network, began in Michigan and has now expanded to 25 states. The Program doubles SNAP benefits when they are redeemed at participating farmers markets and used for fresh fruit and vegetable purchases. Farmers have the incentive to support the program because their bottom line is enhanced by the additional revenue and market participation. Individual states have also used GusNIP grants to realize added incentives for specific communities impacted by food insecurity, such as seniors, to increase purchases of fruits and vegetables from farmers markets. Additional program innovations funded through GusNIP include the establishment of Farm-to-School programs, which remove barriers to local farmers providing local foods to local schools, either through technical assistance to farmers or school food authorities or added funds to incentivize local food purchases.

States, municipalities, not-for-profits like the Fair Field Network, and smaller, community-based organizations can apply for GusNIP grants, but researchers and nutrition advocates have pointed out that equity issues exist. Double Up Food Bucks aims to expand its reach to farmers markets located in underserved areas with limited food access, but it is not a national program. Participation is of course limited by the SNAP participant's access to a farmers market in the first place, as well as knowledge of program availability. Equity issues are acutely faced by smaller-scale, lower-resourced community organizations that may not have the best grant-writing capabilities, leading to a continual outcry from justice-based organizations for the need for more investments and equity in GusNIP program funding (John et al. 2023).

Nutrition Education Programs

Interest in educating Americans on good dietary choices began in the late 1800s with USDA scientists publishing a variety of guidance materials and suggested nutrition requirements for healthy living. Formalization in policy of nutrition education, however, did not begin until 1969, with the permanent establishment of the Expanded Food and Nutrition Education Program (EFNEP). The nation's core nutrition education programs are EFNEP, SNAP-Ed, and WIC. Clinicians should be familiar with how to refer clients to the respective programs (see Table 9.1), when applicable.

Signed into law by President Nixon, EFNEP builds on the longstanding expertise of land-grant universities and is delivered by the Cooperative Extension System administered by the USDA National Institute of Food and Agriculture. Each state has a land-grant university or college, designated to receive funds from the 1862 or 1860 Morrill Acts of Congress or the 1994 Equity in Educational Land-Grant Status Act to provide education and technical training in the areas of agriculture, mechanical arts, military sciences, and classical studies. Cooperative extension systems are administered by each state's land-grant university through the 1914 Smith-Lever Act to transfer knowledge and practical instruction from the land-grant university to local communities. Serving all 50 states and U.S. territories, EFNEP is the longest-serving nutrition education guidance program and focuses on reaching underserved communities: 80% of households receiving EFNEP services are below the poverty line, and 70% are underrepresented minorities, making EFNEP a key delivery vehicle for addressing equity issues in nutrition education (National Institute of Food and

Table 9.1 Major differences between nutrition education programs, and how to find state providers

Program	Description	URL
Expanded Food and Nutrition Education Program (EFNEP)	Administered through land-grant universities; individualized nutrition education focused on reaching underserved participants	https://www.nifa.usda.gov/grants/programs/capacity-grants/expanded-food-nutrition-education-program-efnep
Supplemental Nutrition Assistance Program – Education (SNAP-Ed)	Administered by states, by a variety of providers; accessible to all who qualify for SNAP	https://snaped.fns.usda.gov/state-snap-ed-programs
Special Supplemental Nutrition Program for Women, Infants and Children (WIC)	Administered by states, focused on children's and women's nutritional needs; accessible to all who qualify for WIC	https://www.fns.usda.gov/wic/program-contacts

Agriculture 2023a). EFNEP is unique in that it relies on a paraprofessional model, combining the workforce skills, upward mobility, and cultural relevance of peer educators. Program evaluation is a constant emphasis of EFNEP and helps ensure success. For instance, 90% of adult participants reported improvement in their nutrition after program participation (National Institute of Food and Agriculture 2023b). Although EFNEP is a core element of the nation's nutrition education programs, clinicians should be advised that funding levels from Congress have remained relatively stagnant over the past 20 years, and accessibility varies among states and frequently depends on a potential participant's location.

SNAP-Ed, while not the oldest nutrition education program, serves the largest number, with 1.8 million participants in 2022 (Keller et al. 2024). SNAP-Ed is available not just to SNAP-eligible participants and can be an important referral program for clinicians concerned about client nutrition and well-being. Anyone living at less than 185% of the federal poverty level or residing in a geographic area with half of the population living at less than 185% of the federal poverty level qualifies for SNAP-Ed programming. SNAP-Ed focuses on improving nutrition, reducing obesity and chronic diseases, and encouraging physical activity. Designed to take a holistic approach, SNAP-Ed participants can learn about meal planning and budgeting, as well as healthy culinary preparation skills. Recognizing that chronic diseases from obesity and poor nutrition have a disproportionate impact on food-insecure individuals, a major SNAP-Ed focus is incorporating USDA Dietary Guidelines to reduce obesity. SNAP-Ed over the past decade has emphasized inclusiveness, with bilingual education strategies and curriculum that features culturally relevant foods for different audiences. SNAP-Ed is known for adopting a Policy, Systems, and Environmental Change (PSE) approach and supports a wide array of activities from social marketing campaigns, policy changes to support healthy food procurement in institutional settings, community garden participation and activity, and the more standard nutrition education curriculum. SNAP-Ed relies on an evaluative framework, with each state's providers reporting to USDA on an annual basis. Most statewide evaluations have concluded that SNAP-Ed helps program participants address poor dietary patterns and become less food insecure over time (Keller et al. 2024). SNAP-Ed federal funding was eliminated in the One Big Beautiful Bill Act (2025) adopted by Congress and signed into law by President Trump. Clinicians seeking to refer patients should check availability with their state health or nutrition department after 2026, as some states may continue the educational services at their discretion.

The WIC program provides nutrition education specifically for pregnant and postpartum women (WIC serves these women, infants, and children up to 5 years of age). Unlike other nutrition education programs, participants are encouraged to attend nutrition education sessions through regular, in-person connections with WIC case managers, generally state agency employees. WIC participants also receive counseling on drug use prevention and access to immunizations and other preventive care. The federal government provides training materials for WIC providers, with a variety of curriculum materials focused on the special needs of women and children, also with an emphasis on breastfeeding resources. An interesting point about WIC is the program design, whereby benefit recipients have regular check-ins with an actual person and develop a longer-term relationship, which can help reduce stigma and frustration with bureaucracy and is viewed more positively by program participants than other, more bureaucratic, nutrition programs (Barnes et al. 2023).

Dietary Guidelines for Americans

All federally funded nutrition programs have at their heart a reliance on the Dietary Guidelines for Americans, which make use of the latest nutrition science to encourage healthy eating, advance well-being, and reduce the incidence of diet-related obesity and chronic diseases. Although the first dietary advice was provided to Americans in the early 1900s, formal guidelines were not adopted until 1980, resulting from a partnership between the USDA and what is now HHS. The focus of the first 1980 Dietary Guidelines for Americans (DGAs) was a rather simple listing of seven principles, created by scientists from both agencies (see Table 9.2). The principles encouraged Americans to eat a variety of foods, maintain an "ideal weight," and avoid overconsumption of sugars, sodium, and fats while moderating alcohol consumption (Rowe 2014).

Controversy quickly erupted from the DGAs issuance, and changes were adopted in the NNMRR Act of 1990 to require the release of new guidelines reflecting the latest nutrition science every 5 years (Jahns et al. 2018). Notably, public input is now provided in the form of nominations to what is called the Dietary Guidelines Advisory Committee (DGAC) and is solicited during a public-input process upon release of new draft guidelines. The DGAC relies heavily on peer-reviewed nutri-

Table 9.2 First iteration of the 1980 Dietary Guidelines for Americans

7 Key Principles for Nutrition and Health	Summary of Major Recommendations
1 Eat a variety of foods	Fruits, vegetables, whole grains, cereals, milk, cheese, yogurt, meats, poultry, fish, eggs, and legumes recommended without specific portion sizes
2 Maintain ideal weight	Increase physical activity, maintain an "acceptable weight," don't have seconds, and eat slowly
3 Avoid too much fat, saturated fat, and cholesterol	Protect heart health by avoiding saturated fats, which is especially important for smokers
4 Eat foods with adequate starch and fiber	Increase consumption of complex carbohydrates, and ensure fiber is part of the diet
5 Avoid too much sugar	Learn to read ingredient labels, and eat sugar less frequently to avoid tooth decay
6 Avoid too much sodium	Avoid "hidden" sodium and reduce table salt for reducing dangers of high blood pressure
7 If you drink alcohol, do so in moderation	Heavy alcohol consumption causes ingestion of too many calories and may create nutrient deficiencies; consume in moderation and avoid in pregnancy

tion science compiled and tracked by the USDA Nutrition Evidence Library and provides input and recommendations on the DGAs to the USDA and HHS.

The federal agencies finalize the DGAs and create marketing and communications graphics to help explain the DGAs to the public, as well as to nutrition educators and federally funded food and nutrition providers. With the release of the 1990 version, framing of the DGAs changed from an "avoidance" statement to a more positive "choose" healthier options. Over time, the DGAs have evolved to become more specific in their recommendations for certain dietary intakes as science has changed; for instance, recommending additional consumption of vitamin D and now emphasizing the importance of physical activity, as well as providing specific nutritional advice to pregnant and breastfeeding women (Jahns et al. 2018).

The guidelines are compiled using a variety of evidence-based approaches, focusing on the latest nutrition science while also being cognizant of the need for public input and buy-in. Over time, the DGAs have switched from the 1992 Food Pyramid graphic, which showed categories of foods in a hierarchical fashion, to the more modern My Plate tool deployed in 2011. The purpose of the visuals and associated educational material is, of course, to focus Americans' attention on making healthier choices across their diet.

The DGAs are the building block of all federal nutrition policy, but they are not the only nutrition frameworks designed to encourage healthier eating habits. The American College of Lifestyle Medicine (https://lifestylemedicine.org/), for example, is a professional society of medical professionals dedicated to addressing chronic diseases through six core pillars: nutrition, physical activity, stress management, restorative sleep, social connection, and avoidance of risky substances. As such, the college emphasizes an evidence-based nutritional framework that stresses whole foods, primarily plant-based eating, that emphasizes vegetables, fruits, legumes, seeds, nuts, and fiber—nutrient-dense and antioxidant-rich foods (Frates et al. 2020). Another nutritional framework is the commonly titled EAT-Lancet Commission Report, a science-based framework synergizing planetary health goals and a sustainable approach to food systems with healthy eating (see Chapter 15, "Food Production and Mental Health"). Notably, EAT-Lancet also recommends a diet with fewer meat and dairy products, and with more emphasis on consuming fruits, vegetables, whole grains, and plant-based proteins at the center of each meal (Willett et al. 2019).

State and Local Policy Frameworks and Emergency Food Assistance Programs

Although the bulk of the nation's provision of food assistance is funded at the federal level, there is a role for state and local governments, as well as the not-for-profit sector, in addressing hunger—beyond simply implementing federal programs such as SNAP and WIC. As recent federal restrictions and funding decreases in the nation's nutrition programs come into play, state, local, and philanthropic endeavors will be increasingly critical in addressing food insecurity. Community engagement can be found in a variety of food policy councils, which frequently seek to encourage local and state collaboration. Forming food hubs can be particularly helpful for access to local, healthier, fresh food products to improve nutrition. Emergency or charitable food assistance is frequently provided in communities across the nation. Especially during and after the COVID-19 pandemic, states created several innovative programs designed to alleviate hunger, often linking with the local farm community.

Food Policy Councils

Designed to promote collaboration and coordination, and seeking policy action to address food insecurity and hunger needs, food policy councils can play a key role in leveraging networks. The Johns Hopkins Center for a Livable Future has the most comprehensive listing of food policy councils, and tracks 300 local and statewide councils (Irish et al. 2024). Food policy councils are formally or informally organized networks of community activists, not-for-profit organizations, and academic institutions; they frequently have representation from local or state agencies engaged in food issues or antipoverty efforts. Farmers and farmer associations tend to be engaged in food policy councils, which can result in helpful local organizing activities such as establishing farmers markets in food deserts or forming USDA grant-funded collaborations (like the Double Up Food Bucks program). Frequently, food policy councils serve as informal clearinghouses of information, make policy recommendations for increased services to alleviate food insecurity, and bring forth new ways to innovate in nutritional approaches. During the pandemic, relationships that had formed within these networks proved useful as new food delivery methods were created to address spiking rates of food insecurity and oversupply issues faced by local farmers (Palmer et al., 2020).

Food Hubs

A *food hub* is informally defined by USDA as "a business or organization that actively manages the aggregation, distribution and marketing of source-identified food products, primarily from local and regional producers to strengthen their ability to satisfy wholesale, retail, and institutional demand" (Matson et al. 2013). Food hubs have arguably existed in the agricultural community for decades as farmer-owned and -operated cooperative business structures. Over the past two decades, however, the growth of the local foods movement has encouraged more small-scale farmers to work together. USDA's 2020 local foods survey found that more than 140,000 farmers nationwide sold just over $9 billion in sales direct to consumers through local sales channels, with the top five states for local sales being California, Pennsylvania, New York, Michigan, and Maine (National Agricultural Statistics Service 2022). In addition to farmers markets, farm stands, and community-supported agriculture (CSA) farm shares, some percentage of these local sales are facilitated through food hubs, serving as aggregators. Food hubs can be privately owned, for-profit businesses; not-for-profits designed to aggregate and sell into underserved areas to improve food access; or groups of farmers organized into a cooperative to find efficiencies in processing, marketing, transportation, and logistics of the sale of food. Clinicians should be aware that these structures can be used to improve food access in underserved areas, and that a wide array of federal grant funding is available for business planning, capital improvements, and microloans to encourage small-scale, locally-oriented farm businesses that are primarily producing fresh fruits and vegetables, local meats, and dairy products.

Emergency or Charitable Food Assistance Programs

Charitable food assistance, also referred to as emergency food assistance, can be found in a wide array of communities throughout the United States. Food pantries are generally embedded within communities and run by local nonprofits, including churches and local charities.

Food banks are regional networks set up to "bank" or warehouse food provided through a variety of federal USDA programs (such as the Emergency Food Assistance Program) as well as corporate and local food donations that are then distributed to participating food pantries in a networked fashion. Feeding America, a not-for-profit national network of charitable food assistance organizations, estimated that in 2022, more than 49 million Americans (one of every six) received some form of emergency food assistance (Feeding America 2023). Although charitable food assistance can provide a much-needed supplement to addressing gaps in meals, a justifiable critique cites inconsistencies in availability and accessibility in all communities, and that food assistance provided particularly from corporate donations is not always the most nutritious (as it is often shelf-stable canned and boxed food products). Legitimate policy debates occur as to whether adopting more robust federal and state income-based assistance programs for food purchases—as called for by President Nixon in his opening of the 1969 White House Conference on Food, Nutrition, and Health—might be a better use of the nation's resources and also eliminate dependence on more ad hoc and local charitable feeding assistance (Fisher 2017).

Innovative State Food Insecurity Programs

High rates of food insecurity caused by the COVID-19 pandemic, coupled with the availability of federal dollars through various rounds of federal stimulus packages, enabled a level of innovation in meeting food insecurity needs not seen before or since. New York State paired the dual need to alleviate spiking levels of food insecurity with dire on-farm economic distress faced by farmers, allocating $25 million to food banks for the immediate purchase of surplus fresh fruits, vegetables, and dairy products from local New York producers. Providing a needed lifeline to small-scale farmers and larger dairy cooperatives, the program still exists and has provided more than $147 million, according to the New York State Department of Agriculture and Markets, from a mix of state and federal funds in local food assistance distributed through the charitable feeding assistance networks in New York. The state of Wisconsin, as reported by their Department of Agriculture, took a slightly different approach, preferring to invest more of their stimulus dollars ($50 million) in direct payments to farmers and $65 million to food banks, with $18 million in COVID-19 federal assistance required to be used for local Wisconsin farm products. Like that in New York, this program has lived on after the pandemic, albeit at a much smaller scale, with USDA funding of more than $2 million to establish the Wisconsin Local Food Purchase Assistance Program in 2022. California's Great Plates Delivered program put restaurant and catering facility employees back to work using more than $557 million in Federal Emergency Management Agency pandemic relief funds to provide three meals a day to income-eligible, home-bound, at-risk seniors. Although the program did not outlast the pandemic, it was a lifeline to more than 55,000 seniors, providing more than 22 million meals, although it experienced significant administrative and outreach challenges (Shabazz 2021).

Food Politics

There is no doubt that food is political. Many people have an emotional connection to food, and it is one of the commonalities of everyday life: to sustain ourselves, we must in fact feed our bodies, hopefully with nutritious foods that meet and do not exceed our personal dietary requirements. Reams of work delve into the fraught politics of food—including how food is produced on-farm, manufactured, and distributed—but there are two important points for clinicians to be aware of. First, clients' attitudes toward food policies are not perhaps as polarized as one might assume given the broader context of the divided society in the United States. Second, food is also a business. As such, the corporate sector does in fact seek to broadly influence governmental policies surrounding dietary guidelines, nutrition education, and programs delivering food assistance.

Political Polarization of Food Policy

Political polarization can influence people's reactions to all kinds of wise advice, from policy choices to the time-honored admonition to eat one's vegetables. When it comes to food, recent work has demonstrated that public attitudes—even when viewed through a partisan lens—are becoming more cohesive and less divided over time. Exploring differences in attitudes toward more or less government intervention in food policy between Republicans and Democrats using Pew Survey Research data from 2011 and 2018, economists found greater convergence in political attitudes than expected. Food politics (or people's attitudes in favor of more interventionist government policies in the area of food safety, food quality, and health; support for organic and local food; and food affordability) are becoming less polarized, even in an era of increasing political divisions (Biedny et al. 2020). Why is this point important? Clinicians should take heart that nutrition and food policies may become less contentious over time, despite an often-fraught partisan environment and divisions in elected leaders in Congress over the efficacy and need for emergency feeding assistance programs. A convergence in the electorate about the importance of food affordability and the need for government intervention will, in a democratic society, eventually swing the policy pendulum to ensure greater access to healthy food and income-based nutrition assistance. Federal enactment of the One Big Beautiful Bill Act (2025), which decreases SNAP benefits and other local food-purchase nutrition programs, may perhaps force additional convergence in political attitudes across the partisan divide as the impacts are felt in communities across the nation.

Corporate Influences on Food Policy

Food is necessary for life, but it is also important to recognize that it is a business. The business of growing, processing, distributing, transporting, and marketing food is approximately 5.6% of the U.S. gross domestic product, and according to USDA, is a more than $1.5 trillion dollar industry (Economic Research Service 2024a). Noted nutrition scholars such as Marion Nestle at New York University have extensively chronicled corporate sector lobbying and engagement within food policy decision-making in the halls of Congress and in regulatory agencies, from lobbying to change dietary guidelines to funding academic nutrition research. Notably, "food fights" and high-intensity lobbying campaigns over wording around DGAs have resulted in less prescriptive federal recommendations on limiting consumption of saturated fats, sodium, added sugars, and avoiding overconsumption of meat and high-fat dairy products (Nestle 2007). In a specific example, farm and corporate sector lobbyists teamed up to express consternation around the initial incorporation of environmental sustainability principles in the 2015 DGAs, and as a result, sustainability and planetary health goals were dropped from the finalized DGAs. Corporate sector engagement does not mean clinicians should consider official recommendations to be questionable or corrupt, but it does require that clinicians recognize and understand the influence of global food corporations on the DGAs, food availability, food nutrition and quality, and marketing choices.

Conclusions and Future Research Directions

After more than 50 years, President Biden convened a second White House Conference on Hunger, Nutrition, and Health in 2022 (Biden Harris Administration 2022a). Reflecting the passage of time, the bold goal of the second conference was, again, to end hunger, but also to increase physical activity and healthy eating so that the incidence of chronic disease can be reduced. It is too soon to analyze the long-term impact of the second conference, but the differences in policy recommendations over time are immediately apparent. President Biden's opening remarks and follow-up announcements reflected a focus on private-public-philanthropic sector partnerships and more than $8 billion in commitments by a wide array of partners to act to "end hunger" by 2030 (Biden Harris Administration 2022b). Whereas political beliefs between "regular" citizens over the role of government relating to food policies have converged over time, the belief in government as the primary solution to a problem has clearly waned, given fractures in Congress and an inability to move significant pieces of legislation that would more effectively implement additional income-based approaches to tackling hunger in society today. The political appetite for large-scale, bolder programs to "end hunger"—begun during the Great Depression, carried through World War II and the Johnson Administration's War on Poverty, and honed during the 1969 White House Conference—clearly no longer is the same. Indeed, at the time of this writing, the formerly typical 5-year Farm Bill reauthorization process (critical for both nutrition programs and farm subsidy funding) has been stalled for two years, and actions taken outside of the Farm Bill process in the One Big Beautiful Bill Act (2025) will have significant impacts on the availability of nutrition programs for the nation's hungriest citizens.

Future research into the effectiveness of existing nutrition policies in ending hunger and alleviating food insecurity is warranted. To ensure better public policy, longitudinal studies are needed on the effectiveness of program interventions such as SNAP, WIC, and school meals programs to alleviate food insecurity and increase healthier eating choices to reduce chronic disease (Picciano et al. 2003). Research into the influence of global food corporations as well as nutrition advocates dependent on a plethora of emergency or charitable feeding organizations on policymakers' actions would be helpful. Additional assessments of the general public's appetite for bold, income-based approaches toward ending hunger and creating more equitable food and nutrition security could be relevant to future policymaking endeavors.

Clinical Pearls

- Clinicians should have a basic understanding of the nation's food assistance programs—such as SNAP, WIC, and school meals programs—to make appropriate referrals and should be particularly aware of ongoing inequities in food security.
- The largest nutrition assistance program for adults and families in the United States is SNAP. Clinicians can review state participation requirements and find referral information here: https://www.fns.usda.gov/snap/broad-based-categorical-eligibility.
- SNAP-Ed is federally funded and administered by SNAP state and local implementing agencies until 2026. States conduct needs assessments to ensure that SNAP-Ed is delivered in a hands-on and tailored way for local communities, so SNAP-Ed looks different in every state. Clinicians can view nutrition education resources from SNAP-Ed in multiple languages on the USDA website: https://snaped.fns.usda.gov/resources/nutrition-education-materials.
- Double Up Food Bucks is a nutrition incentive program that matches SNAP EBT purchases of fruits and vegetables dollar for dollar, up to a certain amount per day. Double Up Food Bucks operates in 25 states; referral locations are available here: https://doubleupamerica.org.
- Emergency food assistance can be difficult to find. Clinicians can refer to Feeding America for a nearly complete listing of regional and statewide food banks that link to community-based networks and food pantries: https://regionalfoodbank.net/find-nearest-agency/.

Key Chapter Points

- The evidence-based USDA Dietary Guidelines for Americans form the bulwark of the nation's nutritional science advice but are not absent of political and corporate influence.
- The general qualification for SNAP is 130% of the poverty level for gross income, but eligibility or ease of access varies across the states.

- Charitable food assistance, or emergency food assistance, can be found in a wide array of communities throughout the United States. Food pantries are generally embedded within communities and run by local nonprofits including churches and local charities, whereas food banks are regional networks set up to "bank" or warehouse food that is then supplied to food pantries.
- The local foods movement has helped to stretch the federal food programs' dollars further through purchase incentives (e.g., using SNAP benefits at farmers markets).
- Clinicians and other individuals seeking to become more engaged in food policy and alleviating hunger can seek service opportunities on food policy councils or engage in local not-for-profit charitable feeding organizations.

References

Alma V, Rahimi N: Trends in USDA SNAP Participation Rates: FY 2020 and FY 2022. United States Department of Agriculture, Food and Nutrition Service, 2024. Available at: https://www.fns.usda.gov/research/snap/trends-fy20and22. Accessed November 26, 2024.

Barnes C, Michener J, Rains E: "It's like night and day": how bureaucratic encounters vary across WIC, SNAP, and Medicaid. Soc Serv Rev 97(1):3–42, 2023

Barnes C, Riel V: 'I don't know nothing about that': how "learning costs" undermine COVID-related efforts to make SNAP and WIC more accessible. Adm Soc 54(10):1902–1930, 2022

Biden Harris Administration: National Strategy on Hunger, Nutrition and Health. White House Domestic Policy Council, 2022a, pp. 1–44. Available at: https://bidenwhitehouse.archives.gov/wp-content/uploads/2022/09/White-House-National-Strategy-on-Hunger-Nutrition-and-Health-FINAL.pdf. Accessed November 26, 2024.

Biden Harris Administration: FACT SHEET: The Biden-Harris Administration Announces More Than $8 Billion in New Commitments as Part of Call to Action for White House Conference on Hunger, Nutrition and Health. September 28, 2022b. Available at: https://bidenwhitehouse.archives.gov/briefing-room/statements-releases/2022/09/28/fact-sheet-the-biden-harris-administration-announces-more-than-8-billion-in-new-commitments-as-part-of-call-to-action-for-white-house-conference-on-hunger-nutrition-and-health/. Accessed November 26, 2024.

Biedny C, Malone T, Lusk J: Exploring polarization in US food policy opinions. Appl Econ Perspect Policy 42(3):434–454, 2020

Chriqui JF, Asada Y: The Child and Adult Care Food Program: a critical component of the nutrition safety net for more than 50 years. Am J Public Health 113(S3):S171–S174, 2023 38118098

Compton MT, Suarez JC: Saving farmers and striving for food security: The Agricultural Adjustment Act of 1933, in Struggle and Solidarity: Seven Stories of How Americans Fought for Their Mental Health through Federal Legislation. Edited by Compton MT, Manseau MW. Washington, DC: American Psychiatric Publishing, 17–44, 2023

Economic Research Service: Farm Bill Spending. U.S. Department of Agriculture, December 11, 2018. Available at: https://www.ers.usda.gov/topics/farm-economy/farm-commodity-policy/farm-bill-spending/. Accessed November 26, 2024.

Economic Research Service: Ag and Food Sectors and the Economy. U.S. Department of Agriculture, April 19, 2024a. Available at: https://www.ers.usda.gov/data-products/ag-and-food-statistics-charting-the-essentials/ag-and-food-sectors-and-the-economy/. Accessed November 26, 2024.

Economic Research Service: Key Statistics and Graphics. U.S. Department of Agriculture, September 4, 2024b. Available at: https://www.ers.usda.gov/topics/food-nutrition-assistance/food-security-in-the-u-s/key-statistics-graphics/#foodsecure. Accessed November 26, 2024.

Feeding America: Charitable Food Assistance Participation. Feeding America, 2023. Available at: https://www.feedingamerica.org/research/charitable-food-assistance-participation. Accessed November 26, 2024.

Fisher A: Big Hunger: The Unholy Alliance Between Corporate America and Anti-Hunger Groups (R. Gottlieb, Ed.). Cambridge, MA, MIT Press, 2017

Food and Nutrition Service: A Short History of SNAP. U.S. Department of Agriculture, 2024a. Available at: https://www.fns.usda.gov/snap/history#1939. Accessed November 26, 2024.

Food and Nutrition Service: Program Data Overview. U.S. Department of Agriculture, 2024b. Available at: https://www.fns.usda.gov/pd/overview. Accessed September 15, 2025.

Frates B, Bonnet J, Joseph R, et al: Lifestyle Medicine Handbook, 2nd ed. Monterey, CA, Healthy Learning, 2020

Freeman A: Food oppression in a pandemic. J Law Med Ethics 50(4):711–718, 2022 36883390

Hales LJ, Coleman-Jensen A: Household Food Insecurity Across Race and Ethnicity in the United States, 2016–21. U.S. Department of Agriculture, Economic Research Service, 2024. Available at: http://www.ers.usda.gov/publications/pub-details/?pubid=108904. Accessed November 26, 2024.

Himmelgreen DA, Romero-Daza N: Eliminating "hunger" in the U.S.: changes in policy regarding the measurement of food security. Food Foodways 18(1–2):96–113, 2010

Hirschman J, Chriqui JF: School food and nutrition policy, monitoring and evaluation in the USA. Public Health Nutr 16(6):982–988, 2013 23006629

Hoefer R, Curry C: Food security and social protection in the United States. J Policy Pract 11(1–2):59–76, 2012

Hopkins LC, Gunther C: A historical review of changes in nutrition standards of USDA child meal programs relative to research findings on the nutritional adequacy of program meals and the diet and nutritional health of participants: implications for future research and the Summer Food Service Program. Nutrients 7(12):10145–10167, 2015 26690207

Hoynes HW, Schanzenbach DW: U.S. Food and Nutrition Programs. National Bureau of Economic Research, 2015. Available at: http://www.nber.org/papers/w21057. Accessed November 26, 2024.

Irish A, Clark JK, Bassarab K, et al: Characteristics of regional food policy councils in the United States. Johns Hopkins Center for a Livable Future, 2024. Available at: https://foodpolicynetworks.org/sites/default/files/2024-10/characteristics-of-regional-fpc-in-the-us.pdf. Accessed November 26, 2024.

Ivancic S, Dooling D: Navigating entangled shame: examining the sociomaterialities of food assistance programs. Commun Monogr 90(3):293–316, 2023

Jahns L, Davis-Shaw W, Lichtenstein AH, et al: The history and future of dietary guidance in America. Adv Nutr 9(2):136–147, 2018 29659693

John S, Melendrez B, Leng K, et al: Advancing equity in the farm bill: opportunities for the Gus Schumacher Nutrition Incentive Program (GusNIP). Nutrients 15(23):4863, 2023 38068722

Keller KJM, Bruno P, Foerster S, et al: Thirty years of SNAP-Ed: the transition of the nation's largest nutrition education program into a pillar of the public health infrastructure. J Nutr Educ Behav 56(8):588–596, 2024 38904598

Leung CW, Wolfson JA: Perspectives from supplemental nutrition assistance program participants on improving SNAP policy. Health Equity 3(1):81–85, 2019 30915423

Matson J, Sullins M, Cook C: The Role of Food Hubs in Local Food Marketing. U.S. Department of Agriculture, Rural Development Agency, 2013. Available at: https://www.govinfo.gov/app/details/GOVPUB-A109-PURL-gpo37621. Accessed November 26, 2024.

Moshfegh AJ: The National Nutrition Monitoring and Related Research program: progress and activities. J Nutr 124(9)(Suppl):1843S–1845S, 1994 8089760

National Agricultural Statistics Service: Census of Agriculture—Local Food Marketing Practices. U.S. Department of Agriculture, 2022. Available at: https://www.nass.usda.gov/Publications/AgCensus/2017/Online_Resources/Local_Food/index.php. Accessed November 26, 2024.

National Institute of Food and Agriculture: EFNEP FY 2023 National Report. U.S. Department of Agriculture, 2023a. Available at: https://www.webneers.net/national_report/2023. Accessed November 26, 2024.

National Institute of Food and Agriculture: National Institutes for Food and Agriculture: EFNEP Changing Lives. U.S. Department of Agriculture, March 23, 2023b. Available at: https://www.nifa.usda.gov/about-nifa/impacts/efnep-changing-lives. Accessed November 26, 2024.

National Institute of Food and Agriculture: Gus Schumacher Nutrition Incentive Program (GusNIP). U.S. Department of Agriculture, 2024. Available at: https://www.nifa.usda.gov/grants/programs/hunger-food-security-programs/gus-schumacher-nutrition-incentive-program. Accessed November 26, 2024.

Nestle M: Food Politics: How the Food Industry Influences Nutrition and Health (Revised and Expanded Edition). Oakland, CA, University of California Press, 2007

Newby K, Chen X: Decisions that matter: State Supplemental Nutrition Assistance Program policy restrictiveness limits SNAP participation rate. Soc Sci Q 103(4):868–882, 2022

Nixon R: Remarks at the White House Conference on Food, Nutrition, and Health, December 2, 1969. The American Presidency Project. Available at: https://www.presidency.ucsb.edu/documents/remarks-the-white-house-conference-food-nutrition-and-health. Accessed November 26, 2024.

One Big Beautiful Bill Act, H.R. 1, 119th Cong., July 4, 2025. Available at: https://www.congress.gov/bill/119th-congress/house-bill/1/text. Accessed August 5, 2025.

Palmer A, Atoloye AT, Bassarab K, et al: COVID-19 responses: food policy councils are "stepping in, stepping up, and stepping back." J Agric Food Syst Community Dev 10(1):223–226, 2020

Picciano MF, Coates PM, Cohen BE: History and continued commitment to the nutritional health of the U.S. population. J Nutr 133(6):1949–1952, 2003 12771344

Rowe S: US evidence-based dietary guidelines: the history and the process. Nutr Bull 39(4):364–368, 2014

Shabazz S: Senior nutrition in a pandemic: the California Great Plates Delivered Program. Berkley Food Institute. 1–28, 2021. Available at: https://food.berkeley.edu/wp-content/uploads/2021/05/GREAT-PLATES_WEB_FINAL.pdf. Accessed November 26, 2024.

Willett W, Rockström J, Loken B, et al: Food in the anthropocene: the EAT-Lancet Commission on healthy diets from sustainable food systems. Lancet 393(10170):447–492, 2019 30660336

Woteki CE, Kramer BL, Cohen S, et al: Impacts and echoes: the lasting influence of the White House Conference on Food, Nutrition, and Health. Annu Rev Nutr 40:437–461, 2020 32631144

Wunderlich G, Norwood J: Food Insecurity and Hunger in the United States: An Assessment of the Measure. Washington, DC, National Academies Press, 2006

Part 3

Special Topics on Food and Nutrition

10

Psychotropic Medications, Increased Appetite, and Iatrogenic Weight Gain

Omid Cohensedgh, M.D.

The person who takes medicine must recover twice, once from the disease and once from the medicine.

—Sir William Osler, M.D., Co-Founder of the Johns Hopkins Hospital, 1849–1919

Weight gain, a common side effect of psychotropic medications including antipsychotics, antidepressants, and mood stabilizers, poses a significant challenge in the treatment of mental health disorders. Iatrogenic weight gain can lead to a host of physical health complications, including metabolic syndrome, diabetes, and cardiovascular disease, further burdening patients who are already vulnerable on account of their psychiatric conditions. For clinicians, managing weight gain and related side effects requires a balance between optimizing psychiatric outcomes and mitigating the risk of weight-related comorbidities. This chapter explores the mechanisms, risks, and management strategies for iatrogenic weight gain and provides insight into how best to navigate this frequently complex clinical situation.

Psychotropic Medications Associated With Weight Gain

Antipsychotics

People with serious mental illness (SMI), including schizophrenia and other psychotic disorders, are more likely to die prematurely than those without such disorders. On average, individuals with schizophrenia have a 20% shorter life expectancy than the general population (Laursen 2011). The major driver of the increased risk of mortality is cardiovascular disease, which accounts for approximately 60% of the excess mortality among individuals with schizophrenia (Galletly 2017). Antipsychotic treatment is a significant contributor to weight gain in individuals with SMI, often leading to obesity and increasing the risk of cardiovascular and metabolic complications. Weight gain also increases the risk of disabling conditions such as osteoarthritis and stroke, which can limit physical functioning and perpetuate further weight gain. Beyond physical health complications, antipsychotic-induced weight gain (AIWG) may negatively affect self-image and lead to experiences of stigma and social isolation, often causing poor adherence and treatment discontinuation among patients. Understanding and mitigating AIWG is therefore crucial to improve both physical health and psychiatric outcomes for individuals with SMI.

Before discussing the contribution of antipsychotics to weight gain and metabolic issues, it is important to recognize that individuals with schizophrenia-spectrum disorders are already at an elevated risk for overweight/obesity and cardiometabolic disease, even before treatment initiation. A meta-analysis by Shah et al. (2019) found that compared with healthy controls, treatment-naive individuals with psychosis had greater waist-to-hip ratios, which is a measure of abdominal fat and a strong predictor of cardiovascular disease. This may be partly explained by the negative symptoms of schizophrenia, such as avolition and asociality, which lead to reduced exercise, social isolation, and overall decreased physical activity. Additionally, up to 85% of individuals with schizophrenia smoke cigarettes, which increases the risk of both cardiovascular disease and respiratory disease (Ziedonis et al. 2008).

The debilitating symptoms of SMI often make it difficult to maintain employment and a steady income. As a result, many with schizophrenia reside in low-income neighborhoods where healthy food options are limited and where access to outdoor activities and public spaces is scarce. People with treatment-refractory schizophrenia who reside in long-term-care facilities, such as state hospitals or nursing homes, are at especially high risk of weight gain. In these settings, nutritionally balanced meals are less likely to be offered, and there is often an overreliance on snacks with high sugar and high fat content.

People with SMI also face barriers to accessing regular primary care and engaging effectively with the health care system. Factors such as cognitive impairments and disorganized thinking can make it difficult to make or attend medical appointments or, more broadly, to prioritize one's health. Therefore, adhering to complex treatment plans, including restrained eating, exercise routines, and medication regimens, can be challenging for this patient population.

Individuals with SMI are already predisposed to obesity and metabolic issues, and antipsychotic medications substantially compound these risks. Antipsychotics, especially second-generation antipsychotics (SGAs), are known to significantly affect metabolic health, leading to weight gain, insulin resistance, and dyslipidemia. Patients have described the increased sense of appetite as a feeling of being "completely out of control" and as a "hunger you just can't do anything about … food doesn't satisfy it" (Fitzgerald et al. 2024).

The physiological mechanisms of AIWG are multifactorial and complex and include contributions from genetic susceptibilities, the nervous system, the endocrine system, and the gastrointestinal system (Ye et al. 2023). In the nervous system, the serotonin receptor (5-HT2C) plays a role in regulating appetite and satiety, namely in the hypothalamus. Increased serotonin levels are associated with satiety, and SGAs are potent 5-HT2C antagonists, which disrupt appetite regulation and lead to hyperphagia. Additional neurologic mechanisms for AIWG include increased activity of orexin-producing neurons in the hypothalamus, abnormal expression of brain-derived neurotrophic factor (BDNF) levels in various parts of the brain, and antagonism of the hypothalamic histamine 1 receptor (H1R) leading to reduced energy expenditure and fat accumulation. In the endocrine system, SGAs directly decrease the insulin-stimulated glucose transport rate, inducing insulin resistance, and alter lipogenesis and lipolysis in favor of progressive lipid accumulation and adipocyte enlargement (Vestri et al. 2007).

To stratify risk and tailor treatment decisions, several studies have attempted to identify predictive factors for AIWG. Some studies have found that certain patient characteristics, such as younger age, female sex, and elevated baseline body mass index (BMI), may predict a higher risk of weight gain (Gebhardt et al. 2009); however, a meta-analysis by Fitzgerald et al. (2023) found that these characteristics had no clinically meaningful effect on long-term weight gain. The trend of BMI increase, however, particularly within the first 12 weeks of antipsychotic treatment, does provide strong prognostic information about AIWG (Fitzgerald et al. 2023). Individuals who experience clinically significant weight gain (defined in that meta-analysis as ≥5% increase in baseline body weight) within 12 weeks have a worse long-term prognosis. This underscores the importance of closely monitoring and treating weight gain and metabolic disturbances within the first year of antipsychotic treatment.

The most significant variable in predicting the severity of weight gain is the choice of antipsychotic (Fitzgerald et al. 2023). In a meta-analysis of 100 randomized controlled trials, Pillinger and colleagues (2020) found that among 18 different antipsychotics, chlorpromazine, clozapine, and olanzapine were associated with the most weight gain and had the worst metabolic side effects, including increases in blood glucose, low-density lipoprotein (LDL) cholesterol, and total cholesterol. Quetiapine, risperidone, paliperidone, and asenapine have moderate potential for weight gain, and haloperidol, ziprasidone, aripiprazole, and lurasidone have the lowest potential for weight gain—haloperidol and aripiprazole cause moderate increases in blood glucose and total cholesterol levels, however. The relative risk of AIWG by antipsychotic medication is outlined in Table 10.1.

Interestingly, some studies suggest that treatment response to antipsychotics may correlate with the severity of AIWG. In a meta-analysis by Raben et al. (2018) involving 31 studies, 22 studies found a positive association: treatment responders gained 5.2–9.3 kg more weight on average than nonresponders. This relationship seemingly exists even when controlling for length of treatment, medication adherence, and baseline BMI. The relationship between clinical response and weight gain also may vary depending on the specific antipsychotic used: olanzapine and clozapine demonstrate the strongest association between AIWG and therapeutic benefit (Raben et al. 2018). It is unlikely that

Table 10.1 Levels of risk of antipsychotic-induced weight gain by antipsychotic agent

Risk level	Antipsychotic
Highest risk	Chlorpromazine Clozapine Olanzapine
Moderate risk	Amisulpride Asenapine Brexpiprazole Fluphenazine Paliperidone Quetiapine Risperidone
Lowest risk	Aripiprazole Haloperidol Lurasidone Ziprasidone

weight gain is an actual requirement to observe treatment response, given that not all antipsychotics demonstrate this correlation and that switching from an antipsychotic with a high risk of AIWG to an agent with a lower risk does not necessarily cause clinical deterioration.

Antidepressants

Antidepressants are one of the most prescribed types of medications in the United States, and one of the most common and well-known side effects of antidepressants is weight gain. Those experiencing depression (or other mood or anxiety disorders for which antidepressants are prescribed) may already be prone to changes in baseline weight based on the symptomology of their disease. For example, some patients' depression psychopathologies may involve increases in appetite and weight gain; others may experience low appetite and weight loss. The proportion of depressed individuals who experience weight gain versus weight loss varies significantly across studies, but using appetite as a proxy, Simmons et al. (2020) found that among unmedicated depressed individuals, 43% endorsed increased appetite and 57% endorsed decreased appetite. Depression-related decrease in appetite and weight loss is important to consider when evaluating whether antidepressant treatment is directly causing excess weight gain or simply normalizing a patient's weight and appetite to their pre-illness baseline.

Different classes of antidepressants affect weight in distinct ways over varying timelines. For instance, selective serotonin reuptake inhibitors (SSRIs) and serotonin-norepinephrine reuptake inhibitors (SNRIs) may initially cause weight loss but are likely to lead to long-term weight gain after approximately 6 months of treatment (Lee et al. 2016). In contrast, tricyclic antidepressants (TCAs) tend to cause steady weight gain starting in the first month of treatment. In a meta-analysis by Serretti and Mandelli (2010), SSRIs (fluoxetine, sertraline, citalopram, and paroxetine) and SNRIs (duloxetine and venlafaxine) were associated with an average of 0.5–1 kg weight loss over 4–12 weeks (the "acute phase" of treatment). At time intervals longer than 4 months (the "maintenance phase"), SSRIs/SNRIs were associated with either weight neutrality (fluoxetine and sertraline) or weight gain of 1–3 kg on average (escitalopram, citalopram, paroxetine, and duloxetine). TCAs (amitriptyline, nortriptyline, desipramine, and clomipramine) were associated with approximately 1–2 kg weight gain within 4–12 weeks of treatment, which on average remained stable in studies extending beyond 4 months. Longer-term studies are limited, but one prospective cohort study of approximately 2,500 patients followed over 4 years found that SSRIs and TCAs were associated with a mean increase of BMI of 1 ± 2 kg/m^2 (Mwinyi et al. 2024). Gafoor and colleagues (2018) found that the increased risk of antidepressant-induced weight gain may continue for up to 6 years after the start of treatment.

There is moderate variability in the extent of iatrogenic weight gain between different antidepressants (Gill et al. 2020). Mirtazapine, an atypical tetracyclic antidepressant, has one of the highest potentials for weight gain and is often prescribed for patients who present with loss of appetite and low weight (Serretti and Mandelli 2010). Among SSRIs and SNRIs, there is little clinically significant difference in the propensity for weight gain. Petimar et al. (2024) found that among escitalopram, sertraline, citalopram, paroxetine, fluoxetine, venlafaxine, and duloxetine, the largest difference in weight gain between any two antidepressants was approximately 0.5 kg over 6 months, and the meta-analysis by Serretti and Mandelli (2010) had similar findings. Bupropion, a dual dopamine and norepinephrine reuptake inhibitor, is perhaps the only antidepressant that is associated with weight loss in long-term treatment. In Serreti and Mandelli's report (2010), bupropion was associated with an average loss of 1 kg in the short term and 2 kg in the long term.

The physiological mechanisms of weight changes with antidepressants vary based on their pharmacological profiles (Lee et al. 2016). SSRIs target serotonin (5-HT) receptors, which initially play a role in appetite suppression and can increase plasma leptin levels, an anorexigenic hormone involved in appetite regulation. SSRIs may also reduce impulsivity, leading to decreased food intake. The mechanisms driving weight gain with long-term SSRI use are less clear, although evidence suggests they may involve increased carbohydrate cravings. TCAs contribute to weight gain through antagonism of the histamine H1 receptor, which increases appetite and may cause sedation, reducing physical activity. TCAs also inhibit serotonin and norepinephrine reuptake and block muscarinic receptors, further stimulating appetite and decreasing metabolic rate. Mirtazapine similarly acts on the noradrenergic (α2), histaminergic (H1), and serotonergic (5-HT2 and 5-HT3) systems while also having a low affinity for dopaminergic (D1 and D2) receptors.

Mood Stabilizers

Among mood stabilizers (including valproate, lithium, carbamazepine, and lamotrigine), valproate and lithium are known to cause weight gain. Hayes et al. (2016) found that compared with lithium, valproate had a 1.62 times higher risk of causing greater than 15% weight gain. The study also compared lithium to olanzapine and quetiapine, finding that the hazard ratios for greater than 15% weight gain were 1.84 and 1.67, respectively. This suggests that valproate may rival antipsychotics in the extent of expected weight gain. There also appears to be a dose-dependent increase in weight gain, with one study finding an additional 0.5% increase in weight for each incremental increase in valproate by 500 mg (Grosu et al. 2024).

About 25% of patients on lithium experience weight gain (Torrent et al. 2008). Lithium may cause weight gain through several mechanisms. It can cause thyroid dysfunction, leading to hypothyroidism or subclinical hypothyroidism and subsequent weight gain. This underscores the importance of thyroid function monitoring for patients on lithium. Furthermore, lithium is associated with polydipsia and polyuria secondary to its renal side effects, which can lead to excess intake of liquids, including high-calorie beverages. It may also have a direct effect on hypothalamic centers controlling appetite (Livingstone and Rampes 2006). Studies demonstrate weight gain of 4.5–12 kg associated with lithium, which is likely dose dependent and presents a higher risk in patients with a lithium plasma level higher than 0.8 mmol/L (Torrent et al. 2008).

Weight Gain Prevention and Management Strategies

Weight and Metabolic Monitoring Recommendations

Effective management of iatrogenic weight gain and metabolic complications requires regular monitoring of weight and laboratory values. Prompt detection of weight changes and metabolic disturbances is essential to allow for timely interventions to prevent the progression of overweight/obesity and cardiovascular disease. In 2004, the American Diabetes Association and American Psychiatric Association published a protocol for monitoring patients on SGAs. The guidelines recommend measuring BMI, waist circumference, blood pressure, fasting plasma glucose, and fasting lipid profile at the start of antipsychotic treatment. Mental health clinicians should elicit a detailed medical history during the initial visit and at least annually, including diet, physical activity and exercise habits, family history of metabolic disorders, current medications, and other relevant health information. BMI should be measured once each month during the first 4 months of treatment, then once every 3 months. As discussed previously, weight gain during the first 12 weeks of treatment is strongly predictive of long-term weight gain, so BMI should be closely tracked early in treatment to determine the need for intervention. Blood pressure and fasting blood glucose should also be assessed at 12 weeks and then at least annually. Fasting lipid profile should be measured at 12 weeks and then every 5 years. Waist circumference should be remeasured annually, given that it is considered more predictive of cardiovascular disease risk than BMI (Lee et al. 2008).

Unfortunately, real-world studies demonstrate suboptimal monitoring of metabolic parameters for patients at risk of AIWG. In a large Veterans Affairs study, which included 12,000 patients receiving a newly prescribed antipsychotic medication, only 67% of patients were weighed, 46% had blood glucose or hemoglobin A1c labs, and 32% had LDL cholesterol labs at the initial visit (i.e., within 30 days of initiating an antipsychotic) (Mittal et al. 2013). Follow-up monitoring had even lower rates; only 50% of patients were weighed, 27% had repeat glucose or hemoglobin A1c labs, and 16% had LDL cholesterol labs at any point 60–120 days after antipsychotic initiation. In another study conducted in an inpatient unit at a Canadian tertiary care center, less than one-third of patients starting antipsychotics had at least three cardiometabolic parameters measured (among blood pressure, weight/BMI, lipid profile, fasting glucose/A1C, and waist circumference) and less than 2% of patients had all five parameters measured at baseline (Fontaine et al. 2022). Notably, this study also identified key factors influencing cardiometabolic monitoring, revealing that the specific psychiatrist caring for a patient significantly affected the likelihood of monitoring. As such, monitoring guidelines may not be universally adhered to among mental health clinicians. Additionally, patients with court-ordered treatment (i.e., those who are more severely ill and less treatment adherent) were less likely to be monitored, as were patients with bipolar and related disorders compared with patients with schizophrenia-spectrum disorders.

Mental health clinicians should collaborate with primary care physicians and specialists to ensure that patients with existing or newly found medical comorbidities receive close medical follow-up. As discussed earlier in this chapter, patients with SMI may face substantial challenges engaging with the health care system. Some patients, especially those with significant medical comorbidities, may benefit from receiving their care at an integrated behavioral health care center where they can access both psychiatric and medical care at a single facility. Patients with SMI often report dissatisfaction with medical services because of experiences of stigma, disbelief, or patronizing attitudes from providers, particularly regarding substance use or medication adherence (Lester et al. 2005). Integrated behavioral health clinics, staffed with clinicians trained in SMI care, can foster smoother collaboration between psychiatric and medical providers, streamlining the monitoring and treatment of medical issues and enabling timely medication adjustments when needed. A large study of 16,000 patients demonstrated that patients receiving care at integrated clinics had better outcomes related to blood pressure, A1c, and BMI than patients receiving care at separate institutions (Matthews et al. 2024).

Nonpharmacological Interventions to Address Weight Gain

Nonpharmacologic interventions, including lifestyle and nutritional counseling, may benefit all patients experiencing psychotropic medication-associated weight gain. Mental health clinicians should ideally discuss nonpharmacological interventions with patients at the start of treatment and refer patients to relevant services as appropriate (e.g., a registered dietitian, structured exercise programs, primary care). Patients with mobility issues (e.g., osteoarthritis exacerbated by overweight/obesity) may also benefit from physical therapy, which can help restore physical functioning and reduce pain associated with physical activity and exercise.

Several studies have sought to design, implement, and evaluate behavioral interventions for AIWG. Some examples of treatments include a structured, supervised, facility-based exercise program (Poulin et al. 2007), a 12-session group-based cognitive-behavioral therapy (CBT) intervention (Khazaal et al. 2007), and a series of individualized nutritional counseling sessions by a dietitian (Erickson et al. 2017). A meta-analysis by Alvarez-Jiménez et al. (2008) demonstrated that nonpharmacological interventions, including CBT, nutritional counseling, and exercise programs, were associated with an average weight loss of 2.6 kg compared with treatment as usual in patients with AIWG. Notably, there were no statistically significant differences in efficacy between the different modalities (individual vs. group therapy, CBT vs. nutritional counseling). This suggests that clinicians should recommend interventions that best suit the needs and desires of the individual patient. For example, young patients may be more willing to incorporate exercise into their daily routines through group sports, whereas older patients may require structured programs to incorporate exercise.

Although they are effective, nonpharmacological interventions alone may be insufficient for managing AIWG, particularly when it is moderate or severe. Patients in a qualitative study reported that the recommendation of behavioral interventions as a uniform first-line intervention for AIWG was often frustrating and did not meet their needs (Fitzgerald et al. 2024). The participants noted that several factors, including antipsychotic side effects and fluctuating psychological health, affected their ability to adhere to recommended lifestyle interventions. As one participant stated, "It's easy enough to say you need to lose weight, try diet and lifestyle, but you're saying that at a time when a person is at a low.... It has to be very structured, and what sick person is going to be able to do that?" This underscores the importance of a proactive, individualized, and collaborative approach to treatment that incorporates shared decision-making and contingency planning.

Pharmacologic Interventions for Weight Gain

Several medications show efficacy in treating AIWG, including metformin, topiramate, naltrexone-bupropion, glucagon-like peptide-1 receptor agonists (GLP-1 RAs), and aripiprazole as an adjunctive treatment. Table 10.2 summarizes the mechanisms, efficacy, and side effects of these medications.

Metformin is a relatively safe, well-tolerated, and inexpensive medication that is FDA-approved as a first-line treatment for type 2 diabetes (Nathan et al. 2009). It is one of the most frequently prescribed medications in the United States and the most studied off-label medication for AIWG. Side effects of metformin include nausea, vomiting, and diarrhea, although slow titration may mitigate this. The mechanism of action of metformin is not completely understood, but it has been shown to suppress hepatic gluconeogenesis and promote insulin sensitivity, which reduces blood glucose levels. Metformin also reduces food cravings, and patients describe a "plateauing" effect of AIWG when on metformin (Fitzgerald et al. 2024). In a meta-analysis by de Silva and colleagues (2016), metformin decreased weight by an average of 3.3 kg and BMI by 1.1 kg/m^2 compared with placebo. The follow-up duration of studies included in the analysis ranged from 12 weeks to 6 months, and metformin doses ranged from 500 to 2,250 mg daily. Fitzgerald et al. (2024) developed guidelines for the use of metformin to manage AIWG and recommended metformin as a first-line strategy for patients who find lifestyle interventions unacceptable or inadequate for weight management or for patients who cannot engage in exercise, such as those with physical disabilities. The authors underscored the importance of initiating metformin early during treatment for the best effect, especially for those with existing metabolic comorbidities.

Topiramate is an antiepileptic medication that modulates γ-aminobutyric acid (GABA) and glutamate receptors, which leads to appetite reduction. In a meta-analysis by Correll et al. (2016), topiramate was associated with an average weight loss of 3.6 kg over a mean treat-

Table 10.2 Mechanisms, evidence, and side effects of select medications used in the context of psychotropic medication-associated weight gain

Medication	Mechanism	Evidence	Side Effects
Metformin	Decreases hepatic gluconeogenesis and promotes insulin sensitivity	Strong	Primarily gastrointestinal (nausea, vomiting, diarrhea); lactic acidosis in renal failure
GLP-1 RAs	Promotes insulin secretion, slows gastric emptying, acts centrally in the brain	Strong	Nausea, vomiting, diarrhea; primarily at the start of treatment and during dose increases
Topiramate	Acts on GABA and glutamate receptors to decrease appetite	Strong	Sedation, paresthesias, increased risk of depression/suicidal ideation
Aripiprazole (adjunctive)	Partial D2 receptor agonism; 5-HT2C receptor antagonism	Strong	Akathisia, insomnia, anxiety
Naltrexone-bupropion	Modulates the reward pathway subserved by dopamine and norepinephrine	Low to moderate	Nausea, constipation, headache

ment duration of 14 weeks, similar to metformin. Naltrexone-bupropion has shown mixed results, with one study (Lee et al. 2022) demonstrating a reduction in weight by an average of 11% over 52 weeks of treatment and other studies showing no significant difference between the treatment and control groups. Aripiprazole at doses of 5–15 mg has also been shown to reduce weight by an average of 2.5 kg over 12 weeks with good tolerability when added to a clozapine regimen (Fleischhacker et al. 2010).

Recently, GLP-1 RAs have emerged as a promising pharmacologic option for the management of psychotropic-induced weight gain (Trott et al. 2024). GLP-1 RAs, such as semaglutide and liraglutide, are currently approved by the FDA for type 2 diabetes and obesity in the general population. Formulations include subcutaneous injections, typically administered once a week, or oral pills taken once a day.

GLP-1 is a peptide hormone produced in the intestines following food intake and acts on multiple targets to help regulate blood sugar and weight gain. For example, it promotes insulin secretion and decreases glucagon release, which lowers blood glucose levels. It targets receptors in the gut to slow gastric emptying, which promotes satiety. It also acts on specific brain regions to control appetite and reduce food cravings. In areas such as the dorsomedial hypothalamus and lateral septum, it decreases appetite, whereas in the nucleus accumbens and ventral tegmental area, it reduces the activation of reward pathways triggered by high-calorie foods.

Preliminary studies on GLP-1 RAs in the treatment of psychotropic drug-related weight gain have been encouraging. Trott et al. (2024) reviewed six completed trials of GLP-1 RAs, ranging from 12 to 30 weeks in duration. Four of the six studies have been published; of those four, two investigated exenatide (weekly injection) and the other two investigated liraglutide (daily injection). Among the inclusion criteria were having schizophrenia and being on antipsychotics, as well as the presence of either overweight or obesity, with one study including only participants with prediabetes. GLP-1 RAs significantly reduced body weight, waist circumference, LDL cholesterol, and fasting blood glucose levels compared with placebo. Participants lost on average 4.2 kg (on exenatide) to 6.0 kg (on liraglutide), both with 24-week follow-up, compared with participants receiving placebo. Ongoing trials are investigating semaglutide, which has shown superior efficacy in reducing body weight compared with liraglutide and exenatide in the general population (Stretton et al. 2023).

Although GLP-1 RAs show promise, they come with limitations. Their high cost and limited insurance coverage, especially for patients without type 2 diabetes, can make access challenging. Patients who solely meet the FDA-approved indication of obesity may have difficulty obtaining coverage. In addition to access issues, gastrointestinal side effects—such as nausea, vomiting, and diarrhea—are common, especially when starting or increasing the dose; these side effects generally subside over time. A meta-analysis by Patoulias et al. (2023) found, among patients on antipsychotics, no significant difference in the rate of treatment discontinuation due to adverse events with GLP-1 RAs compared with control treatments.

Notably, no trial has yet explored GLP-1 RAs as a preventive measure for AIWG. Starting GLP-1 RA treatment alongside antipsychotics—for example, in first-episode psychosis—could potentially prevent weight gain before it begins. This proactive approach may help preserve physical health and support long-term adherence to antipsychotic medication. Research in this and related areas is needed.

Future Research Directions

Future research on AIWG should focus on expanding the evidence for pharmacologic interventions, particularly GLP-1 RAs, which have shown promise in mitigating weight gain in this population. Additionally, evidence from clinical trials shows that novel antipsychotics with different mechanisms of action, such as xanomeline-trospium, may have a lower risk of weight gain and warrant further investigation as potential alternatives to second-generation antipsychotics. Long-term studies are needed to assess the durability of these interventions, their impact on psychiatric outcomes, and their accessibility in real-world settings. Understanding genetic and metabolic predictors of weight gain could also help personalize treatment approaches and improve patient outcomes.

Clinical Pearls

- Clinicians should closely monitor weight and metabolic parameters before starting an antipsychotic and at set intervals during treatment to determine the need for weight loss interventions. This is especially important in the first 12 weeks of treatment, as increases in BMI during this period are a strong predictor of longer-term weight gain.

- Although clozapine and olanzapine may be the most effective antipsychotics, they are also associated with the highest rates of antipsychotic-induced weight gain.
- Clinicians should expect patients to experience antipsychotic-induced weight gain and initiate weight management treatments, including lifestyle counseling.
- Clinicians should ensure that patients follow up with their primary care providers and relevant specialists to optimize the treatment of overweight/obesity and metabolic disorders at the start of treatment with antipsychotics. Referral to integrated care centers may benefit patients with significant medical comorbidities.
- For patients with depression and weight or metabolic concerns, bupropion may be favored as first-line treatment, given its association with weight loss. However, short-term therapy (e.g., 6 months) with SSRIs or SNRIs is not associated with weight gain.

Key Chapter Points

- People with serious mental illness face elevated risks of overweight/obesity and cardiometabolic disease owing to diverse baseline factors and antipsychotic-induced weight gain, driving stigma, poor treatment adherence, comorbidities, and increased cardiovascular morbidity and mortality.
- The severity of antipsychotic-induced weight gain is primarily influenced by the choice of antipsychotic medication, with clozapine and olanzapine causing the most significant weight and metabolic changes.
- Patients on second-generation antipsychotics should be monitored regularly for weight gain and changes in metabolic parameters.
- Among antidepressants, mirtazapine is likely to cause the greatest weight gain, SSRIs and SNRIs cause moderate weight gain, and bupropion is associated with weight loss.
- Metformin is the most extensively studied and effective agent for weight loss in patients with antipsychotic-induced weight gain; GLP-1 receptor agonists represent a promising emerging class of medications.

References

Alvarez-Jiménez M, Hetrick SE, González-Blanch C, et al: Non-pharmacological management of antipsychotic-induced weight gain: systematic review and meta-analysis of randomised controlled trials. Br J Psychiatry 193(2):101–107, 2008 18669990

American Diabetes Association, American Psychiatric Association, American Association of Clinical Endocrinologists, et al: Consensus development conference on antipsychotic drugs and obesity and diabetes. Diabetes Care 27(2):596–601, 2004 14747245

Correll CU, Maayan L, Kane J, et al: Efficacy for psychopathology and body weight and safety of topiramate-antipsychotic cotreatment in patients with schizophrenia spectrum disorders: results from a meta-analysis of randomized controlled trials. J Clin Psychiatry 77(6):e746–e756, 2016 27337425

de Silva VA, Suraweera C, Ratnatunga SS, et al: Metformin in prevention and treatment of antipsychotic induced weight gain: a systematic review and meta-analysis. BMC Psychiatry 16(1):341, 2016 27716110

Erickson ZD, Kwan CL, Gelberg HA, et al: A randomized, controlled multisite study of behavioral interventions for veterans with mental illness and antipsychotic medication-associated obesity. J Gen Intern Med 32(Suppl 1):32–39, 2017 28271424

Fitzgerald I, Crowley EK, Ní Dhubhlaing C, et al: Informing the development of antipsychotic-induced weight gain management guidance: patient experiences and preferences—qualitative descriptive study. BJPsych Open 10(5):e136, 2024 39086041

Fitzgerald I, Sahm LJ, Byrne A, et al: Predicting antipsychotic-induced weight gain in first episode psychosis: field-wide systematic review and meta-analysis of non-genetic prognostic factors. Eur Psychiatry 66(1):e42, 2023 37278237

Fleischhacker WW, Heikkinen ME, Olié JP, et al: Effects of adjunctive treatment with aripiprazole on body weight and clinical efficacy in schizophrenia patients treated with clozapine: a randomized, double-blind, placebo-controlled trial. Int J Neuropsychopharmacol 13(8):1115–1125, 2010 20459883

Fontaine J, Chin E, Provencher JF, et al: Assessing cardiometabolic parameter monitoring in inpatients taking a second-generation antipsychotic: the CAMI-SGA study—a cross-sectional study. BMJ Open 12(4):e055454, 2022 35414553

Gafoor R, Booth HP, Gulliford MC: Antidepressant utilisation and incidence of weight gain during 10 years' follow-up: population based cohort study. BMJ 23;361:k1951, 2018

Galletly CA: Premature death in schizophrenia: bridging the gap. Lancet Psychiatry 4(4):263–265, 2017 28237638

Gebhardt S, Haberhausen M, Heinzel-Gutenbrunner M, et al: Antipsychotic-induced body weight gain: predictors and a systematic categorization of the long-term weight course. J Psychiatr Res 43(6):620–626, 2009 19110264

Gill H, Gill B, El-Halabi S, et al: Antidepressant medications and weight change: a narrative review. Obesity 28(11):2064–2072, 2020 33022115

Grosu C, Hatoum W, Piras M, et al: Associations of valproate doses with weight gain in adult psychiatric patients: a 1-year prospective cohort study. J Clin Psychiatry 85(2):23m15008, 2024

Hayes JF, Marston L, Walters K, et al: Adverse renal, endocrine, hepatic, and metabolic events during maintenance mood stabilizer treatment for bipolar disorder: a population-based cohort study. PLoS Med 13(8):e1002058, 2016 27483368

Khazaal Y, Fresard E, Rabia S, et al: Cognitive behavioural therapy for weight gain associated with antipsychotic drugs. Schizophr Res 91(1–3):169–177, 2007 17306507

Laursen TM: Life expectancy among persons with schizophrenia or bipolar affective disorder. Schizophr Res 131(1–3):101–104, 2011 21741216

Lee CM, Huxley RR, Wildman RP, et al: Indices of abdominal obesity are better discriminators of cardiovascular risk factors than BMI: a meta-analysis. J Clin Epidemiol 61(7):646–653, 2008 18359190

Lee K, Abraham S, Cleaver R: A systematic review of licensed weight-loss medications in treating antipsychotic-induced weight gain and obesity in schizophrenia and psychosis. Gen Hosp Psychiatry 78:58–67, 2022 35863294

Lee SH, Paz-Filho G, Mastronardi C, et al: Is increased antidepressant exposure a contributory factor to the obesity pandemic? Transl Psychiatry 6(3):e759, 2016 26978741

Lester H, Tritter JQ, Sorohan H: Patients' and health professionals' views on primary care for people with serious mental illness: focus group study. BMJ 330(7500):1122, 2005 15843427

Livingstone C, Rampes H: Lithium: a review of its metabolic adverse effects. J Psychopharmacol 20(3):347–355, 2006 16174674

Matthews EB, Lushin V, Macneal E, et al: The impact of structural integration on clinical outcomes among individuals with serious mental illness and chronic illness. Community Ment Health J 60(7):1372–1379, 2024 38850504

Mittal D, Li C, Williams JS, et al: Monitoring veterans for metabolic side effects when prescribing antipsychotics. Psychiatr Serv 64(1):28–35, 2013 23117285

Mwinyi J, Strippoli MF, Kanders SH, et al: Long-term changes in adiposity markers during and after antidepressant therapy in a community cohort. Transl Psychiatry 14(1):330, 2024 39138155

Nathan DM, Buse JB, Davidson MB, et al: Medical management of hyperglycemia in type 2 diabetes: a consensus algorithm for the initiation and adjustment of therapy: a consensus statement of the

American Diabetes Association and the European Association for the Study of Diabetes. Diabetes Care 32(1):193–203, 2009 18945920

Patoulias D, Michailidis T, Dimosiari A, et al: Effect of glucagon-like peptide-1 receptor agonists on cardio-metabolic risk factors among obese/overweight individuals treated with antipsychotic drug classes: an updated systematic review and meta-analysis of randomized controlled trials. Biomedicines 11(3):669, 2023 36979648

Petimar J, Young JG, Yu H, et al: Medication-induced weight change across common antidepressant treatments: a target trial emulation study. Ann Intern Med 177(8):993–1003, 2024 38950403

Pillinger T, McCutcheon RA, Vano L, et al: Comparative effects of 18 antipsychotics on metabolic function in patients with schizophrenia, predictors of metabolic dysregulation, and association with psychopathology: a systematic review and network meta-analysis. Lancet Psychiatry 7(1):64–77, 2020 31860457

Poulin MJ, Chaput JP, Simard V, et al: Management of antipsychotic-induced weight gain: prospective naturalistic study of the effectiveness of a supervised exercise programme. Aust N Z J Psychiatry 41(12):980–989, 2007 17999270

Raben AT, Marshe VS, Chintoh A, et al: The complex relationship between antipsychotic-induced weight gain and therapeutic benefits: a systematic review and implications for treatment. Front Neurosci 11:741, 2018 29403343

Serretti A, Mandelli L: Antidepressants and body weight: a comprehensive review and meta-analysis. J Clin Psychiatry 71(10):1259–1272, 2010 21062615

Shah P, Iwata Y, Caravaggio F, et al: Alterations in body mass index and waist-to-hip ratio in never and minimally treated patients with psychosis: a systematic review and meta-analysis. Schizophr Res 208:420–429, 2019 30685395

Simmons WK, Burrows K, Avery JA, et al: Appetite changes reveal depression subgroups with distinct endocrine, metabolic, and immune states. Mol Psychiatry 25(7):1457–1468, 2020 29899546

Stretton B, Kovoor J, Bacchi S, et al: Weight loss with subcutaneous semaglutide versus other glucagon-like peptide 1 receptor agonists in type 2 diabetes: a systematic review. Intern Med J 53(8):1311–1320, 2023 37189293

Torrent C, Amann B, Sánchez-Moreno J, et al: Weight gain in bipolar disorder: pharmacological treatment as a contributing factor. Acta Psychiatr Scand 118(1):4–18, 2008 18498432

Trott M, Arnautovska U, Siskind D: GLP-1 receptor agonists and weight loss in schizophrenia: past, present, and future. Curr Opin Psychiatry 37(5):363–369, 2024 38847529

Vestri HS, Maianu L, Moellering DR, et al: Atypical antipsychotic drugs directly impair insulin action in adipocytes: effects on glucose transport, lipogenesis, and antilipolysis. Neuropsychopharmacology 32(4):765–772, 2007 16823387

Ye W, Xing J, Yu Z, et al: Mechanism and treatments of antipsychotic-induced weight gain. Int J Obes 47(6):423–433, 2023 36959286

Ziedonis D, Hitsman B, Beckham JC, et al: Tobacco use and cessation in psychiatric disorders: National Institute of Mental Health report. Nicotine Tob Res 10(12):1691–1715, 2008 19023823

11

Eating Disorders and Disordered Eating

Ashley Andreou, M.D.

"I ate to numb the pain, to fill the emptiness that I felt inside. I ate to feel something, anything, other than the gnawing ache of loneliness and the weight of the world on my shoulders."

—Roxane Gay, *Hunger: A Memoir of (My) Body*

Food, a key part of our daily lives, contains macronutrients and micronutrients critical to health and survival. Although eating is second nature for many, certain eating behaviors—restriction, excess, and imbalance—can have detrimental effects on physical and mental health. Before psychiatrists characterized disordered eating in the third edition of the *Diagnostic and Statistical Manual of Mental Disorders* (DSM-III) in 1980 (American Psychiatric Association 1980), physicians understood that patients' health was linked, at least in part, to the food they ate. For decades, medical literature has described the physical effects of nutrition from hyperlipidemia to hypoglycemia. More recently, eating patterns have been recognized not only as disorders but also as a potential symptom of and risk factor for other psychiatric illnesses (Stice 2002). Roxane Gay's book, *Hunger: A Memoir of (My) Body*, provides a narrative account of how psychological disturbances, such as the repercussions of trauma, can shape a person's food intake (Gay 2017).

Throughout the DSM's evolution of defining eating disorders, the field of psychiatry has advanced its understanding of the underlying neurobiology, increased recognition of the diversity of clinical presentations, and honed its focus on behavioral patterns rather than specific phenotypes. This chapter aims to sharpen clinicians' understanding of disordered eating and increase awareness of the complex, bidirectional relationship between mental health and nutrition. The chapter also explores how food insecurity can shape eating disorders. Clinicians' understanding of eating patterns and nutrition is integral not only to identifying and treating categorical eating disorders but also to providing thoughtful and comprehensive care to all psychiatric patients.

DSM Eating Disorders

DSM-5 recognizes anorexia nervosa, bulimia nervosa, binge-eating disorder (BED), avoidant/restrictive food intake disorder (ARFID), pica, rumination disorder, and other specified feeding or eating disorder (OSFED). OSFED includes atypical anorexia nervosa (AAN), purging disorder, and night eating syndrome (NES) (American Psychiatric Association 2022). DSM-5 criteria are given in Table 11.1. Diagnostic clarification is critical not only for early intervention, appropriate treatment, prognostication, risk assessment, and insurance coverage, but also for patients to understand their illness, fostering psychological mindedness and agency. In addition, many eating disorders co-occur with other psychiatric illnesses (Hambleton et al. 2022). Although the rates vary across each disorder, the most well-defined comorbidities include depression, anxiety disorders, substance use disorders, obsessive-compulsive disorder (OCD), borderline and obsessive-compulsive personality disorders, and posttraumatic stress disorder (PTSD) (Hudson et al. 2007). The temporal relationship and mediating and moderating factors between eating disorders and other psychiatric comorbidities is complex. All DSM eating disorders can lead to malnutrition—a state of imbalance between the body's needs and the nutrients it receives, potentially leading to weight loss, muscle wasting, growth stunting, weakened immunity, organ dysfunction, and increased risk of chronic diseases (American Psychiatric Association 2022). Malnutrition, in

Table 11.1 DSM eating disorders: prevalence, diagnostic threshold, common nutritional and medical impacts, and common psychiatric comorbidities

Eating disorder	Lifetime prevalence	Diagnostic threshold	Common medical sequelae	Common psychiatric comorbidities
Anorexia nervosa	0.80%	Restriction of energy intake leading to significantly low body weight (BMI <18.5); intense fear of gaining weight or becoming fat; disturbance in the way one's body weight or shape is experienced; includes restrictive and binge-purge subtypes depending on primary behavior driving disorder	Malnutrition; electrolyte imbalances; reduced metabolic rate; cardiovascular problems (e.g., low heart rate, arrhythmias); GI issues (e.g., constipation, delayed gastric emptying); low thyroid levels (e.g., sick euthyroid syndrome); hematologic changes (e.g., anemia and leukopenia); menstrual disturbance/amenorrhea; osteopenia and osteoporosis	Depression; anxiety disorders; OCD; substance use disorders; personality disorders (OCPD being most prevalent)
Atypical anorexia nervosa (AAN)	3.96% for OSFED	Restriction of energy intake without significantly low body weight (BMI ≥18.5); intense fear of gaining weight or becoming fat; disturbance in the way one's body weight or shape is experienced	Malnutrition; electrolyte imbalances; reduced metabolic rate; cardiovascular problems (e.g., low heart rate, arrhythmias); GI issues (e.g., constipation, delayed gastric emptying); low thyroid levels (e.g., sick euthyroid syndrome); hematologic changes (e.g., anemia and leukopenia)	Depression; anxiety disorders; OCD; substance use disorders (may be more prevalent than in anorexia nervosa); personality disorders (OCPD being most prevalent)

Table 11.1 DSM eating disorders: prevalence, diagnostic threshold, common nutritional and medical impacts, and common psychiatric comorbidities (*continued*)

Eating disorder	Lifetime prevalence	Diagnostic threshold	Common medical sequelae	Common psychiatric comorbidities
Bulimia nervosa	0.28%	Recurrent episodes of binge eating; recurrent inappropriate compensatory behaviors to prevent weight gain (e.g., vomiting, laxative misuse, fasting, excessive exercise); occurring at least once a week for 3 months; self-evaluation unduly influenced by body shape and weight	Malnutrition; electrolyte imbalances; GI problems (e.g., esophageal damage, gastroesophageal reflux disease, gastritis, gastroparesis, functional colonic impairment); dental problems; dehydration; menstrual disturbance/ oligomenorrhea	Depression; anxiety disorders; PTSD; substance use disorders; impulsivity; personality disorders (BPD being most prevalent)
Binge-eating disorder (BED)	0.85%	Recurrent episodes of binge eating; binge eating episodes associated with three or more of the following: eating much more rapidly than normal; eating until feeling uncomfortably full; eating large amounts of food when not feeling physically hungry; eating alone because of feeling embarrassed by how much one is eating; feeling disgusted with oneself, depressed, or very guilty afterward; marked distress regarding binge eating; occurs at least once a week for 3 months; no regular compensatory behaviors	Obesity; type 2 diabetes; cardiovascular disease; metabolic syndrome; GI problems (e.g., gastroesophageal reflux disease, constipation, diarrhea); sleep apnea	Depression; anxiety disorders; PTSD; substance use disorders

Table 11.1 DSM eating disorders: prevalence, diagnostic threshold, common nutritional and medical impacts, and common psychiatric comorbidities (*continued*)

Eating disorder	Lifetime prevalence	Diagnostic threshold	Common medical sequelae	Common psychiatric comorbidities
Avoidant/ restrictive food intake disorder (ARFID)	3.96% for OSFED; disorder-specific prevalence unclear, more common in children and adolescents	Eating disturbance manifested by persistent failure to meet appropriate nutritional or energy needs associated with one or more of the following: significant weight loss (or failure to achieve expected weight gain in children) or nutritional deficiency; dependence on enteral feeding or oral nutritional supplements; marked interference with psychosocial functioning; not better explained by lack of available food or by an associated culturally sanctioned practice; not attributable to a concurrent medical condition or better explained by another mental disorder	Malnutrition; growth retardation; delayed puberty	Anxiety disorders; autism spectrum disorder; OCD; intellectual disability

Table 11.1 DSM eating disorders: prevalence, diagnostic threshold, common nutritional and medical impacts, and common psychiatric comorbidities (*continued*)

Eating disorder	Lifetime prevalence	Diagnostic threshold	Common medical sequelae	Common psychiatric comorbidities
Pica	3.96% for OSFED	Persistent eating of nonnutritive, nonfood substances over a period of at least 1 month; eating of nonnutritive, nonfood substances inappropriate to the developmental level of the individual; behavior is not part of a culturally supported or socially normative practice	Malnutrition; poisoning; GI blockages; infections	Autism spectrum disorder; intellectual disability; schizophrenia; OCD
Rumination disorder	3.96% for OSFED; disorder-specific prevalence unclear, more common in infants and individuals with intellectual disability	Repeated regurgitation of food over a period of at least 1 month; regurgitation is not attributable to an associated gastrointestinal or other medical condition; eating disturbance does not occur exclusively with anorexia nervosa, bulimia, BED, or ARFID; if the symptoms occur in the context of another mental disorder (e.g., intellectual disability, autism spectrum disorder), they likely warrant additional clinical attention	Malnutrition; esophageal damage; digestive issues; dental problems	Intellectual disability; autism spectrum disorder; anxiety disorders; OCD

Table 11.1 DSM eating disorders: prevalence, diagnostic threshold, common nutritional and medical impacts, and common psychiatric comorbidities (*continued*)

Eating disorder	Lifetime prevalence	Diagnostic threshold	Common medical sequelae	Common psychiatric comorbidities
Night eating syndrome (NES)	3.96% for OSFED	Eating at night, insomnia, morning anorexia	Obesity; disrupted sleep; digestive issues	Mood disorders; anxiety disorders; substance use disorders; personality disorders
Purging disorder	3.96% for OSFED	Recurrent purging behaviors without binge eating	Malnutrition; electrolyte imbalances; GI issues (e.g., esophageal damage, gastroesophageal reflux disease, gastritis, gastroparesis, functional colonic impairment); dental problems	Mood disorders; anxiety disorders; substance use disorders; personality disorders

Binge eating is defined as eating large amounts of food in a discrete period with a sense of lack of control. BMI = body mass index; BPD = borderline personality disorder; GI = gastrointestinal; OCD = obsessive-compulsive disorder; OCPD = obsessive-compulsive personality disorder; OSFED = other specified feeding or eating disorder; PTSD = posttraumatic stress disorder.

turn, can exacerbate psychiatric symptoms (e.g., low mood, irritability, mood lability) (Kaye et al. 2004).

With such a high rate of psychiatric comorbidities, mental health professionals should know how to evaluate and develop an initial treatment plan, given the likelihood that they will encounter patients with eating disorders in their practice. Furthermore, awareness of how an eating disorder may affect co-occurring conditions (e.g., managing lithium levels in a patient with both bipolar disorder and bulimia nervosa) is critical to treatment planning and collaboration with other providers.

Eating disorders primarily affect adolescent girls and young women, but they can occur in all gender identities and at all ages (Becker et al. 2017). The number of men with eating disorders is increasing (Strother et al. 2012), and growing evidence suggests that transgender and gender-nonconforming individuals are more likely to experience eating disorders than cisgender individuals (Nagata et al. 2020). Eating disorders typically emerge during adolescence or early adulthood (Accurso et al. 2024), but they can develop at any age, including childhood and older adulthood. The estimated lifetime prevalences are: 0.80% for anorexia nervosa, 0.28% for bulimia, and 0.85% for BED (Udo and Grilo 2018); that of OSFED is 3.96% (Galmiche et al. 2019).

Recently, there has been an alarming surge in eating disorders among children and adolescents (Pastore et al. 2023). Development of an eating disorder is multifactorial, with driving factors spanning genetics (e.g., family history of eating disorders or other mental health conditions), psychology (e.g., low self-esteem, perfectionism, stress, trauma), biology (e.g., neurotransmitter imbalances, hormonal changes), and sociocultural factors (e.g., media portrayals of thinness, societal pressure to be thin, cultural ideals of beauty) (Barakat et al. 2023).

Anorexia Nervosa and Atypical Anorexia Nervosa

Anorexia nervosa is characterized by a persistent restriction of energy/caloric intake leading to significantly low body weight (BMI <18.5 kg/m^2 in adults, <5th BMI percentile in youth). Individuals with anorexia nervosa have an intense fear of gaining weight and a disturbance in their perception of body weight and shape. There are two subtypes of anorexia nervosa: the restrictive subtype (AN-R), in which the primary behavior is severe calorie restriction, and the binge-purge subtype (AN-BP), in which individuals additionally experience binge eating and/or purging (e.g., self-induced vomiting, laxative abuse). Binge eating and purging do not equal a diagnosis of bulimia but may reflect AN-BP if a person is significantly underweight.

Individuals with anorexia nervosa engage in severe, persistent, and maladaptive dietary restriction characterized by a specific avoidance of dietary fat (Steinglass et al. 2015). Eating behavior in anorexia nervosa is highly stereotyped, including rearranging food on the plate, cutting food into small pieces, hiding food, slowing or frequently pausing eating, limiting food variety, and excessively consuming water during meals (Gianini et al. 2015). The weight loss and malnourishment resulting from persistent dietary restriction in anorexia nervosa are associated with a range of medical sequelae, including widespread disturbances in endocrine function, metabolism, and bone health. Common issues include electrolyte abnormalities (e.g., hypokalemia and hyponatremia), cardiovascular issues (e.g., bradycardia and arrhythmias), gastrointestinal problems (e.g., gastroparesis and constipation), orthostatic hypotension, low thyroid levels, hematologic changes (e.g., anemia and leukopenia), menstrual irregularities in females (e.g., amenorrhea), and osteopenia/osteoporosis (Walsh et al. 2023).

In addition to the deleterious physical effects of anorexia nervosa, the disorder also erodes psychological health. Compared with the general population, individuals with anorexia nervosa experience increased rates of anxiety, depression, OCD, and obsessive-compulsive personality disorder (OCPD) (Juli et al. 2023). For instance, OCPD has a general population prevalence of 8%, compared with 22% among patients with AN-R (Sansone and Sansone 2011). The characteristics of OCPD, such as a need for order, perfectionism, and excessive devotion to work, often align with and reinforce the symptoms of AN-R. This includes rigid dieting rules, meticulous calorie counting, and an unwavering focus on weight loss, often at the expense of social connections and overall well-being. In essence, the personality traits associated with OCPD can exacerbate the restrictive behaviors and rigid thinking patterns seen in AN-R (Sansone and Sansone 2011).

In the acute illness phase, anorexia nervosa can also contribute to emotional dysregulation; social isolation and relationship issues; cognitive impairments in memory, concentration, and decision-making; and suicide risk (Moskowitz and Weiselberg 2017). Anorexia nervosa has one of the highest mortality rates of all psychiatric illnesses, second only to opioid use disorder (Moskowitz and Weiselberg 2017). Clinicians should be aware of how patients' eating disorders are affecting their overall psychiatric presentation.

Atypical anorexia nervosa (AAN) was first incorporated by DSM-5 in 2013 and is categorized within DSM's Other Specified Feeding or Eating Disorders (OSFEDs). In AAN, patients maintain a normal or above-normal weight despite significant weight loss, and they meet all other criteria of anorexia nervosa, including fear of gaining weight and a disturbance in one's view of body weight or shape. Contrary to its "atypical" designation, accumulating evidence indicates that AAN is becoming increasingly prevalent, with a lifetime prevalence rate that is two to three times higher than that of anorexia nervosa; such prevalence is increasing youth psychiatric hospitalization rates (Kramer 2023).

Because of restrictive eating, individuals with AAN frequently experience the same physical health risks as patients with anorexia nervosa, presenting with similar rates of medical sequelae (e.g., bradycardia, electrolyte disturbances). With the caveat that research into AAN is in its infancy, both types can be equally dangerous, but the severity of vital sign abnormalities (e.g., bradycardia and hypotension) and complications may differ (Walsh et al. 2023). For instance, menstrual irregularities in females and osteopenia/osteoporosis are more common in anorexia nervosa.

Importantly, patients with higher body weight are at an almost 2.5-fold increased risk for disordered eating and tend to score higher on psychopathology as measured by the Eating Disorder Examination–Questionnaire (EDE-Q); nonetheless, they are less likely to be accurately diagnosed and treated (Forbes et al. 2014). This issue may be particularly salient for patients with AAN, whose clinicians may neglect to screen for—or who may even reinforce—weight loss; that is, when patients with higher BMI disclose that they are losing weight, many clinicians may reflexively encourage it because of the training that has ingrained the health risks of obesity. Such biases may lead to missed diagnoses and preventable health consequences, particularly in light of evidence that earlier treatment for eating disorders is associated with higher rates of remission (Nazar et al. 2017).

Bulimia Nervosa

Bulimia nervosa involves recurrent episodes of binge eating—consuming significantly more food than most people would in a short period (<2 hours), accompanied by a sense of loss of control over one's eating—followed by compensatory behaviors, at least once a week for 3 months (American Psychiatric Association 2022). Compensatory behaviors can involve self-induced vomiting, excessive exercise, fasting, or laxative use.

In terms of food choice, individuals with bulimia may consume large quantities of foods high in caloric content and dietary fat, with diminished regard for nutritional content during binges (e.g., sweets, desserts, sugary beverages, fast foods) (Gianini et al. 2019). Bulimia behaviors result in malnutrition as well as severe electrolyte abnormalities (e.g., individuals who vomit can develop hypokalemia and hypochloremic metabolic alkalosis; individuals who abuse laxatives can develop hyperchloremic metabolic alkalosis), sialadenosis (i.e., salivary gland hypertrophy), gastrointestinal issues (e.g., esophageal damage, gastroesophageal reflux disease, gastritis, gastroparesis, functional colonic impairment), dental problems (e.g., enamel erosion, cavities, dry mouth), and dehydration (Gibson et al. 2019). Even when bulimia is in remission, the physical effects of the disease on dentition (Nijakowski et al. 2023) and damage to the digestive tract (e.g., Barrett's esophagus dysplasia) may persist and continue to impact health (Denholm and Jankowski 2011). Bulimia is associated with an increased frequency of anxiety, depression, substance use disorders, and borderline personality disorder (Juli et al. 2023). For instance, borderline personality disorder—characterized by impulsivity and self-harm, among other features—has a general population prevalence of 6%, compared with 28% among patients with bulimia (Sansone and Sansone 2011). Impulsivity is evident in both binge-eating episodes and the subsequent counterregulatory behaviors, such as self-induced vomiting and the misuse of laxatives or diuretics, which can be considered forms of self-harm (Sansone and Sansone 2011).

Binge Eating Disorder

Binge eating disorder (BED) involves repeated episodes of binge eating at least once a week for at least 3 months, characterized by consuming large quantities of food in a short period and feeling a loss of control (American Psychiatric Association 2022). Although research is limited on food choices among patients with BED, current evidence demonstrates that binges involve a wide array of foods that are typically highly processed (Ayton et al. 2021). Accumulating evidence suggests that recurrent binge eating may alter the brain's reward system by altering food preferences and cravings (Gearhardt et al. 2009). These behaviors impact nutritional status and overall health. Individuals with BED can experience malnutrition due to a combination of food choices and irregular eating patterns that disrupt nutrient absorption and utilization (Ayton et al. 2021). Although binge eating episodes may involve consuming sizable quantities of food, the nutritional quality is often poor, largely consisting of ultraprocessed and carbohydrate-rich food (Ayton et al. 2021). The most prevalent medical complications of BED are chronic diseases related to obesity, including cardiovascular disease, type 2 diabetes, metabolic syndrome, and sleep apnea (Kessler et al. 2013). Psychologically, BED is associated with many of the same mental health comorbidities as bulimia (e.g., depression, anxiety disorders, substance use disorders) but may be less associated with personality disorders (Juli et al. 2023).

Avoidant/Restrictive Food Intake Disorder

Avoidant/restrictive food intake disorder (ARFID) is defined as a consistent failure to meet nutritional needs because of a lack of interest in eating, sensory sensitivity, or fear of adverse consequences, rather than a disturbance in body image or fear of weight gain (American Psychiatric Association 2022). Specifically, fear of adverse consequences (e.g., choking or vomiting); sensory sensitivities to certain flavors, smells, textures, or temperatures; and low appetitive drive may lead to reduced food intake and associated malnutrition (Fisher et al. 2014). Whereas anorexia nervosa and bulimia typically present in adolescence and overwhelmingly affect females (Hudson et al. 2007), ARFID commonly occurs in childhood and affects males and females similarly (Fisher et al. 2014). Diagnosis of ARFID may be delayed, as many patients will initially present to medical services (e.g., gastroenterology) out of concern for failure to thrive (Fisher et al. 2014).

Pica

Pica is the persistent eating of nonfood substances (e.g., dirt, clay, sand, paint chips, soap, hair, paper, cloth, ice, ash, detergent) over at least 1 month, not otherwise explained by a culturally supported or socially normative practice (American Psychiatric Association 2022). The preferential consumption of nonnutritive substances can replace nutritious foods and lead to inadequate intake of essential nutrients such as vitamins, minerals, and protein. Excessive ingestion of nonfood substances can also impair nutrient absorption of other foods and cause constipation, diarrhea, and intestinal obstruction (Rose et al. 2000). Additionally, nutritional status may be compromised by toxic exposures from paint chips or dirt contaminated with heavy metals. Such exposures can also increase the risk of psychosis (American Psychiatric Association 2022). Other psychiatric manifestations of pica include pica as an OCD-related compulsion. Pica is associated with higher rates of schizophrenia, trichotillomania, anxiety disorders, depression, and intellectual disability (Rose et al. 2000).

Rumination Disorder

Rumination disorder consists of food regurgitation followed by repeated chewing, swallowing, or spitting for a period of greater than 1 month (American Psychiatric Association 2022) and is often comorbid with intellectual disability, autism spectrum disorder, anxiety disorders, and OCD (Chial et al. 2013). Repeated regurgitation can lead to malnutrition, weight loss, gastrointestinal issues, and dental erosion (Chial et al. 2013).

Other Specified Feeding or Eating Disorder: Purging Disorder and Night Eating Syndrome

DSM-5 includes several diagnoses within the other specified feeding or eating disorder (OSFED) category, including AAN (discussed earlier), purging disorder, and night eating syndrome (NES). OSFED, the most common eating disorder, is a heterogeneous category, encompassing a variety of eating disorders with varying symptoms and severity (Fisher et al. 2014).

Purging disorder involves recurrent purging behavior (e.g., self-induced vomiting, laxative misuse, diuretic misuse) to control weight in the absence of binge eating. The physical sequelae of recurrent purging are similar to those observed in bulimia, including electrolyte imbalances (e.g., hypokalemia, hyponatremia), cardiac arrhythmias, esophageal tears, dental erosion, salivary gland enlargement, and gastrointestinal problems (Keel et al. 2005). A comprehensive evaluation to rule out alternative eating disorder diagnoses (e.g., AN-BP, bulimia, AAN), discussion of the dangerous physical symptoms associated with purging behavior, and referral to primary care for medical monitoring are integral aspects of care for individuals with purging disorder. Psychiatric comorbidities are similar to those of bulimia, including mood and anxiety disorders (Juli et al. 2023).

NES is defined by consuming a significant portion of daily calories late in the evening or during nighttime awakenings. Disruption of consistent daytime meal patterns and the natural rhythm of digestion can cause acid reflux, heartburn, and indigestion and can impair nutrient absorption (Allison et al. 2010). Individuals with NES also experience higher rates of mood disturbances, and insomnia can be associated with nighttime eating (Allison et al. 2010). Research shows that nighttime eating often includes highly processed foods (Allison et al. 2010). Because of the association between NES and circadian disruption and insomnia, it is crucial to screen for underlying mood, anxiety, substance use, and sleep disorders. In addition, it may be helpful to discuss sleep hygiene and work with patients to establish regular mealtimes.

Screening for Eating Disorders

The American Psychiatric Association (2023) recommends screening for eating disorders as part of any initial psychiatric evaluation, using validated tools like the SCOFF questionnaire (named for initialisms in its five questions) (Morgan et al. 2000) and the Eating Disorder Assessment for DSM-5 (EDA-5) (American Psychiatric Association 2016). Clinicians should conduct screening universally because well-documented blind spots exist, including diagnostic biases surrounding patients who have normal to high BMI (e.g., AAN) (Golden et al. 2016) or who do not fit the societal stereotype of eating disorders, including patients with diverse, minoritized identities (e.g., LGBTQ+; Black, Indigenous, People of Color [BIPOC]; low socioeconomic status) (Becker et al. 2017). Eating disorders are equally prevalent across socioeconomic status as well as racial and ethnic groups (Moreno et al. 2023), and individuals with multiple marginalized identities may be at higher risk, including low-income and LGBTQ+ individuals (Burke et al. 2023). Low-income patients and BIPOC are also more likely to have missed diagnoses and not receive treatment (Accurso et al. 2024).

When clinicians suspect an eating disorder is present based on initial screening, they should conduct a further assessment that includes evaluation of physical health (current BMI and longitudinal weight history); eating behaviors (food restrictions, avoidance, binge eating, compensatory behaviors, changes in food preferences or diet); psychological factors (preoccupation with food, weight, and body shape); family history; and eating disorder treatment history. The American Psychiatric Association additionally recommends a comprehensive evaluation for patients with a possible eating disorder, including assessment of physical health to measure vital signs, body weight, and signs of malnutrition; laboratory tests to assess electrolyte levels, liver function, kidney function, and micronutrient levels; psychiatric evaluation to identify co-occurring mental health conditions, eating patterns, weight control behaviors, and body image concerns; and a medical history review, identifying any medical conditions that are associated with or exacerbated by an eating disorder (American Psychiatric Association 2022). Electrocardiograms should be obtained in patients with restrictive or purging behaviors, as well as those receiving QTc-prolonging medications (American Psychiatric Association 2022).

Food Insecurity and Eating Disorders

Food insecurity, which is defined as limited or uncertain access to adequate amounts of safe and nutritious food, may mimic an eating disorder (Gundersen and Ziliak 2015). For instance, individuals may demonstrate an overreliance on certain foods because they are less expensive, may appear to binge eat when Supplemental Nutrition Assistance Program benefits come in, and may restrict food intake so that their children or other dependents have enough food. Clinicians should consider screening using tools such as the Hunger Vital Sign questions or others described in Chapter 6 ("Food- and Nutrition-Related Rating Scales and Assessment in the Clinical Setting"). Although food insecurity can impact nutrition separately, patients can be both food insecure and have an eating disorder. Notably, experiencing food insecurity can increase the risk for certain eating disorders, particularly bulimia and BED (Accurso et al. 2024). Moreover, a positive screening for food security alone is associated with significant mental health impacts (Cain et al. 2022) and is important to address when thinking more broadly about a patient's differential diagnosis and treatment.

Treating eating disorders in individuals experiencing food insecurity presents unique challenges, including limited resources, difficulty establishing regular eating patterns, and the psychological impacts of scarcity. Therefore, clinicians should prioritize the individual's needs and preferences, considering their cultural background, socioeconomic status, and personal experiences. Clinicians may collaborate with a multidisciplinary team, including social workers and dietitians, to help patients access regular, nutritious meals through food pantries, other community organizations, or government assistance programs; secure stable housing to provide a safe and supportive environment for recovery; and develop meal plans that are affordable, accessible, nutritious, and culturally appropriate. Alternatively, patients who do not screen positive may continue to have an elevated risk of developing an eating disorder and should continue to be monitored as their treatment evolves.

Outside of eating disorders, the presence of a serious mental illness raises the probability of individuals being food insecure (Smith et al. 2024). Psychiatric symptoms can be functionally impairing, limit people's livelihoods, and result in low socioeconomic status. With the stereotype of eating disorders being more prevalent in higher socioeconomic groups, providers should counteract their diagnostic bias by jointly using tools like the SCOFF or EDA-5 alongside the Hunger Vital Sign. Chapter 5 ("Food Insecurity and Mental Health") provides more information on food insecurity.

Clinical Considerations for Patients With Eating Disorders

Eating disorders, especially anorexia nervosa, often lead to malnutrition because of restricted food intake and impaired nutrient absorption. Significant weight loss results in a decreased basal metabolic rate (Hanachi et al. 2019), which improves with weight restoration (Schebendach et al. 1995). Individuals with anorexia nervosa are also at a higher risk of heart arrhythmias, bradycardia, prolonged QT interval, and seizures due to electrolyte imbalances from restriction and purging. Along with increased suicide risk, these serious effects on various organ systems underpin the staggering mortality rate associated with anorexia nervosa (Moskowitz and Weiselberg 2017).

Nutrient deficiencies can extend beyond macronutrients (i.e., carbohydrates, protein, fats) to deficiencies of essential vitamins and minerals (i.e., micronutrients) that can cause a host of medical issues. Micronutrient deficiencies predominantly affect individuals with anorexia nervosa and include deficiencies in vitamin B12, folate, iron, calcium, vitamin D, zinc, and iodine (Achamrah et al. 2017). Poor micronutrient status secondary to eating disorders can impair red blood cell production, tissue oxygenation, nerve function, immune system strength, wound healing, bone health, and thyroid function (Achamrah et al. 2017). Clinicians treating patients with eating disorders should monitor for signs and symptoms of these medical issues.

Providers should weigh the risks and benefits when considering medications that could increase the risk of medical complications in low-weight individuals or those who purge, such as arrhythmias (e.g.,

QTc-prolonging antipsychotics, selective serotonin reuptake inhibitors [SSRIs], antihistamines), bradycardia (e.g., clonidine), electrolyte imbalances (e.g., hyponatremia from SSRIs, serotonin norepinephrine reuptake inhibitors [SNRIs], and lithium), and seizures (e.g., bupropion, clozapine, clomipramine, and benzodiazepine withdrawal). For example, medications such as lithium, with a narrow therapeutic window, should be used cautiously in patients with active purging behavior, as dehydration could result in supratherapeutic lithium levels. Other medications require food intake for optimal absorption, which may render them suboptimal for patients with a restrictive eating disorder. For example, absorption of medications such as ziprasidone and lurasidone is reduced by approximately 50% if they are taken without sufficient food (Gandelman et al. 2009). In addition, the body's energy conservation during caloric deficit can lead to hormonal imbalances, most commonly resulting in amenorrhea in anorexia nervosa and oligomenorrhea in bulimia, both of which can result in reduced bone density (Robinson et al. 2017). Clinicians may consider avoiding medications that increase the risk of infertility (e.g., risperidone through prolactin increase) or falls and resulting fractures (e.g., benzodiazepines). Clinicians should use shared decision-making with patients to assess medication initiation and longitudinal monitoring.

Altogether, clinicians are likely to encounter patients with eating disorders that have far-reaching effects on their nutritional status and metabolism, which should be accounted for when providing care. The clinical considerations discussed above are summarized in Table 11.2. Not all patients will have each of the above complications from their disorder. However, awareness is the critical first step in facilitating informed discussions with patients and ensuring safe, effective, and holistic psychiatric treatment.

Non-DSM Disordered Eating Patterns

Although DSM identifies the most ubiquitous and severe eating disorders, it is helpful to have a clinical awareness of disordered eating patterns that do not meet diagnostic thresholds, especially given their prevalence in the media and potential adverse health effects. Research is emerging around patterns of disordered eating, including food addiction, orthorexia, and emotional eating (Table 11.3). The eating patterns discussed here are not included in DSM or American Psy-

Table 11.2 Key clinical considerations when treating patients with eating disorders

Clinical consideration	Detailed guidance
Medication choice	Avoid QTc-prolonging medications (e.g., certain antipsychotics, SSRIs, antihistamines, clonidine) in patients at risk for arrhythmias due to electrolyte imbalances and bradycardia. In patients who purge, use caution with medications that depend on fluid balance for therapeutic levels (e.g., lithium). In the presence of electrolyte imbalances and malnutrition, consider alternatives to medications that can lower the seizure threshold (e.g., bupropion, clozapine, clomipramine, benzodiazepine withdrawal). In patients with amenorrhea and oligomenorrhea, use shared decision-making when considering medications that increase the risk of infertility (e.g., risperidone). In patients with reduced bone density, consider avoiding medications that increase fall and fracture risk (e.g., benzodiazepines).
Medical monitoring	Monitor for signs and symptoms of electrolyte imbalance (e.g., weakness, fatigue, irregular heartbeat, seizures). Regularly assess weight and BMI trends. Assess for medical sequelae through lab work (e.g., complete blood count, iron panel, vitamin levels, electrolytes, renal function, liver function).
Psychiatric monitoring	Screen for co-occurring mental health conditions (e.g., depression, anxiety, substance use disorders). Be aware of the increased risk of suicide in patients with eating disorders.
Patient education and counseling	Educate patients about the physical and psychological effects of eating disorders. Provide support and encouragement for recovery. Encourage patients to seek nutritional counseling and medical care as needed. Engage in shared decision-making regarding treatment options.

Table 11.2 Key clinical considerations when treating patients with eating disorders (*continued*)

Clinical consideration	Detailed guidance
Collaboration	Collaborate with other health care professionals (e.g., primary care physicians, dietitians, therapists) to provide comprehensive care. Refer patients to specialized eating disorder treatment programs when necessary.

BMI = body mass index; SSRI = selective serotonin reuptake inhibitor.

chiatric Association treatment guidelines because research is nascent and mixed. As research on disordered eating grows, clinicians should understand their patients' eating behaviors to discern whether they meet DSM diagnostic thresholds and be able to discuss how patients' food intake may be affecting their nutritional status and mental health.

Much debate exists surrounding eating patterns not included in DSM. The controversy is multifaceted. One salient issue is that eating patterns such as orthorexia and food addiction have symptoms that overlap with those of eating disorders clearly defined in the DSM—orthorexia with anorexia nervosa, OCD, and anxiety disorders; food addiction with binge-eating disorder, bulimia nervosa, and substance use disorders—thus complicating differential diagnosis. Second, there is substantial subjectivity in what constitutes "healthy" eating, which applies a narrow sociocultural lens and risks pathologizing eating, altogether complicating the identification of overeating or orthorexia. Additionally, the neurobiological mechanisms underlying eating patterns such as food addiction remain unclear. Some studies suggest that certain foods may activate reward pathways, but the relationship between food intake and psychological factors remains complex. Finally, the limited and often low-quality research on these conditions hinders the development of robust, evidence-based diagnostic and treatment practices. This lack of clarity and evidence creates significant barriers to effectively addressing these eating patterns. Ultimately, the lack of ideological and research consensus has led to the exclusion of these eating behaviors from recognition in DSM, which creates challenges in diagnosis, research, and treatment.

It is worth noting that this exploration is not aimed at pathologizing eating patterns that are outside of the well-delineated DSM disorders.

Table 11.3 Emerging concepts pertaining to disordered eating

Eating pattern	Key characteristics	Potential impact	Clinical considerations
Emotional eating	Eating in response to emotions rather than hunger	Weight gain; nutrient deficiencies; digestive issues	Identify emotional triggers; develop coping mechanisms; promote mindful eating
Food addiction	Compulsive food intake, loss of control, cravings	Nutrient deficiencies; obesity; metabolic disorders	Assess for binge eating disorder; consider behavioral interventions; monitor for co-occurring mental health conditions
Orthorexia	Obsessive focus on healthy eating, rigid dietary rules	Malnutrition; nutrient deficiencies; social isolation	Screen for anorexia nervosa or atypical anorexia nervosa; address distorted thinking patterns; encourage a balanced diet

Note. These non-DSM disordered eating patterns are emerging areas of research, and related clinical information is evolving.

Like emotional states, eating patterns can vary day to day, minute to minute, and it is not until there are negative health consequences or functional impairment that clinicians may wish to address such issues. Clinicians should remember that general scientific consensus does not yet exist around the diagnostic definitions, prevalence, risk factors, management, or treatment of the eating patterns discussed next. Rather than guiding clinical decision-making, this section can aid clinicians in discussing eating habits with patients by informing them about the spectrum of disordered eating that is increasingly present online (and may be raised by patients).

Emotional Eating

The interplay between emotions and eating is a visceral, universal truth—people are all too familiar with the trope of wanting to consume a tub of ice cream after a relationship breakup. Emotional eating is not a new concept, but its scientific study is more recent. As defined in research, emotional eating is the propensity to consume food in response to emotional states rather than hunger (Reichenberger et al. 2020). Hunger is an evolutionary response. Thus, it is unsurprising that research has identified both neurobiological and psychological factors that mediate the development of feeling hungry. Emotional eating is not a problem in and of itself—it's human—but eating more frequently in response to emotional rather than hunger stimuli may disrupt regular meal patterns. These behaviors can lead to difficulties in maintaining balanced diets and appropriate caloric intake in relation to the body's energy needs, with some studies identifying emotional eating as a risk factor for recurrent weight gain (Konttinen et al. 2019).

Like food addiction described below, research has also found that emotional eating may be correlated with dysregulation of the brain's reward system and driven by stress, anxiety, depression, and boredom (Reichenberger et al. 2020). If a client brings up their eating and how it relates to their emotions, a clinician may first assess the frequency, severity, and distress of emotional eating episodes to understand if it may better be characterized as BED or another DSM disorder. In addition to screening for clinical mood disorders and prior trauma, clinicians may work with patients to identify emotional triggers for eating, explore emotion regulation strategies (e.g., dialectical behavioral therapy distress tolerance skills focused on temperature change, intense exercise, and paced breathing), and develop adaptive coping skills.

Food Addiction

A controversial subject within the scientific community, food addiction has been postulated as compulsive food intake that is associated with a loss of control, intense cravings, and continued use despite negative consequences, while not meeting criteria for BED (Whatnall et al. 2022). Food addiction is receiving increased focus in scientific literature and the media, especially with growing research on glucagon-like peptide 1 (GLP-1) receptor agonists and their potential to decrease "addictive" eating behaviors (Bruns Vi et al. 2024). Some research has demonstrated that overeating may not be defined by "choice" but instead may have overlapping properties with substance addiction (Gordon et al. 2018). In 2013, gambling disorder was the first behavioral addiction included in DSM owing to the body of research demonstrating parallel behavioral symptoms and neurophysiology (i.e., how stress and biological risk factors impact predisposition) to substance use disorders (American Psychiatric Association 2022). The Yale Food Addiction Scale (YFAS) is a self-report questionnaire that operationalizes the criteria for DSM substance use disorders to capture the loss of control, cravings, physical dependence, and tolerance some people may feel when eating (Gearhardt et al. 2009). Initial evidence regarding the physical impacts of food addiction shows potential impaired nutrition due to preferential consumption of processed and ultraprocessed foods rather than fresh fruits and vegetables, whole grains, and other nutritious foods that contain a multitude of vital nutrients (Whatnall et al. 2022).

Some research has proposed that the concept of food addiction is closely related to consuming ultraprocessed foods, may involve changes to the reward system neurocircuitry via serotonin and dopamine modulation, and can result in symptoms emblematic of other addictive disorders (e.g., cravings, loss of control, withdrawal symptoms) (Whatnall et al. 2022). However, the level of physical, mental, and social impairment needs to be further investigated to better understand whether it is a disorder distinct from BED, as someone experiencing binge episodes would be diagnosed with BED. In light of the robust evidence on the health effects of BED versus the varied literature on food addiction, clinicians need to be able to discern whether eating patterns meet DSM criteria and offer patients appropriate, evidence-based treatment. Further research on the hypothesized idea of food addiction will uncover how it is different from BED and inform the treatment of medical comorbidities that may result when patients chronically consume food in higher quantities than their daily caloric needs (e.g., diabetes, cardiovascular disease) (World Health Organization 2024).

Orthorexia

The rise of wellness influencers and social media posts touting "clean eating" has led to increased attention to a subclinical pattern of irregular eating called orthorexia: the preoccupation with clean or "healthy" eating (Turner and Lefevre 2017). Orthorexia encompasses a spectrum of behaviors and attitudes toward eating that involve rigid dietary rules and extreme fixation on food quality and purity, which can lead to digestive issues, malnutrition, and functional or psychological impairment. Orthorexia can range from avoiding processed foods, artificial additives, and genetically modified organism (GMO)-containing foods to eliminating entire food groups. At its extreme, making mindful dietary choices can shift into consuming only foods perceived as pure. These restrictive behaviors may share properties with anorexia nervosa, and individuals should be screened appropriately; unhealthy restrictive eating should not be rebranded as clean eating. Clinicians should do a comprehensive clinical evaluation to determine whether a patient has lost weight, is underweight, or is engaging in restricting, binge eating, or purging. Clinicians can also complete the SCOFF or EDA-5 to ensure that they are not missing a DSM eating disorder diagnosis while additionally screening for potential OCD and OCPD given coinciding traits (e.g., excessive meal planning, ritualistic eating).

If individuals do not meet clinical thresholds for an eating disorder, it is still important for clinicians to discuss with patients how strict dietary choices may impact their nutritional status and psychological or social functioning. For instance, in the same way that a patient adhering to a strict vegan diet may become iron or vitamin B12 deficient, someone adhering to a ketogenic diet and avoiding carbohydrates may similarly develop deficiencies in B vitamins, fiber, and specific minerals (Patikorn et al. 2023) or may not have sufficient energy. In addition, a person eating a limited range of foods may disrupt their gut microbiome and experience constipation, bloating, and irritable bowel syndrome (Marano et al. 2025). Clinicians may refer patients for nutritional counseling if they are concerned that patients' subclinical eating patterns are harming their nutritional status; a dietitian may assist in developing a more balanced and flexible eating plan. Additional clinical considerations for mental health providers include examining how a patient's sustained focus on consuming certain foods may lead to anxiety/depression, body image issues, lack of socializing, and reduced enjoyment from food or activities such as cooking together or eating together.

Psychiatric Symptoms and Disordered Eating

Regardless of diagnosis, food is imperative to all patients' functioning, health, and well-being. From psychotic illnesses to mood disorders, patients' psychiatric symptomology may contribute to irregular eating and suboptimal nutrition. Although patients' consumption patterns may not meet clinical thresholds, clinicians should be aware of the potential impact of patients' disordered eating that may result from their primary psychiatric illness. Following is a nonexhaustive list of disorders most likely to influence appetite or eating patterns.

Psychotic illnesses, characterized by disturbances in thought, perception, and behavior, can profoundly impact eating habits and nutritional status. Delusional beliefs about food safety or contamination may lead to restrictive eating patterns, resulting in malnutrition (Seeman 2014). Cognitive impairments and disorganized thinking can hinder meal planning and preparation, leading to irregular eating patterns and poor food choices (Addington and Addington 2000). Additionally, negative symptoms, such as reduced motivation and anhedonia, can diminish interest in food or the healthfulness of one's diet and can decrease appetite (Kirkpatrick et al. 2006).

Similarly, mood disorders can have significant negative effects on eating. Depressive symptoms such as amotivation and low energy may lead to a reduced ability to grocery shop and prepare meals; lack of appetite, social isolation, and anhedonia may limit food enjoyment and engagement in opportunities for social eating (American Psychiatric Association 2022). Alternatively, individuals with atypical depression may experience increased appetite with overeating or emotional eating. Both depression and mania can disrupt daily routines and circadian rhythm, which can lead to irregular meal patterns (Akbar and Shi 2024). Mood disorders also often co-occur with substance use (Conway et al. 2006), and most clinicians are familiar with the impact of chronic alcohol or illicit substance use on nutrition.

Certain substances, such as stimulants, can suppress appetite, leading to reduced food intake and potential weight loss. On the other hand, other substances, including alcohol, stimulants, cannabis, and opioids, can stimulate appetite and lead to poor food choices, with individuals opting for high-calorie, low-nutrient foods, such as ultra-processed foods and snacks, as well as fast food (Mahboub et al. 2021). In addition, substance use can interfere with nutrient absorption and metabolism, leading to malnutrition (Mahboub et al. 2021). Alcohol, for example, can both acutely (e.g., alcohol-associated hepatitis) and chronically (e.g., alcoholic fatty liver disease and cirrhosis) damage the liver, which is crucial for nutrient processing (Louvet and Mathurin 2015). In addition, chronic alcohol use can cause electrolyte imbalances (e.g., hypokalemia, hypomagnesemia, hyponatremia) and deplete key micronutrients, including thiamine, folate, magnesium, zinc, and vitamins B6, C, A, and D (Lieber 1975). Substance use can disrupt regular mealtimes, leading to irregular eating patterns. Substance use, such as heavy alcohol or methamphetamine consumption, can also lead to dental problems, making it difficult to eat and enjoy food.

Patients with borderline personality disorder are also more likely to exhibit substance use or disrupted eating patterns (Trull et al. 2000). For instance, they may use food to cope with negative emotions, stress, boredom, or loneliness. During periods of emotional distress, individuals with borderline personality disorder may restrict their food intake and, during periods of impulsivity, they may engage in binge-eating episodes.

OCD can also influence eating and create nutrient deficiencies through food contamination fears, rigid meal rituals, and compulsive eating behaviors (e.g., binge eating or restrictive eating) that do not meet criteria for a DSM eating disorder (American Psychiatric Association 2022). Finally, autism spectrum disorder may be a risk factor for nutrient deficiencies given the high prevalence of restrictive eating patterns, picky eating due to sensory sensitivities, and gastrointestinal issues (e.g., constipation, diarrhea, irritable bowel syndrome) (Bandini et al. 2010).

Psychiatric Medications and Disordered Eating

In addition to psychiatric symptoms, medications used to treat certain psychiatric disorders—including second-generation antipsychotics—may increase appetite, and stimulants used to treat ADHD may cause appetite suppression. Bupropion may decrease appetite, whereas mirtazapine, SNRIs, valproic acid, and lithium can increase appetite. Using well-documented medication side effect profiles, clinicians should discuss how medications may influence appetite and eating habits and, in turn, nutritional status. The impact of antipsychotics, antidepressants, and mood stabilizers on appetite—and the potential for iatrogenic weight gain and related consequences—is discussed further in Chapter 10 ("Psychotropic Medications, Increased Appetite, and Iatrogenic Weight Gain").

Eating disorders often co-occur with other mental illnesses. As discussed above, patients' psychiatric presentations, levels of functioning, and medications can affect their eating in the absence of a DSM eating disorder diagnosis. If a clinician is concerned about a patient's nutrition, it may be appropriate to follow weight, BMI, and waist circumference; pursue lab work (e.g., A1C, glucose, complete blood count, vitamin levels, mineral levels, electrolytes, renal function, liver function, lipids); consider nutrient supplementation; and make a referral to an internist and registered dietitian.

Future Research Directions

Based on the content presented in this chapter, several key areas emerge as crucial directions for research in the field of eating disorders and disordered eating. AAN is a growing concern, with increasing diagnoses and hospitalizations. To better understand this condition, longitudinal studies on health outcomes are needed. Research should focus on identifying risk factors and comparing the long-term physical and psychological impacts of AAN to those of anorexia nervosa, which would inform the development of more effective treatment strategies and improve prognosis. Furthermore, considering the trend toward personalized medicine and the higher likelihood of missed diagnoses in AAN, research into biological markers is essential. Studies should aim to identify hormonal, genetic, and neurological markers with high sensitivity and specificity to aid in the identification of eating disorders.

With growing research highlighting the diverse impacts of eating disorders, there is a clear need to counteract diagnostic bias. This requires the development and validation of culturally sensitive screening tools that are effective for diverse populations, including LGBTQ+, BIPOC, and individuals from low socioeconomic backgrounds. Moreover, a deeper understanding of the prevalence, specific manifestations, and unique risk factors of eating disorders in understudied populations is essential. Finally, research is needed to adapt existing therapies and develop new interventions tailored to address the specific needs and challenges faced by these diverse populations.

This chapter also reviews "subclinical" patterns of disordered eating being explored by researchers, such as orthorexia and food addiction. However, more research is required regarding the definitions and differences from DSM eating disorders, distinct pathophysiology, and potential long-term physical and psychological health impacts of these behaviors. This research would help to clarify the trajectory and potential clinical significance of these patterns, informing prevention and early intervention efforts.

Future research should also investigate the shared neurobiological and psychological mechanisms that underlie eating disorders and co-occurring conditions such as depression, anxiety, OCD, and substance use disorders. This will help in developing and testing integrated treatment approaches that effectively address both eating disorders and the co-occurring mental health conditions. Furthermore, it is essential to conduct further research on the multifactorial relationship between psychiatric medications and eating disorders and explore how these medications may influence appetite, weight, and eating behaviors.

Finally, research should focus on designing and evaluating interventions that concurrently address food insecurity and eating disorders, recognizing the potential synergistic effects of these conditions. Research is also needed on eating disorder treatment that addresses the unique challenges faced by those with food insecurity. Moreover, it is important to research the impact of social policies and programs aimed at alleviating food insecurity on the prevalence and treatment of eating disorders and other psychiatric conditions.

Clinical Pearls

- Clinicians should screen universally for eating disorders, using validated tools such as the SCOFF questionnaire and the Eating Disorder Assessment for DSM-5 (EDA-5) as part of any initial psychiatric evaluation. Eating disorders are prevalent in psychiatric patient populations and often go undetected, undiagnosed, and untreated.
- Clinicians should be mindful of diagnostic biases. Implicit biases about weight, gender, race, ethnicity, or socioeconomic status can influence assessment. Eating disorders can affect anyone. Pay close attention to atypical presentations, such as those with normal or high BMI, as seen in atypical anorexia nervosa. Given higher remission with earlier diagnosis, missed diagnoses have significant consequences.
- Clinicians should tailor medication management to the individual's needs. When prescribing psychiatric medications for patients with eating disorders, carefully consider the potential for drug interactions, adverse effects, and the impact on physical and mental health. Consider avoiding medications that heighten risks of arrhythmias (e.g., QTc-prolonging antipsychotics, selective serotonin reuptake inhibitors [SSRIs], antihistamines), bradycardia (e.g., clonidine), electrolyte imbalances (e.g., hyponatremia from SSRIs, serotonin norepinephrine reuptake inhibitors [SNRIs], and lithium), and seizures (e.g., bupropion, clozapine, clomipramine, and benzodiazepine withdrawal). Assess for purging behavior when using medications such as lithium, as serum levels can widely fluctuate based on fluid balance.

- Patients may engage in disordered eating patterns that do not meet DSM criteria. Clinicians should be prepared to assess these disordered eating patterns—such as emotional eating, food addiction, orthorexia, night eating syndrome, and purging disorder—with their patients and screen them for DSM eating disorders.
- Clinicians should recognize the complex interplay between eating disorders and other mental health conditions. Eating disorders frequently co-occur with conditions such as depression, anxiety, substance use disorders, OCD, and PTSD. These conditions can influence each other, so it is essential to consider both when developing a treatment plan.

Key Chapter Points

- Eating disorders are prevalent and can have serious physical and psychological consequences that influence nutritional status and, in turn, psychiatric treatment (e.g., medication choices).
- Irregular eating patterns that do not meet diagnostic thresholds (e.g., emotional eating, food addiction, orthorexia) can still affect nutritional status and psychiatric treatment.
- Patients with eating disorders do not fit a unitary profile. Clinician bias regarding who gets eating disorders and the diverse patient populations afflicted necessitate universal screening and methodical monitoring for the physical and psychological effects of disordered eating: nutritional deficiencies, electrolyte imbalances, organ damage, metabolic changes, and psychological impacts.
- Food insecurity can impact eating patterns by negatively affecting mental health (e.g., increasing stress, depression, and anxiety) and mimicking eating disorders (e.g., patients may exhibit an overreliance on less expensive foods, appear to binge eat when Supplemental Nutrition Assistance Program benefits come in, and restrict food intake so that their children or other dependents have enough food). Food insecurity can also co-occur with eating disorders. Binge-eating disorders are higher in populations facing food insecurity, highlighting the importance of screening patients for eating disorders and food insecurity (using tools such as the Hunger Vital Sign to assess for food insecurity) and the potential impact on a patient's eating patterns and nutritional status.

- From delusions to compulsions to disorganized behavior, a complex interplay exists between psychiatric disorders and irregular eating that can shape nutritional status.

References

Accurso EC, Cordell KD, Guydish J, Snowden LR: Exploring demographic and clinical characteristics of racially and ethnically diverse youth with eating disorders using California Medicaid claims data. J Am Acad Child Adolesc Psychiatry 63(6):615–623, 2024 37992854

Achamrah N, Coëffier M, Rimbert A, et al: Micronutrient status in 153 patients with anorexia nervosa. Nutrients 9(3):225, 2017 28257095

Addington J, Addington D: Neurocognitive and social functioning in schizophrenia: a 2.5 year follow-up study. Schizophr Res 44(1):47–56, 2000 10867311

Akbar Z, Shi Z: Unfavorable mealtime, meal skipping, and shiftwork are associated with circadian syndrome in adults participating in NHANES 2005–2016. Nutrients 16(11):581, 2024 38892514

Allison KC, Lundgren JD, O'Reardon JP, et al: Proposed diagnostic criteria for night eating syndrome. Int J Eat Disord 43(3):241–247, 2010 19378289

American Psychiatric Association: Diagnostic and Statistical Manual of Mental Disorders (3rd ed.), Washington, DC, American Psychiatric Association Publishing, 1980

American Psychiatric Association: Eating Disorder Assessment for DSM-5 (EDA-5). Washington, DC, American Psychiatric Association Publishing, 2016

American Psychiatric Association: Diagnostic and Statistical Manual of Mental Disorders (5th ed., Text Revision). Washington, DC, American Psychiatric Association Publishing, 2022

American Psychiatric Association: The American Psychiatric Association Practice Guideline for the Treatment of Patients with Eating Disorders, 4th edition. Washington, DC, American Psychiatric Association Publishing, 2023

Ayton A, Ibrahim A, Dugan J, et al: Ultra-processed foods and binge eating: a retrospective observational study. Nutrition 84:111023, 2021 33153827

Bandini LG, Anderson SE, Curtin C, et al: Food selectivity in children with autism spectrum disorders and typically developing children. J Pediatr 157(2):259–264, 2010 20362301

Barakat S, McLean SA, Bryant E, et al; National Eating Disorder Research Consortium: Risk factors for eating disorders: findings from a rapid review. J Eat Disord 11(1):8, 2023 36650572

Becker AE, Kleinman KP, Sonneville KR: Eating disorders in diverse populations. Curr Opin Psychiatry 30(6):423–429, 2017 28777107

Bruns Vi N, Tressler EH, Vendruscolo LF, et al: IUPHAR review: Glucagon-like peptide-1 (GLP-1) and substance use disorders: an emerging pharmacotherapeutic target. Pharmacol Res 207:107312, 2024 39032839

Brytek-Brykalska A, Baran A, Harasym J, et al: The gut microbiome in eating disorders. Nutrients 15(12):2748, 2023

Burke NL, Hazzard VM, Schaefer LM, et al: Socioeconomic status and eating disorder prevalence: at the intersections of gender identity, sexual orientation, and race/ethnicity. Psychol Med 53(9):4255–4265, 2023 35574702

Cain KS, Meyer SC, Cummer E, et al: Association of food insecurity with mental health outcomes in parents and children. Acad Pediatr 22(7):1105–1114, 2022 35577282

Chial HJ, Camilleri M, Williams DE: Rumination syndrome: diagnosis, treatment, and pathophysiology. Am J Gastroenterol 108(5):603–610, 2013

Conway KP, Compton W, Stinson FS, et al: Lifetime comorbidity of DSM-IV mood and anxiety disorders and specific drug use disorders: results from the National Epidemiologic Survey on Alcohol and Related Conditions. J Clin Psychiatry 67(2):247–257, 2006 16566620

Denholm M, Jankowski J: Gastroesophageal reflux disease and bulimia nervosa: a review of the literature. Dis Esophagus 24(2):79–85, 2011 21276151

Fisher MM, Rosen DS, Ornstein RM, et al: Characteristics of avoidant/restrictive food intake disorder in children and adolescents: a "new disorder" in DSM-5. J Adolesc Health 55(1):49–52, 2014 24506978

Forbes B, Cooper Z, Shafran R: Psychological treatments for anorexia nervosa: a systematic review and meta-analysis. Int J Eat Disord 47(7):683–695, 2014

Galmiche M, Déchelotte P, Lambert G, et al: Prevalence of eating disorders over the 2000–2018 period: a systematic literature review. Am J Clin Nutr 109(5):1402–1413, 2019 31051507

Gandelman K, Alderman JA, Glue P, et al: The impact of calories and fat content of meals on oral ziprasidone absorption: a randomized, open-label, crossover trial. J Clin Psychiatry 70(1):58–62, 2009 19026256

Gay R: Hunger: A Memoir of (My) Body. New York, Harper, 2017

Gearhardt AN, Corbin WR, Brownell KD: Preliminary validation of the Yale Food Addiction Scale. Appetite 52(2):430–436, 2009 19121351

Gianini L, Foerde K, Walsh BT, et al: Negative affect, dietary restriction, and food choice in bulimia nervosa. Eat Behav 33:49–54, 2019 30903862

Gianini L, Liu Y, Wang Y, et al: Abnormal eating behavior in video-recorded meals in anorexia nervosa. Eat Behav 19:28–32, 2015 26164671

Gibson D, Workman C, Mehler PS: Medical complications of anorexia nervosa and bulimia nervosa. Psychiatr Clin North Am 42(2):263–274, 2019 31046928

Golden NH, Schneider M, Wood C: Preventing obesity and eating disorders in adolescents. Pediatrics 138(3):e20161649, 2016 27550979

Gordon EL, Ariel-Donges AH, Bauman V, et al: What is the evidence for "food addiction"? A systematic review. Nutrients 10(4):477, 2018 29649120

Gundersen C, Ziliak JP: Food insecurity and health outcomes. Health Aff (Millwood) 34(11):1830–1839, 2015 26526240

Hambleton A, Pepin G, Le A, et al: Psychiatric and medical comorbidities of eating disorders: findings from a rapid review of the literature. J Eat Disord 10(1):132, 2022 36064606

Hanachi M, Dicembre M, Rives-Lange C: Micronutrients deficiencies in 374 severely malnourished anorexia nervosa inpatients. Nutrients 11(4):792, 2019

Hudson JI, Hiripi E, Pope HG, et al: The prevalence and correlates of eating disorders in the National Comorbidity Survey Replication. Biol Psychiatry 61(3):348–358, 2007 16815322

Juli R, Juli MR, Juli G, et al: Eating disorders and psychiatric comorbidity. Psychiatr Danub 35(Suppl 2):217–220, 2023 37800230

Kaye WH, Bulik CM, Thornton L, et al: The complex interplay between eating disorders and psychiatric comorbidity. CNS Spectr 9(6):435–445, 2004

Keel PK, Haedt A, Edler C: Purging disorder: an ominous variant of bulimia nervosa? Int J Eat Disord 38(3):191–199, 2005 16211629

Kessler RC, Berglund PA, Chiu WT, et al: The prevalence and correlates of binge eating disorder in the World Health Organization world mental health surveys. Biol Psychiatry 73(9):904–914, 2013 23290497

Kirkpatrick B, Fenton WS, Carpenter WT, et al: The NIMH-MATRICS consensus statement on negative symptoms. Schizophr Bull 32(2):214–219, 2006 16481659

Konttinen H, van Strien T, Männistö S, et al: Depression, emotional eating and long-term weight changes: a population-based prospective study. Int J Behav Nutr Phys Act 16:28, 2019

Kramer R: Considerations in evidence-based treatment of adolescents with atypical anorexia nervosa. J Health Serv Psychol 49(1):41–51, 2023 36811063

Lieber CS: Alcohol and malnutrition in the pathogenesis of liver disease. JAMA 233(10):1077–1080, 1975 1174154

Louvet A, Mathurin P: Alcoholic liver disease: mechanisms of injury and targeted treatment. Nat Rev Gastroenterol Hepatol 12(4):231–242, 2015 25782093

Mahboub N, Rizk R, Karavetian M, et al: Nutritional status and eating habits of people who use drugs and/or are undergoing treatment for recovery: a narrative review. Nutr Rev 79(6):627–635, 2021 32974658

Marano G, Rossi S, Sfratta G, et al: Gut microbiota in women with eating disorders: a new frontier in pathophysiology and treatment. Nutrients 17(14):2316, 2025

Moreno R, Buckelew SM, Accurso EC, et al: Disparities in access to eating disorders treatment for publicly-insured youth and youth of color: a retrospective cohort study. J Eat Disord 11(1):10, 2023 36694235

Morgan JF, Reid F, Lacey JH: The SCOFF questionnaire: a new screening tool for eating disorders. West J Med 172(3):164–165, 2000 18751246

Moskowitz L, Weiselberg E: Anorexia nervosa/atypical anorexia nervosa. Curr Probl Pediatr Adolesc Health Care 47(4):70–84, 2017 28532965

Nagata JM, Ganson KT, Austin SB: Emerging trends in eating disorders among sexual and gender minorities. Curr Opin Psychiatry 33(6):562–567, 2020 32858597

Nazar BP, Gregor LK, Albano G, et al: Early response to treatment in eating disorders: a systematic review and a diagnostic test accuracy meta-analysis. Eur Eat Disord Rev 25(2):67–79, 2017 27928853

Nijakowski K, Jankowski J, Gruszczyński D, et al: Eating disorders and dental erosion: a systematic review. J Clin Med 12(19):6161, 2023 37834805

Pastore M, Indrio F, Bali D, et al: Alarming increase of eating disorders in children and adolescents. J Pediatr 263:113733, 2023 37717906

Patikorn C, Saidoung P, Pham T, et al: Effects of ketogenic diet on health outcomes: an umbrella review of meta-analyses of randomized clinical trials. BMC Med 21(1):196, 2023 37231411

Reichenberger J, Schnepper R, Arend AK, et al: Emotional eating in healthy individuals and patients with an eating disorder: evidence from psychometric, experimental and naturalistic studies. Proc Nutr Soc 79(3):290–299, 2020 32398186

Robinson L, Micali N, Misra M: Eating disorders and bone metabolism in women. Curr Opin Pediatr 29(4):488–496, 2017 28628540

Rose EA, Porcerelli JH, Neale AV: Pica: common but commonly missed. J Am Board Fam Pract 13(5):353–358, 2000 11001006

Sansone RA, Sansone LA: Personality pathology and its influence on eating disorders. Innov Clin Neurosci 8(3):14–18, 2011 21487541

Schebendach J, Golden NH, Jacobson MS, et al: Indirect calorimetry in the nutritional management of eating disorders. Int J Eat Disord 17(1):59–66, 1995 7894454

Seeman MV: Eating disorders and psychosis: Seven hypotheses. World J Psychiatry 4(4):112–119, 2014 25540726

Smith J, Stevens H, Lake AA, et al: Food insecurity in adults with severe mental illness: A systematic review with meta-analysis. J Psychiatr Ment Health Nurs 31(2):133–151, 2024 37621069

Steinglass J, Foerde K, Kostro K, et al: Restrictive food intake as a choice—a paradigm for study. Int J Eat Disord 48(1):59–66, 2015 25130380

Stice E: Risk and maintenance factors for eating pathology: a meta-analytic review. Psychol Bull 128(5):825–848, 2002 12206196

Strother E, Lemberg R, Stanford SC, et al: Eating disorders in men: underdiagnosed, undertreated, and misunderstood. Eat Disord 20(5):346–355, 2012 22985232

Trull TJ, Sher KJ, Minks-Brown C, et al: Borderline personality disorder and substance use disorders: a review and integration. Clin Psychol Rev 20(2):235–253, 2000 10721499

Turner PG, Lefevre CE: Instagram use is linked to increased symptoms of orthorexia nervosa. Eat Weight Disord 22(2):277–284, 2017 28251592

Udo T, Grilo CM: Prevalence and correlates of DSM-5-defined eating disorders in a nationally representative sample of US adults. Biol Psychiatry 84(5):345–354, 2018 29859631

Walsh BT, Hagan KE, Lockwood C: A systematic review comparing atypical anorexia nervosa and anorexia nervosa. Int J Eat Disord 56(4):798–820, 2023 36508318

Whatnall M, Skinner JA, Leary M, et al: Food addiction: a deep dive into "loss of control" and "craving." Curr Addict Rep 9(3):318–325, 2022

World Health Organization: Noncommunicable Diseases. World Health Organization, 2024. Available at: https://www.who.int/news-room/fact-sheets/detail/noncommunicable-diseases. Accessed March 27, 2025

12

The Gut–Brain Connection and the Microbiome

Stephanie E. Langlois, M.B.A.

All disease begins in the gut.
—Hippocrates

Throughout human evolution, agriculture and culinary-based socialization patterns, including how food is obtained and consumed, have charted our course. In synchrony with these external macroscale events, a more subtle, yet vital human relationship was underway: the development of the modern human gut microbiome. Although the human species has always understood the importance of food—even fought wars over it for millennia—our mutualistic relationship with our gut microbiome and its effect on our health and evolution have been largely overlooked, until very recently. In modern times, we have challenged our microbial ecosystems with antibiotics, refined our diets until they lack variation, performed cesarean sections, created formula for feeding babies, and imposed strict hygiene standards, before understanding the depth and complexity of this mutualistic relationship. Almost unfathomable even a few years ago, modern science has now coined terms such as the "gut–brain connection" to explain how our gut microbiome influences our brain health. Now we must develop preventive and holistic health recommendations that support our microbiome as a critical element of our health.

The Human Gut Microbiome and Its Impact on Health

The human microbiome is the collection of microbes including bacteria, viruses, and fungi, as well as their genes and metabolic outputs, that naturally live on and inside our bodies (National Institute of Environmental Health Sciences 2024). Our human-cell-to-microbe ratio is greatly dominated by our microbes, meaning most of "us" is actually not human at all (Yi and Li 2012). It is unsurprising, then, that our microbes play such an influential role in our internal processes and environmental stimuli responses.

Throughout the body, the type and prevalence of microbes vary. For instance, ears, nose, skin, the digestive tract, and other organs have different microbes specialized for purposes that aid the functionality of those body systems. We all have a different microbial makeup that can change over time because of a variety of factors, leaving the potential for clinical treatment interventions and preventive measures.

The human microbiome, specifically the gut microbiome, has extensive effects on our long-term health outcomes. Mental health–related outcomes will be discussed later in this chapter, but first is a highlight of the sheer scope of the gut microbiome's influence. Vaginal delivery introduces an infant to its first dose of gut flora, whereas cesarean delivery occurs in a more sterile environment that drastically changes the composition of the infant's gut microbiome. Cesarean births have been linked to an increased risk of food allergy, asthma, diabetes, obesity, and other autoimmune and metabolic diseases, illnesses mediated in part by an altered gut microbiome in infancy (Zhang et al. 2021). Gut microbiome imbalances are linked to chronic diseases such as autoimmune, cardiovascular, respiratory, neurological, psychological, metabolic, inflammatory, intestinal, and kidney diseases (Zhang et al. 2021). The importance of microbiota to health has been long established through studies on germ-free animal models (animals without a microbiome) that show catastrophic systemic deficits in the areas of immune function, neurological development, cancer, diabetes, obesity, and cardiovascular disease (Yi and Li 2012). As evident in examples such as these, gut microbiota play a mediating effect between our bodily systems and our environment that influences the long-term trajectory of our health and wellness.

The relation between chronic illness and the gut microbiome is important in the psychiatric setting because people with serious mental illnesses have high rates of comorbid chronic diseases that significantly lower their life expectancy. In discussing how to leverage knowledge of the gut microbiome to improve psychiatric health, it is critical to note that chronic illness comorbidities may be addressed with changes to the gut microbiome.

Development and Maintenance of the Gut Microbiome

Our microbial ecosystem develops in conjunction with our immune system in infancy and early childhood, with far-reaching effects on our lifelong health and wellness (Laue et al. 2022). This process begins in utero with effects from the mother's medications, diet, stress, vaccinations, and chemical exposures. It continues during birth, influenced by mode of delivery—either vaginal or cesarean—and into early infancy with breastfeeding, antibiotics, infant vaccinations, and environmental exposures. Gut microbiome development reaches an adult-like stage characterized by relative stasis by the age of 12–36 months (Laue et al. 2022). As we age, dietary and environmental changes may shift the ecology of our microbiome, but the critical foundations are set early on. This emphasizes the importance of maternal and infant diet and environmental exposures to toxins that can affect the microbiome.

The relationship between our gut microbiome and the food we eat is both direct and complex. Our gut microbiota feed on what we ingest while also processing it for our own digestion and metabolic needs. Research has struggled to elucidate the causal directionality of good nutrition and gut microbiome effects in randomized, controlled trials. However, it is compelling that healthy dietary guidelines around the world are consistent: at least 50% of the diet should be fruits, vegetables, legumes, and whole grains; a smaller portion should be animal-based protein; and sugar, salt, saturated fat, and processed/packaged foods should be avoided (Armet et al. 2022). Studies have found that changing the diet for 1 day from entirely plant-based or entirely animal-based can affect microbial gene expression; however, other studies did not find consistent results even after weeks or months of dietary changes (David et al. 2014). Consistent and long-term dietary change, especially increasing fiber intake, does alter overall ratios of beneficial microbes, highlighting the need for preventive, long-term, holistic actions for a healthy gut microbiome. These actions can include high fiber intake or *prebiotics* (nondigestible plant fiber that feed beneficial gut bacteria, found in many fruits, vegetables, and whole grains) and *probiotics* (live microorganisms, typically bacteria or yeast, that increase the population of beneficial gut bacteria, such as those found in fermented foods), as well as optimizing the prenatal maternal diet and prioritizing breastfeeding of infants. Because this is a long-term process, our society needs to prioritize lifelong healthy diets in school systems, hospitals, workplaces, local grocery stores, assisted living facilities, and nursing homes.

Our gut microbiome has become integral to our functioning because we have evolved together. There is inherent risk in ingesting external material and incredible complexity in the process that makes food bioavailable to meet our nutritional needs. First, our gut microbiota must ensure the food we consume is safe, acting in conjunction with our immune system to rid us of potentially harmful material (e.g., in the mucosa). Then the gut microbiome begins breaking down our food into usable byproducts, or metabolites. Because our food serves as energy and nutrition for our entire body and all its functions, disruptions in this process can have far-reaching effects. This is where we begin to see associations between the genus and species composition of an individual's gut microbiome, the function or dysfunction of this system, and systemic health effects. The complexity of the digestive process, including host/environment immune and microbe interactions with food, emphasizes the synchrony between our microbes and our body's processes.

The Gut Microbiome and Influences on Psychiatric Disorders: The Basics

The gut microbiome has a considerable influence on our digestive function, but it also has a surprisingly impactful relationship with our higher-order cognitive functioning via the gut–brain axis. This recipro-

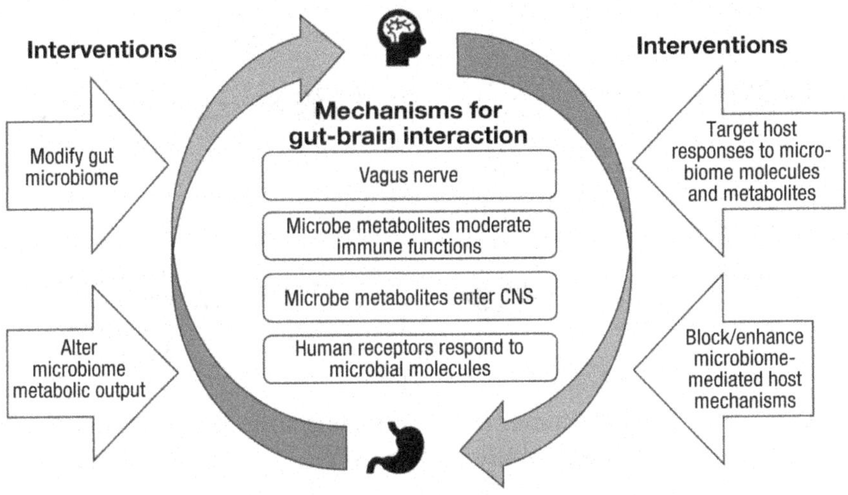

Figure 12.1 Mechanisms for gut–brain interactions and potential therapeutic interventions.

CNS = central nervous system.

cal pathway has several mechanisms that enable connections between the gut microbiome and the central nervous system (CNS): 1) direct activation of the vagus nerve, 2) microbe metabolic byproducts (metabolites) that can leave the intestine and cross the blood–brain barrier or interact with our immune system, and 3) recognition of microbial molecules by human receptors (Laue et al. 2022) (Figure 12.1). Intestinal bacteria can also produce important neurologically active molecules such as γ-aminobutyric acid (GABA), dopamine, noradrenaline, and histamines (Laue et al. 2022). The immune system plays a critical mediation role in these gut–brain interactions via systemic inflammatory signaling pathways. Altogether, this system represents a gut–brain connection that is pervasive, specific, and highly coevolved.

The highly coevolved nature of these interactions makes it difficult to ascertain directionality of the associations between gut microbes and health outcomes. A common method for determining directionality of these interactions is to transfer gut microbes from a host with a psychological or neurological pathology to a germ-free animal model (Shoubridge et al. 2022). One way to do that is fecal microbiota transplantation (FMT) because feces consistently contain samples of the microbes present in the gut. If the recipient begins displaying the

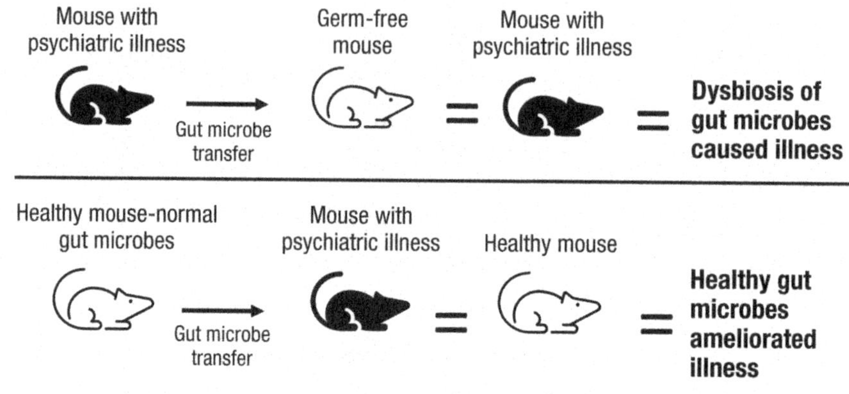

Figure 12.2 **Psychiatric changes resulting from gut microbe transfer in murine models.**

A common method for testing causality between the microbiome and psychiatric and neurological illnesses (it should be noted that the results do not always prove true for the illnesses described in this chapter, in that causality has not been determined in some instances).

pathology associated with the host, then the pathology is caused by the gut microbes that were not present until FMT (Figure 12.2).

The following sections address stress/anxiety/depression, psychotic disorders, autism-spectrum disorder (briefly), and bipolar disorder. Neurodegenerative disorders like Alzheimer's disease, Parkinson's disease, Huntington's disease, and multiple sclerosis are beyond the scope of this brief overview, although they also have significant interactions with the gut microbiome with implications for prevention, detection, and treatment (Hirschberg et al. 2019; Shoubridge et al. 2022; Wasser et al. 2020).

The Microbiome and Interactions With the HPA Axis: Stress, Anxiety, and Depression

The hypothalamic-pituitary-adrenal (HPA) axis regulates the stress response and plays a large role in stress, depression, and anxiety disorders. Stress can alter the composition of gut microbiota to a state of imbalance, or *dysbiosis*, where certain species are overrepresented and others are underrepresented. Several factors during pregnancy, including stress, can trigger gut microbe imbalances and other hormonal and immune changes that affect the development of the HPA axis in the fetus (Frankiensztajn et al. 2020). After birth, the infant can continue to experience gut microbial imbalances from their own stress that further inhibits normal development of the HPA axis. This can lead to an increased incidence of stress, anxiety, depression, and PTSD in childhood and adulthood (Frankiensztajn et al. 2020).

The relationship between food, stress, the microbiome, HPA axis development, and anxiety and depressive disorders is exemplified by the effects of a high-fat diet. A high-fat diet can lead to obesity and an imbalanced gut microbiome. Obesity is associated with an increased risk of anxiety and depressive disorders through functional changes in the HPA axis, primarily due to insulin resistance. Causality is determined in mouse models by feeding mice a high-fat diet resulting in insulin resistance and observing alterations in the HPA axis and subsequent depressive and anxious behaviors (Frankiensztajn et al. 2020). The depressive and anxious behaviors, however, can be improved with antibiotics that affect the imbalances of the gut microbiome associated with obesity. Additionally, germ-free mice on a normal diet exhibited insulin resistance, HPA axis alterations, and anxiety/depression symptoms after being transferred the imbalanced microbes (via FMT) from the pathological host mice (Frankiensztajn et al. 2020). This shows that the altered gut microbiome induced symptoms even in the absence of the high-fat diet, proving the causal influence of the gut microbiome on these behaviors. In humans, obesity and a high-fat diet in pregnant mothers can lead to developmental brain abnormalities in the fetus that result in anxiety and depressive disorders in the child later in life, likely as a result of the causal pathway just described, in which gut microbes of the mother play a significant role.

The Gut Microbiome and Early Psychosis and Schizophrenia

The gut microbiome has associations with many aspects of the schizophrenia disease course, including onset, development, pathology, symptom severity, global functioning, disease progression, and treatment response (Tsamakis et al. 2022). People who experience first-episode psychosis have a lower diversity of gut microbiota and dysbiosis of several specific species of microbes (Figure 12.3), compared with controls. These imbalances can predict the development of symptoms, and which symptoms will be more severe throughout the disease course. Dysbiosis indications in first-episode psychosis psychopathology include low

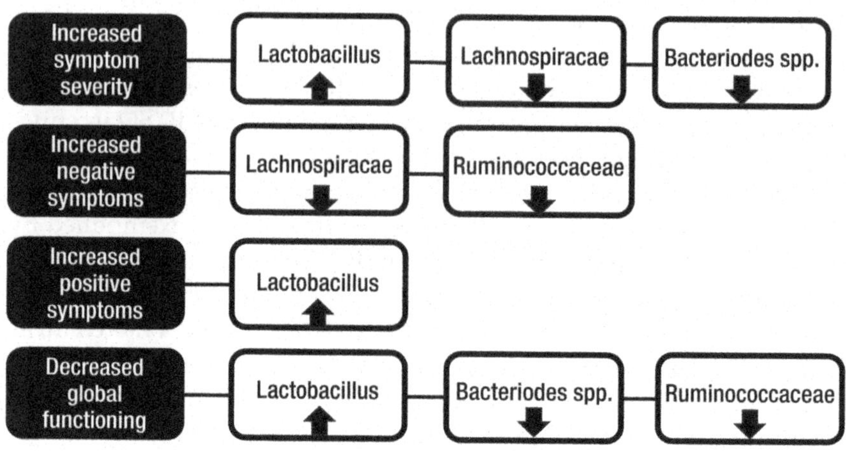

Figure 12.3 Gut microbiome abnormalities that correlate with first-episode psychosis symptoms.

tryptophan levels, high kynurenic acid levels, metabolic changes, and regional changes in gray matter volume in the brain (Tsamakis et al. 2022). First-episode psychosis patients with more microbiome abnormalities versus controls had worse treatment responses and much lower rates of remission after 1 year. Treatment with risperidone significantly altered the gut microbiome composition compared with treatment-naive psychotic patients. Taken altogether, these data show that the gut microbiome plays an important role in the psychopathology of first-episode psychosis. Identifying clinical indicators such as these could potentially result in a better long-term prognosis.

The gut microbiome also plays a mediating role in schizophrenia. Schizophrenia is often comorbid with autoimmune, gastrointestinal, and inflammatory diseases, all of which are influenced by the gut microbiome. As with anxiety and depression, causality has been demonstrated by FMT in mouse models resulting in the development of schizophrenia-like symptomology. Some proposed mechanisms for the gut microbiome's influence on schizophrenia pathology include increased intestinal permeability, systemic low-level inflammation, disruptions in tryptophan-kynurenine metabolism, alterations in amino acid and lipid metabolism, disruptions in GABA and glutamate cycles, changes in several crucial metabolic pathways, and differences in brain structure (Tsamakis et al. 2022).

The Gut Microbiome and Autism-Spectrum Disorder

Autism-spectrum disorder (ASD) is a psychological disorder thought to have one of the most direct associations with gut microbiome dysbiosis. In a case study among children, dysbiosis of *Clostridium* gut bacteria could trigger ASD symptoms, which were resolved with antibiotic treatment (Saurman et al. 2020). The symptoms, which returned soon after stopping the antibiotic, indicate a relationship between the bacteria and ASD symptoms. Gluten-free or low-carbohydrate diets, a ketogenic diet, and probiotics may also improve ASD symptoms through their impact on the gut microbiome, although this result has not always been replicable (Saurman et al. 2020). Furthermore, gut microbiota can synthesize serotonin, which is elevated in children with ASD (Saurman et al. 2020). Tryptophan is a building block of serotonin (a hormone and neurotransmitter) that has wide-ranging effects on the nervous and digestive systems, including effects on sleep, digestion, and mood. Disruptions to this system and its effects on the behavioral symptomatology of ASD likely parallel the mechanistic pathways by which these factors influence the behavioral symptoms of schizophrenia, since inflammation and disruptions in tryptophan metabolism are also hallmark comorbidities in schizophrenia pathology.

The Gut Microbiome and Bipolar Disorder

Gut microbe dysbiosis and inflammation have also been found in bipolar disorder, and changes correspond to whether symptomatology is in a depressive versus euthymic state. Specifically, whereas gut microbe diversity was lower overall in people with bipolar disorder, it was consistently also lower within the bipolar disorder population during depressive states (Sublette et al. 2021). Lower microbial diversity is associated with higher systemic inflammation, which has been associated with increased severity of the behavioral health disorders discussed thus far.

Diet also has an influence on bipolar disorder symptomatology. A diet high in nitrates (in cured meats) with an effect on specific sets of gut microbes has been correlated with an increased rate of acute mania in people with bipolar disorder (Sublette et al. 2021). Bipolar disorder has also been associated with a lower intake of polyunsaturated fatty acids, which affects bacteria's ability to adhere to the intestinal wall and increases its permeability (Sublette et al. 2021). A dietary pattern with low fiber, high fat, and refined sugars correlates with microbiome dysbiosis specific to bipolar disorder, although the directionality of these associations has not been determined, since clinical symptoms of bipolar disorder may include carbohydrate cravings and hyperphagia in the depressive stage. Species of *Clostridiales* that feed from fermentation of fiber in the colon and produce byproducts including butyrate (known for anti-inflammatory properties) are found in lower ratios in bipolar disorder (Sublette et al. 2021). This same pattern is also found in first-episode psychosis and schizophrenia (Sublette et al. 2021).

Treatment of Psychiatric Conditions With the Gut Microbiome as a Mediator

The treatment of psychiatric disorders via interventions targeting the gut microbiome are complex. There are four main categories of therapeutic pathways to consider: 1) modifying gut microbiota (probiotics and FMT), 2) altering microbiome metabolic output, 3) targeting host responses to microbiome-derived factors, or 4) blocking or enhancing microbiome-mediated host mechanisms (Shoubridge et al. 2022).

The first therapeutic pathway is most relevant for nutrition or diet-based interventions. Modification of the gut microbiome includes using probiotics (beneficial microorganisms introduced to the digestive system in yogurt, kefir, sauerkraut, kombucha, or probiotic capsules) or prebiotics (nondigestible foods that promote the growth of beneficial gut bacteria: high-fiber foods such as oats and other whole grains, garlic and many other vegetables, almonds and other nuts, and flaxseed and other seeds). Prebiotics/probiotics that affect mental health have been termed *psychobiotics*. Success in using probiotics or prebiotics to influence mental health outcomes has varied, and the results have been largely unsustainable (Shoubridge et al. 2022). In the FMT method, fecal material from an unaffected individual is encapsulated and swallowed. This method has had several successes, especially in treating *Clostridioides difficile* infections, but needs much more research before being used to treat mental health conditions. The Mediterranean diet has resulted in an improvement of symptoms in autism, Parkinson's disease, Alzheimer's disease, and depression through beneficial effects on the gut microbiome. It is important to note that all treatment potentials discussed here are in their infancy and require much more research and in-depth understanding. In particular, the directionality of the associations between medication effects, the gut microbiome, and disease etiology remains largely unestablished.

It is important to note that gut microbiome interactions can enhance or decrease the efficacy of psychotropic drugs by altering the drug's bioavailability, toxicity, or bioactivity. Some examples include effects on duloxetine and ketamine (Shoubridge et al. 2022). There are also correlations between specific gut microbes and psychiatric treatment resistance, leaving the potential for treatment resistance to be addressed via therapies that integrate options to promote a healthy gut microbiome.

Stress, Anxiety, and Depression

The Mediterranean diet—characterized by healthy fats and high fiber—can result in higher gut microbe diversity, lower inflammation, and increased integrity of the intestinal barrier, which positively affects depression symptoms (Liu et al. 2023). FMT also improves depression and anxiety symptoms and decreases comorbid gastrointestinal issues. One study found significant improvement in depressive symptoms after 4 weeks of using oral FMT capsules as an add-on therapy in patients with major depressive disorder (Liu et al. 2023). This effect has been replicated in preclinical studies, and the treatment option is gaining traction in scientific research. Using probiotics as a treatment option for depression (and any psychiatric illness) requires in-depth knowledge of relevant gut microbiota and the many confounding factors that influence the disease course, making it difficult to develop as a therapy. However, there are studies showing that probiotics can alleviate depressive symptoms. A group of microorganisms called *next-generation probiotics* have proven even more effective, but much more research is needed (Liu et al. 2023). Similarly, prebiotics have shown some potential but have had inconsistent results in research studies. Combining prebiotics and probiotics is often recommended to optimize the effects of both.

Schizophrenia

Studies leveraging the gut microbiome to treat schizophrenia have been largely negative. A meta-analysis of 28 studies investigating antibiotics, antimicrobials, and prebiotics/probiotics found that none of them affected symptomology beyond that of placebo (Minichino et al. 2021). However, other studies have shown some antipsychotic effects related to the use of prebiotics/probiotics that are hypothesized to have an effect by inducing vagal nerve stimulation or having anti-inflammatory effects (Munawar et al. 2021). Clinical applications of the gut microbiome on treatment options for schizophrenia may still be relevant, because the gut microbiome can have effects on treatment resistance (although the directionality of this association has not been established). Prebiotics and probiotics can also be used in conjunction with antipsychotics to reduce gastrointestinal symptoms commonly associated with antipsychotic medications.

Autism-Spectrum Disorder

There has been significant ASD symptom improvement with specific diets including gluten-free, casein-free, soy-free, and ketogenic diets, though interactions with gut microbiota have not been established in these diets (Saurman et al. 2020). Probiotics and FMT can improve symptoms of the gastrointestinal issues typically seen in ASD but do not bring about sustained behavioral changes. As noted earlier, although antibiotics to treat *Clostridium* infection decreased the behavioral symptoms of ASD, this was not a long-term effect. Other studies on using antibiotics to treat ASD have not shown promise (Saurman et al. 2020). One issue with the current research is the diversity of clinical characteristics and phenotypes seen in ASD. Further research needs to diagnose and categorize various cohorts of ASD based on clinical characteristics and phenotypes to target treatments toward specific ASD groups with more homogeneous symptomologies.

Bipolar Disorder

As in schizophrenia, mood-stabilizing medications used to treat bipolar disorder can affect the gut microbiome. For example, on risperidone, the resulting gut microbe dysbiosis is associated with beneficial changes in the short-chain fatty acids butyrate and propionate (created by the gut microbiota when they break down indigestible carbohydrates such as fiber in the large intestine) as well as tryptophan metabolism, which all affect the course of bipolar illness (Sublette et al. 2021). Again, however, the direction of the causal effect was not determined. Similar patterns may occur with mood-stabilizing medications, although the research is limited. Fiber-rich diets can lower the risk of depressive symptoms by increasing production of short-chain fatty acids that can improve cognitive processes in multiple ways. Prebiotics and probiotics have demonstrated some efficacy in improving cognitive performance, reducing rumination, improving mood, and lowering rehospitalization rates in patients with bipolar disorder (Lucidi et al. 2021). One study of FMT showed improvements in bipolar disorder symptoms, particularly in sleep regulation (Lucidi et al. 2021). These results are very similar to patterns seen in depression and schizophrenia. Our understanding of the gut microbiome's effect on mental illnesses largely follows similar patterns: healthy foods diversify the gut microbiome, reduce inflammation, and lead to the production of beneficial psychoactive metabolites.

Looking Ahead

Overall, there is a significant dearth of randomized, controlled trials studying the effects of microbiome interventions as treatment options for psychiatric disorders. Research is accumulating for neurodegenerative disorders as well, but it is beyond the scope of this chapter. There have been promising psychiatric preclinical trials in animal models, but few clinical trials in humans. In the studies that do exist, the probiotics commonly contain the same few strains of microbes, giving a very limited understanding of the range of therapeutic options. The beginning of this section reviewed four types of treatment options, but it is clear that nearly all studies target the first (altering the gut microbiome directly) and have been met with limited success that does not appear to be sustainable long term, especially in the absence of a continuous dose of prebiotics or probiotics.

The commonalities for all of the interventions noted underscore that treatment options are in their infancy. This is due to limited understanding of the mechanisms by which the gut microbiome mediates these illnesses, a way to culture various strains of probiotics for human consumption (further highlighted by FMT—which has been used since the fourth century BC in China—still being one of the most effective methods of microbial transfer) (Zhang et al. 2023), and major clinical variation in the presentations of these illnesses.

Nutritional Factors Affecting the Gut Microbiome

When we eat, we feed not only ourselves but our gut microbiota as well. What we do not absorb directly is processed by our gut microbiota and turned into metabolites that have many effects on our health. These metabolites can range from neuroactive molecules such as serotonin, dopamine, and GABA that directly affect our brain functioning, but these metabolites can also regulate our gene expression, hormones, and immune response, resulting in systemic health effects. In this way, our gut microbiome acts as a mediating factor between the food we eat and how it affects us. Healthy nutrition guidelines outline the foods we should eat to optimize health, in part by promoting gut microbe diversity, and result in beneficial ratios of the "right" gut microbial colonizers. For example, high fiber intake "feeds" *Clostridiales* gut bacteria that produce anti-inflammatory byproducts that may improve symptoms of bipolar disorder and schizophrenia (Sublette et al. 2021). Fortunately, nutrition-based prevention of mental health disorders and neurodegenerative disorders via the gut microbiome aligns with existing widespread nutritional guidelines, which have been discussed extensively in other chapters of this book. As a result, we do not need to rethink our nutritional advice to accommodate our new understanding of the gut microbiome. However, the importance of proper nutrition and access to it assumes a new vitality as we understand the complexity and interconnectedness of these systems.

Our best chances for leveraging our gut microbiome for lifelong brain health occur prenatally and in the first 3 years of a child's life. Our gut microbiome develops in conjunction with our nervous system and our immune system, reaching a mostly developed stage by age 3 (Laue et al. 2022). This is also a pivotal time for neurodevelopment, laying the foundation for lifelong brain health. The mother's microbiome is the sole source of the fetal microbiome until delivery, highlighting the importance of her prenatal nutrition as well as other factors in the mother's lifestyle that affect her microbiome. As such, food programs such as the Supplemental Nutrition Assistance Program (SNAP) or the Special Supplemental Nutrition Program for Women, Infants, and Children (WIC) that support the nutrition of pregnant mothers and young children take on critical importance far beyond that of dietary sustenance. However, they also highlight barriers to proper nutrition faced by many, especially those with a history of psychiatric illness.

Barriers to optimal nutrition exist for all populations but are exacerbated in people with psychiatric conditions. Common widespread barriers include lack of healthy food options (e.g., nearby stores not carrying fresh foods, no transportation to grocery stores, no kitchen to cook in), low socioeconomic status resulting in financial constraints

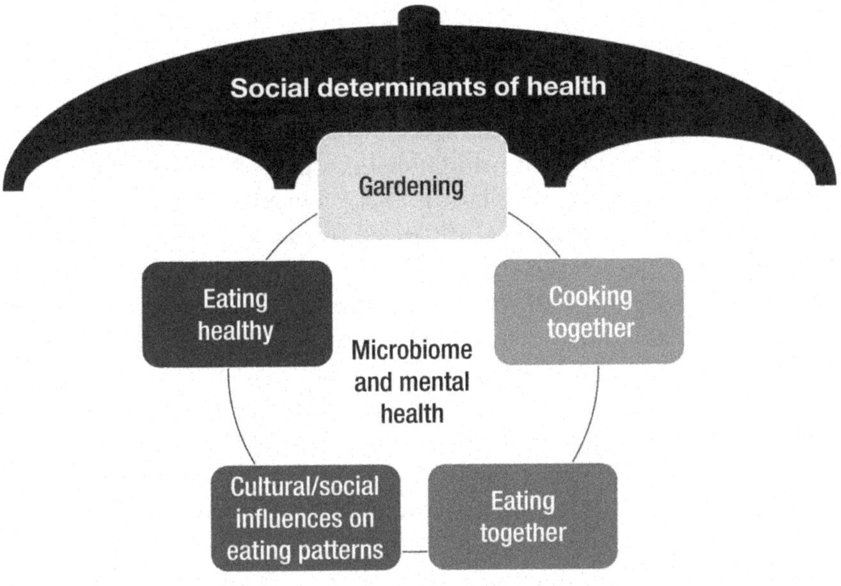

Figure 12.4 **Layers of influence on the gut microbiome and mental health.**

for buying healthy foods, limited nutrition literacy, and long-standing taste preferences (Figure 12.4). People with serious mental illness (SMI) are often more likely to experience all of these barriers, in addition to illness-specific barriers such as psychotropic medication–induced appetite changes, reduced motivation or cognitive changes that inhibit cooking or shopping habits, and decreased capacity to understand and use nutritional information (Hotzy et al. 2022). Personality traits modified as a result of psychiatric disease course can also affect eating behaviors. For instance, agreeableness and extraversion are linked with healthy eating behaviors, whereas neuroticism coincides with unhealthy or disordered eating behaviors (Hotzy et al. 2022). Emotion regulation and sociability also strongly influence eating behaviors and are highly variable or potentially limited in persons with psychiatric conditions. Combined, the intersection of these barriers, eating habits, the gut microbiome, and mental illness suggests that the mental health field should remain vigilant in addressing eating behaviors as part of routine care and be mindful of the negative effects of some psychotropic medications on eating behaviors and nutrition.

Socialization Patterns and Their Effect on the Gut Microbiome

Nutrition and dietary choices affect our gut microbiome, which in turn affects our mental health, but holistic approaches to overall health include addressing social determinants of health and mental well-being. The gut microbiome is influenced in many ways by our social behavior and close relationships and interactions with other humans. Delivery method and breastfeeding serve as the foundation for our gut microbiome. New evidence shows that socialization continues to influence our gut microbiome into adulthood. Evidence for this comes from the 60-year Wisconsin Longitudinal Study, with more than 10,000 participants. In a sample of 408 fecal samples from this group, married couples were found to have more similar microbes than their siblings or unrelated people, and siblings showed no more similarity than unrelated people (Dill-McFarland et al. 2019). These results indicate that the composition of our gut microbes continues to develop over our lifetime and in conjunction with that of our partners and close relationships. This finding underscores the importance of our social relationships in the development of our gut microbiome and widens the potential for corrective dietary and supplementary efforts to modify our microbiome into adulthood.

Additionally, increased diversity in the gut microbiome could be predicted by a self-reported high level of close relationships (Dill-McFarland et al. 2019). Human health and mortality is negatively affected by social isolation, whereas social integration has more significant positive effects than individual behaviors such as weight management or smoking cessation (Dill-McFarland et al. 2019). Potential mediators of this association include modifying stress levels, introducing psychosocial resources, reinforcing healthy habits, and reducing dependence on self-medicating behavior such as alcohol, tobacco, or drug use (Dill-McFarland et al. 2019). This social benefit highlights the possibility that gardening and culinary-based socialization practices (e.g., growing, cooking, and eating together) influence our gut microbiome and our health far more than a culmination of digestion and metabolic byproducts (Figure 12.4).

People with psychiatric conditions have barriers to health and well-being that are further confounded by an increased incidence of negative socialization patterns. Disease symptoms such as paranoia, apathy, depression, anxiety, and cognitive impairments often lead to reduced social opportunities and difficulty maintaining positive close relationships. Social isolation, low diversity in the gut microbiome, and SMI have all been independently linked to significantly increased risk of morbidity and mortality. From a clinical perspective, these associations may offer new pathways to treat medication-resistant pathologies from a holistic perspective that leverages socialization opportunities as well as new therapies that directly influence the gut microbiome, such as FMT and the use of prebiotics and probiotics.

Future Research Directions

Although there is an abundance of evidence that the gut microbiome mediates mental health, many of the specific mechanisms behind the associations are unknown. It has been difficult to untangle these processes from confounding factors such as genetics, lifestyle changes, medication interactions, and normal disease course. The great variation in the spectrum of illness in many psychiatric disorders also complicates diagnoses and the ability to attribute specific microbes to specific illnesses or behaviors. The future of gut microbiome therapeutic research will likely be highly individualistic—consistent with the goals of personalized, precision medicine. Finally, because the gut microbiome is inextricable from the context and social determinants of health environment in which it exists, population-level outcomes and improvements are unlikely unless there is translational social science research and implementation addressing these external influences.

Clinical Pearls

- Optimizing nutrition among young children and mothers may hold promise in preventing mental health disorders based on growing knowledge of the gut microbiome.
- People with psychiatric conditions may benefit from nutrition counseling and behavioral strategies tailored to the limitations of their illness. Clinicians should collaborate with nutritionists or registered dietitians to address the needs of clients in promoting a healthy diet and a healthy gut microbiome.
- Clinicians can recommend optimal intake of prebiotics, which are nondigestible plant fiber that feed beneficial gut bacteria, by encouraging intake of fruits, vegetables, legumes, oats and other

whole grains, seeds, and nuts to aid in the prevention and potential treatment of psychiatric illness.
- Clinicians can recommend intake of probiotics, which are live microorganisms, typically bacteria or yeast, that increase the population of beneficial gut bacteria. These are found in fermented foods, yogurt, kefir, sauerkraut, and kombucha, to aid in the prevention and potential treatment of psychiatric illness.
- Leveraging good nutrition and knowledge of the gut microbiome to address psychiatric illnesses will be a holistic endeavor involving behavioral adaptation, reduction of negative social determinants of health, large-scale policy change, and food system adaptation to promote accessibility of healthy foods.

Key Chapter Points

- The gut microbiome and our bodies exist as a highly coevolved system; as such, disruptions can cause far-reaching health effects. There needs to be much more research on causal relationships between the microbiome and our health, especially randomized, controlled trials and human clinical studies.
- Microbiome therapies for mental illnesses are in their infancy, and clinical efforts would be better focused on prevention during critical neurodevelopmental phases. This includes maternal and infant nutrition, stress reduction, and encouraging breastfeeding, to promote optimal microbiome development during this critical stage.
- Maintenance of a healthy gut microbiome is a holistic process that must occur continuously over the lifetime, with a focus on prevention of dysbiosis through diet, optimizing socialization, and addressing social determinants of health.
- Agricultural practices and culinary-based socialization opportunities affect our microbiome and mental health holistically through activities such as gardening, cooking together, eating together, eating healthy, eating local, and recognizing cultural and social influences on eating patterns.
- Comorbid chronic illnesses and negative social determinants of health are especially prevalent among individuals with SMI, and these contribute significantly to gut microbiome dysbiosis, with effects that worsen outcomes for both chronic illnesses and mental health.

References

Armet AM, Deehan EC, O'Sullivan AF, et al: Rethinking healthy eating in light of the gut microbiome. Cell Host Microbe 30(6):764–785, 2022 35679823

David LA, Maurice CF, Carmody RN, et al: Diet rapidly and reproducibly alters the human gut microbiome. Nature 505(7484):559–563, 2014 24336217

Dill-McFarland KA, Tang ZZ, Kemis JH, et al: Close social relationships correlate with human gut microbiota composition. Sci Rep 9(1):703, 2019 30679677

Frankiensztajn LM, Elliott E, Koren O: The microbiota and the hypothalamus-pituitary-adrenocortical (HPA) axis, implications for anxiety and stress disorders. Curr Opin Neurobiol 62:76–82, 2020 31972462

Hirschberg S, Gisevius B, Duscha A, et al: Implications of diet and the gut microbiome in neuroinflammatory and neurodegenerative diseases. Int J Mol Sci 20(12):3109, 2019 31242699

Hotzy F, Risch L, Mötteli S: Nutritional Needs in Mental Healthcare: study protocol of a prospective analytic observational study assessing nutritional status, eating behavior and barriers to healthy eating in psychiatric inpatients and outpatients compared to healthy adults. Front Psychiatry 13:906234, 2022 35774087

Laue HE, Coker MO, Madan JC: The developing microbiome from birth to 3 years: the gut–brain axis and neurodevelopmental outcomes. Front Pediatr 10:815885, 2022 35321011

Liu L, Wang H, Chen X, et al: Gut microbiota and its metabolites in depression: from pathogenesis to treatment. EBioMedicine 90(90):104527, 2023 36963238

Lucidi L, Pettorruso M, Vellante F, et al: Gut microbiota and bipolar disorder: an overview on a novel biomarker for diagnosis and treatment. Int J Mol Sci 22(7):3723, 2021 33918462

Minichino A, Brondino N, Solmi M, et al: The gut-microbiome as a target for the treatment of schizophrenia: a systematic review and meta-analysis of randomised controlled trials of add-on strategies. Schizophr Res 234:1–13, 2021 32295752

Munawar N, Ahsan K, Muhammad K, et al: Hidden role of gut microbiome dysbiosis in schizophrenia: antipsychotics or psychobiotics as therapeutics? Int J Mol Sci 22(14):7671, 2021 34299291

National Institute of Environmental Health Sciences: Microbiome. National Institute of Environmental Health Sciences, 2024. Available at: https://www.niehs.nih.gov/health/topics/science/microbiome. Accessed February 25, 2025.

Saurman V, Margolis KG, Luna RA: Autism spectrum disorder as a brain-gut-microbiome axis disorder. Dig Dis Sci 65(3):818–828, 2020 32056091

Shoubridge AP, Choo JM, Martin AM, et al: The gut microbiome and mental health: advances in research and emerging priorities. Mol Psychiatry 27(4):1908–1919, 2022 35236957

Sublette ME, Cheung S, Lieberman E, et al: Bipolar disorder and the gut microbiome: a systematic review. Bipolar Disord 23(6):544–564, 2021 33512753

Tsamakis K, Galinaki S, Alevyzakis E, et al: Gut microbiome: a brief review on its role in schizophrenia and first episode of psychosis. Microorganisms 10(6):1121, 2022 35744639

Wasser CI, Mercieca EC, Kong G, et al: Gut dysbiosis in Huntington's disease: associations among gut microbiota, cognitive performance and clinical outcomes. Brain Commun 2(2):fcaa110, 2020 33005892

Yi P, Li L: The germfree murine animal: an important animal model for research on the relationship between gut microbiota and the host. Vet Microbiol 157(1–2):1–7, 2012 22079217

Zhang C, Li L, Jin B, et al: The effects of delivery mode on the gut microbiota and health: state of art. Front Microbiol 12:724449, 2021 35002992

Zhang T, Gao G, Kwok LY, et al: Gut microbiome-targeted therapies for Alzheimer's disease. Gut Microbes 15(2):2271613, 2023 37934614

Part 4

Cooking, Gardening, and Growing Food

13

Cooking, Cooking Together, Eating Together, and Mental Health

Liana Lau, M.D., M.S.

The table is a meeting place, a gathering ground, the source of sustenance and nourishment, festivity, safety, and satisfaction. A person cooking is a person giving: even the simplest food is a gift.

—Laurie Colwin, American author, 1944–1992

Globalization and a multitude of modern amenities and services have made home cooking simultaneously much more accessible and much more inconvenient. We now have unprecedented, inexpensive access to ingredients that our ancestors could have only dreamt of; yet we also have fast food conglomerates and delivery apps at our fingertips. Why spend several hours grocery shopping and laboring over a stovetop to make a chicken tikka masala from scratch when it can conveniently arrive at your door, fresh and piping hot, with just a few clicks? Or perhaps even be microwaved from a frozen prepackaged meal, ready within a few minutes? During the COVID-19 pandemic, rates of home cooking rose but have fallen again postpandemic; a survey of 12,000 Americans in 2023 revealed that 81% cook more than half of their meals at home, and 59% use precut frozen fruits and vegetables or frozen entrées (Atomik Research 2023). Economic considerations aside, home cooking has significant potential for improving both physical and mental health. The ability to choose recognizable ingredients, bypassing the mystery ingredient list of ultraprocessed foods, increases the likelihood of healthier dietary intake. The act itself of cooking is often somewhat exertional, promoting physical activity. Whether cooking alone or cooking for a group and dining together as a shared social activity, cooking offers many mental health benefits.

Home Cooking

Home cooking, at its core, entails assembling edible ingredients and altering them for a specific purpose: consumption. Simple home cooking can include a broad array of activities, from boiling an egg to mixing arugula with hazelnuts, roasted beets, goat cheese, olive oil, and vinegar. The use of the word "cook" is somewhat of a misnomer, as heat is not necessary for a meal to be considered home cooked. Although the ingredients used for cooking at home can include shortcuts, such as pasta sauce from a jar or frozen dumplings, for the purposes of this chapter, home cooking refers to cooking with individual ingredients, such as flour, fresh or frozen vegetables, meat, and canned anchovies. This distinction is not meant to condemn cooking with shortcuts as unhealthy but rather to focus on cooking with whole foods: recognizable ingredients without preservatives or ultraprocessed ingredients. Home cooking is not necessarily healthier, as it is certainly possible to douse a would-be healthy dish in butter, cream, and salt at home; however, there is significantly more control over the choice and quantity of ingredients, as opposed to eating out at restaurants or microwaving a frozen entrée.

Throughout millennia, people have engaged in home cooking for necessity, pleasure, or both. Home cooking has always been the most economical choice, although potentially also the most time-consuming. For those with dietary restrictions or medical issues, home cooking may also be the safest way to guarantee appropriate food. For many, home cooking also provides great joy in its apparent, easy-to-achieve alchemy;

within minutes or hours, disparate ingredients can transform into something much greater than the sum of their parts, delightful to all the senses, especially taste. Home cooking can promote flow state and mindfulness in its use of focused tasks and grounding through the senses. It also reinforces various cognitive skills, such as attention, planning, reasoning, calculation, problem solving, adaptation, and memory, as well as fine motor skills.

Cooking and Physical Health

Although not all home cooking is necessarily healthy, the ability to select for healthier ingredients, decrease the amount of unhealthy ingredients, and cook with whole foods contributes to improved nutrition. As depicted in Figure 13.1, cooking has been associated with various physical health benefits, including lower body mass index (BMI), lower adiposity, lower diastolic blood pressure, and higher high-density lipoprotein (HDL) cholesterol. These health benefits are likely mediated through improved nutrition, including increased vegetable and fruit consumption, decreased neophobia (fear of new foods), increased breakfast eating, decreased snack intake, and increased whole grain consumption.

Home cooking has been shown through population-based studies to be associated with physical health benefits. Studies on home cooking define frequent home cooking as more than five times a week and infrequent home cooking as fewer than three times a week. In a population-based study in the United Kingdom of 11,396 adults, frequent home cooking was associated with lower BMI, less excess body fat, and higher adherence to the Dietary Approaches to Stop Hypertension (DASH) diet and Mediterranean diet (Mills et al. 2017). In a study in Tokyo involving 293 adolescents, infrequent home cooking was associated with higher diastolic blood pressure and lower HDL cholesterol (Tani et al. 2020). In a cross-sectional study of 5,311 elementary school students, also in Tokyo, a lower frequency of home cooking was associated with less vegetable intake, skipping breakfast, and more snacking (Tani et al. 2021). In multiple systematic reviews examining the impact of home cooking, the majority of studies have shown frequent home cooking to be associated with improvements in fruit and vegetable intake, other beneficial dietary behavior changes, reduced weight, and cooking confidence (Hasan et al. 2019; Hersch et al. 2014; Reicks et al. 2018).

Even short cooking interventions can make a difference; studies have shown varying levels of success in changing dietary behav-

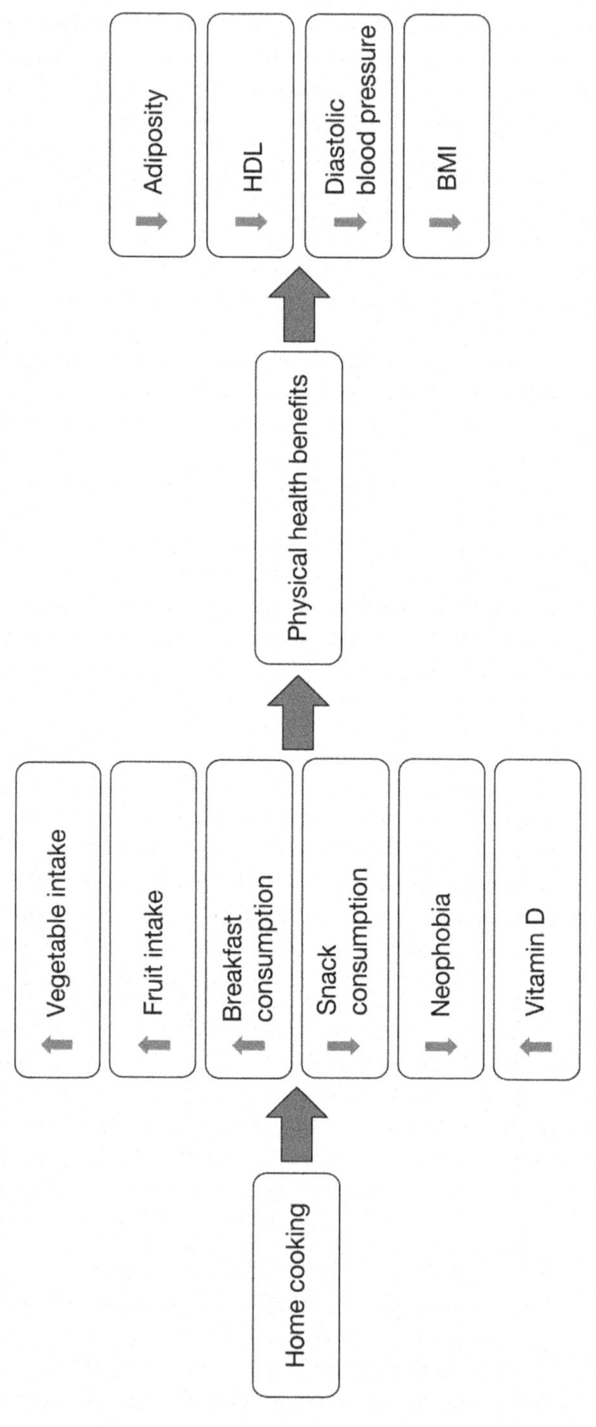

Figure 13.1 Some of the potential physical health benefits of cooking.

BMI = body mass index; HDL = high density lipoprotein cholesterol.

iors through cooking programs, likely dependent on the medium of delivery and length of the intervention. Many studies have focused on cooking programs for children as an approach to early intervention, as children have greater difficulty with vegetable consumption in the context of the current food environment. In a study in Flint, Michigan, 246 children ages 8–18 participated in a children-only or virtual family cooking program for 9 total hours over 6 consecutive weeks to prepare two recipes in small groups each week. Participants reported improved cooking self-efficacy, intake of vegetables, health-related quality of life, and physical functioning (Saxe-Custack et al. 2023). In a study comparing nutrition workshops and a 3-hour hands-on cooking workshop in children ages 8–9, children who were active participants were more likely to choose healthy foods, such as spinach, and had reduced neophobia. Children who participated in home cooking more frequently were more likely to eat fruit and vegetables (Maiz et al. 2021).

Although individuals with serious mental illness (SMI) have higher rates of obesity, cardiovascular disease, cancer, and respiratory disease, most cooking programs do not target this population despite their need for improved nutrition and behavioral changes. In an exploratory study of 18 individuals with SMI, a 6-week nutrition education cooking class showed significant increases in calcium, vitamin D, grains, and fruit consumption, as well as cooking self-efficacy and grocery shopping skills (Clark et al. 2015). The results suggest that clinicians should consider referring their clients to cooking programs, as many would likely benefit from such dietary interventions.

Cooking and Mental Health

Home cooking contributes to improved mental health through two distinct pathways: improved nutrition and the act of cooking itself. It has been well established that the effect of nutrition on mood is mediated in part through the gut microbiome, which produces mood-regulating transmitters, affects the body's stress response, and communicates with the brain via the vagus nerve. Consumption of healthy food, including prebiotics (nondigestible plant fiber that feed beneficial gut bacteria, found in many fruits, vegetables, and whole grains) and probiotics (live microorganisms, typically bacteria or yeast, that increase the population of beneficial gut bacteria, such as those found in fermented foods), can improve mental health, whereas consumption of fast food and other types of lower-quality food contributes to higher rates of depression (Hamad et al. 2024).

Cooking provides a tangible reward after some effort, which can improve self-esteem and independence. There is a low barrier to entry into the activity of cooking, as anyone can learn how to cook. For a seasoned chef, there is always more to learn. Cooking together can be an enjoyable social activity even if two people have different capabilities, as the labor is easily divisible and teachable. It can be self-soothing to cook a familiar, comforting dish, or challenging and intellectually stimulating to create a fusion dish inspired by particular cuisines. Some of the potential pathways linking home cooking to mental health are shown in Figure 13.2. Lack of confidence and safety concerns, however, can be significant barriers to home cooking.

Most studies on cooking interventions last only several weeks, as basic cooking skills are teachable within that time frame and are sufficient for most people to cook a variety of foods. A study of 657 Australian adults in a 7-week cooking intervention program showed improvement in cooking confidence, ability to change eating habits and overcome lifestyle barriers, subjective vitality, and sense of well-being (Rees et al. 2022). The improvement in subjective vitality and well-being are likely mediated by increased sense of self-efficacy and hope for positive dietary changes.

Research has shown that home cooking can have positive effects on children and adolescents, although this effect may be mediated through family meals. In a cross-sectional study of 5,311 elementary school students in Tokyo, lower frequency of home cooking was associated with more behavioral problems, peer relationship problems, and emotional symptoms and lower frequency of caregiver involvement, even after adjusting for eating with caregivers (Tani et al. 2021). Lower frequency of home cooking itself may be attributable to family-level factors, such as caregiver fatigue or unavailability. A study examining the relationship between maternal mood and meal frequency showed that higher scores of maternal anxiety and depression were associated with irregular, infrequent family meals (Helle et al. 2024). Although mothers should not be held solely accountable for meal preparation in the family, this study suggests that maternal anxiety and depression may be a confounding factor for the adverse outcomes associated with infrequent family meals.

College students are especially vulnerable to poor diets due to food insecurity and a shift in eating patterns and meal preparation activities. They may have a meal plan provided by the college or university, have an increased risk of unhealthy eating, or struggle to provide food for themselves if they had previously been dependent on their parents.

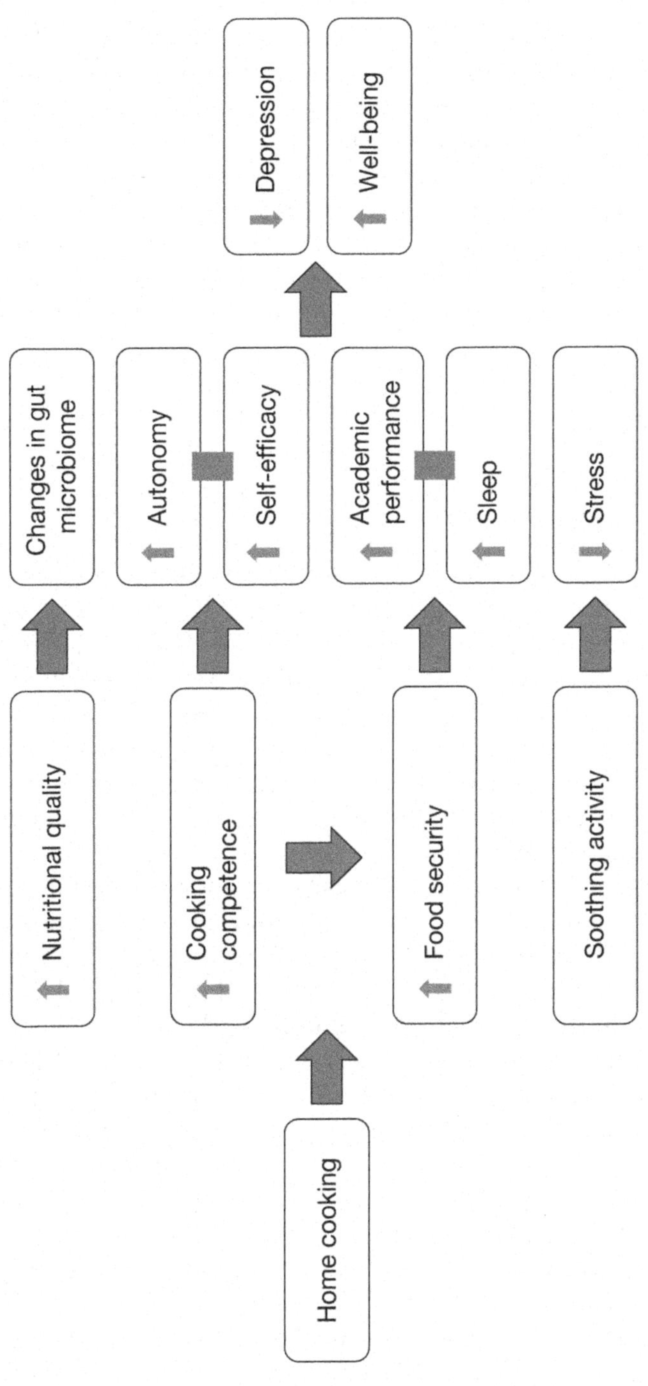

Figure 13.2 Some of the potential pathways mediating mental health benefits of cooking.

High levels of food insecurity have been associated with higher levels of stress, poor sleep quality, disordered eating, decreased intake of fruits and vegetables, difficulty focusing in class, and poor academic performance. A community-based cooking and texting intervention at the University of Kentucky and the University of Maine led to better diet quality, including increased vegetable intake, as well as lower rates of anxiety and depression (Barr-Porter et al. 2024). This intervention comprised cooking classes led by nutritionists and frequent text messages to disseminate information. The cooking classes encompassed various topics, including meal planning, knife skills, budgeting, and nutrients. The text messages between the classes reminded students of farmers market hours and locations, food pantry resources, and wellness resources.

Cooking Together

Home cooking already confers significant benefits as a solitary activity, but it can be further enhanced as a social activity. Whether as a parent-child bonding activity, in cookbook clubs or themed dinner parties, or to decrease the labor with a roommate or partner, cooking together as a social activity offers an easy opportunity to share an experience. Cooking classes abound, allowing friends to engage in a new activity and reflect afterward over a shared meal. Cooking as a hobby is readily accessible; despite varying skill levels, it is easy to share cooking videos, recipes, and experimental creations.

As depicted in Figure 13.3, studies have shown that cooking together can improve mental health. A systematic review of inpatient and community-based cooking interventions showed a positive effect on socialization, self-esteem, quality of life, and mood (Farmer et al. 2018). In a family cooking intervention, parents expressed that they enjoyed cooking with other parents for the social interaction and inspiration around modeling parent-child interactions (Tørslev et al. 2021).

In older adults, several factors may contribute to significant detrimental changes in cooking and enjoyment of food: living alone, bereavement, changes in taste and smell, and poor dentition. Changes in taste, smell, and ability to chew food limit some older adults' ability to consume previously familiar foods. Living alone may contribute to decreased motivation to shop and to prepare and eat meals. Without companionship, an older adult may choose to eat less diverse foods, skip meals, and eat more snacks. A systematic review of culinary nutri-

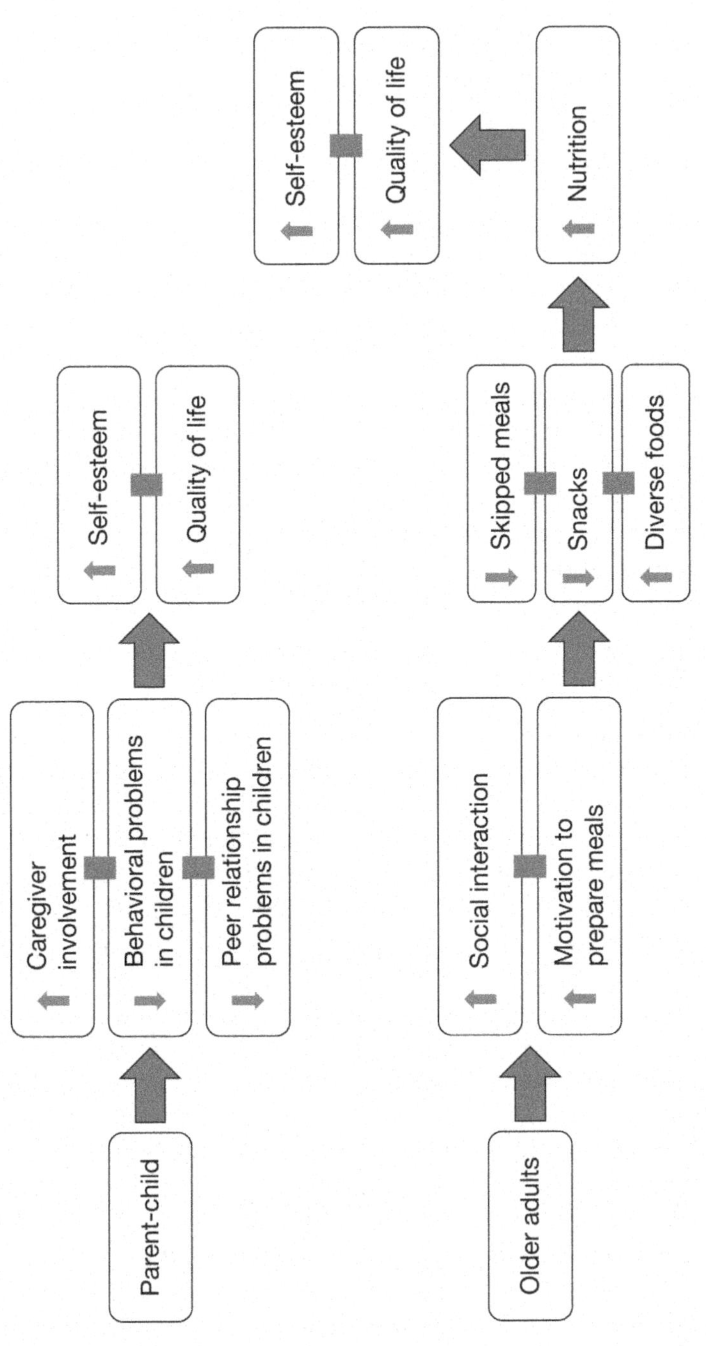

Figure 13.3 Some of the potential benefits of cooking together.

tion education programs in community-dwelling older adults showed that such programs can improve dietary habits and health literacy but would benefit from greater accessibility, such as virtual options instead of face-to-face only (Alghamdi et al. 2023).

Eating Together

Whether cooking alone or cooking together, the natural outcome of cooking is eating. When the goal is to cook for others, as opposed to cooking for one, the focus shifts significantly. Parents may be more cognizant of nutritional quality when cooking for their children and put more effort into a balanced meal. Busy college students or adults may be more likely to slow down and think about their dietary choices when eating with peers, as opposed to grabbing something to go. The main benefits of eating together are mediated through the positive effects of social interaction. As depicted in Figure 13.4, eating together confers a heightened sense of well-being, opportunities for bonding and communication, fewer depressive symptoms, fewer adolescent health risk factors, and marital satisfaction.

Family Meals and Mental Health

Most studies on eating together have focused on family meals and their effects on children and parents. When children are at school and apart from their parents during the day, family meals at the end of the day can serve as a comforting ritual to look forward to. Family routines have been associated with better health and well-being, parental competence, and marital satisfaction (Utter et al. 2018). The routine provides stability and grounds family members. Family meals provide an opportunity for communication and family bonding. Over food, family members can organically process any emotional turmoil from across the day, reflect together, and reinforce shared values.

In a study of 4,746 high school students in Minnesota, having frequent family meals was associated with greater family connection, parental monitoring and communication, and fewer health risk behaviors. Parents who had maintained regular family meals since adolescence or started regular family meals with their own children had better self-esteem and fewer depressive symptoms (Utter et al. 2018). Another study in Minnesota found a correlation between infrequent family meals and tobacco, alcohol, and marijuana use; poor academic performance; depressive symptoms; and suicidal thoughts and actions, after

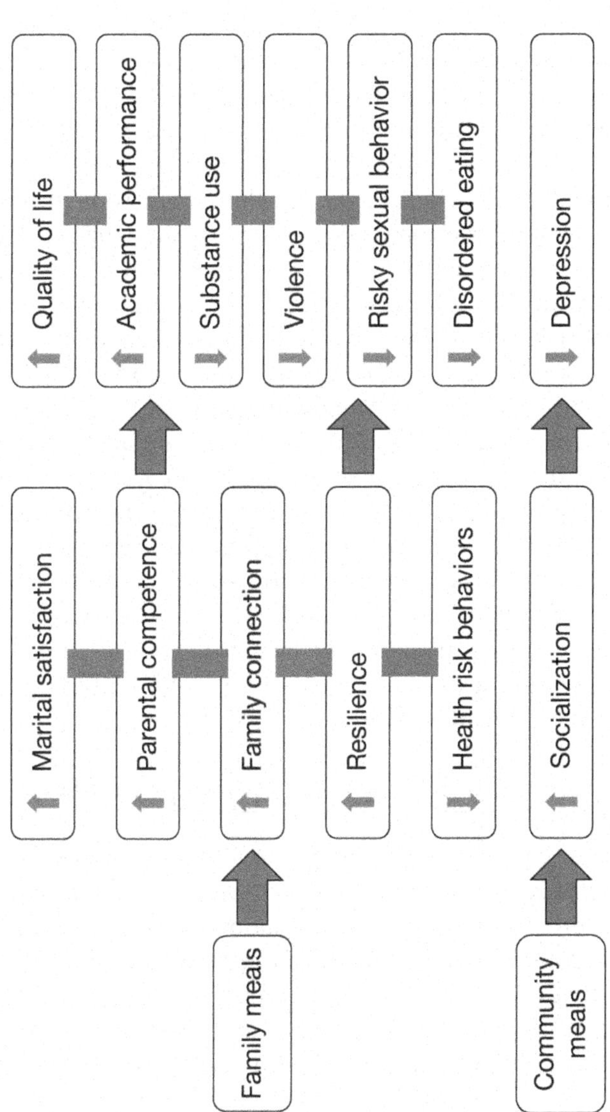

Figure 13.4 Some of the potential benefits of eating together.

controlling for family connectedness (Eisenberg et al. 2004). In a systematic review exploring the association between family meals and adolescent risk outcomes, having frequent family meals was associated with decreased alcohol use, disordered eating, aggressive and violent behavior, sexual activity, poor academic performance, depression, and suicide attempts (Skeer and Ballard 2013). In a study of 8,500 secondary school students in New Zealand, having infrequent family meals was associated with household poverty and the students being older; having frequent family meals was associated with fewer depressive symptoms, with a greater effect in girls (Utter et al. 2016). Older students may prefer to avoid their parents for meals if they are already feeling depressed, leading to a cascading effect. In a cross-sectional study of elementary school students in Tokyo, lower frequency of home cooking was associated with lower prosocial behavior and lower levels of resilience, but this association was attenuated by eating together (Tani et al. 2021).

Through the China Family Panel Studies (CFPS), 14,960 households from 25 provinces were surveyed to assess the impact of systemic factors affecting diet on adults over the age of 50. One study assessed the impact of rural versus urban settings and the social dimension of diet on older adults. In this population, a greater frequency of eating together as a family was associated with decreased depressive symptoms in rural residents (Zhou et al. 2023). The lack of correlation in urban residents may be attributed to increased socialization with non-family members in an urban setting or a greater emphasis on traditional values in the rural setting.

Community Meals and Mental Health

As meals punctuate the day regularly, solitary meals can exacerbate feelings of loneliness and loss. In a systematic review of community shared meal programs for older populations, significant associations were observed between shared meal programs and improved dietary intake (Middleton et al. 2022). The programs also had a positive impact on participants' social networks and perceived well-being. Participants reported choosing to attend these shared meal programs for access to a hot meal, eating a meal outside the home, eating a home-style cooked meal, not having to cook a meal, low cost of meals, making new friends, and socializing with others (Middleton et al. 2022). These factors suggest a longing for home cooking, possibly due to decreased ability to cook independently or decreased motivation to cook alone.

Structured Cooking Programs

Although some learn to cook from observing or assisting their parents with home cooking, there is no universal cooking curriculum. Many parents do not necessarily feel comfortable guiding their children to cook, and they may not necessarily know what is nutritionally appropriate. Although some schools have home economics classes that impart basic cooking skills, many home cooks learn independently through trial and error. Structured cooking programs offer an opportunity for children and adults to build cooking self-confidence and nutritional knowledge in a safe environment. For the vast majority of individuals who do not attend culinary school, there are various options in the community, including short-term cooking classes, therapeutic cooking programs, and culinary medicine programs.

Therapeutic Cooking Programs

Most cooking programs have been designed to improve dietary outcomes and physical health; even when not designed to target mental health specifically, they offer mental health benefits. In our increasingly digitized world, children often lack appropriately stimulating activities that can rival the appeal of the screen. Their fixation on the internet, coupled with decreased independent play, has contributed to apathy and amotivation to learn and achieve (Hari 2021). Cooking programs targeted at children provide an excellent means for instilling curiosity, engagement, and autonomy. Therapeutic cooking programs are rare but show great potential.

There are currently several established cooking programs for children. LA Sprouts in Los Angeles provides 12 weeks of 90-minute culturally tailored gardening, nutrition, and cooking classes to third through fifth graders, and a randomized, controlled trial has shown improved identification of vegetables, greater nutrition and gardening knowledge, and increased likelihood of gardening at home (Davis et al. 2016). Cooking with Kids is an experiential food education curriculum that exposes elementary school children to fresh foods through multiple 2-hour multicultural cooking lessons and 1-hour fruit and vegetable tasting lessons. It was initially developed in low-income, predominantly Hispanic schools in a Southwestern U.S. city and was expanded to four elementary schools in Colorado with predominantly White students (Cunningham-Sabo and Lohse 2013).

The Family Cooking Classes project in Copenhagen aims to promote health and prevent type 2 diabetes by providing families with children ages 8–12 with five 4-hour afternoon or evening classes over 4 weeks. This project focuses not only on cooking healthy food, but also on social interactions, playful cooking and creativity, and eating together to support positive parenting strategies (Tørslev et al. 2021). Based on the premise that children's healthy behaviors are associated with positive parenting strategies, this unique program facilitates parental encouragement and monitoring through visual recipes such that children have more ownership of the cooking process. Parents expressed that before the cooking program, significant barriers to cooking with their children included stress and concern for safety. The guidance of professionals allowed the parents to trust their children and delegate tasks appropriately to lighten the load of cooking at home.

Cooking Matters for Adults in the United States is a nationally recognized 6-week hands-on nutrition education cooking class that covers cooking on a budget, grocery shopping skills, food safety, and ways to increase fruit, vegetable, and calcium intake and decrease sodium and fat consumption. Its focus on low-income populations, simple messages, weekly incentives, and take-home ingredients to practice healthy recipes allows it to be used broadly in various populations, including those with SMI (Clark et al. 2015).

For individuals with autism-spectrum disorder (ASD), occupational therapy is crucial for improving quality of life through skill-building in activities of daily living, leisure, and social activities. Il Tortellante in Modena, Italy, established in 2016, is a novel therapeutic cooking program for adolescents and young adults with ASD that focuses on producing fresh pasta while addressing other therapeutic goals, including money and pantry management, social skills, emotion recognition, and independent living. Participants attend the program 5 days a week for 3–6 hours a day; a pilot study, despite a long period of interruption due to the pandemic, showed improvement in daily living skills and socialization (Veneruso et al. 2022). The program is still ongoing and is accessible for nonverbal individuals.

Culinary Medicine

Over the past few decades, there has been increasing interest in the intersection of food and the field of medicine. Culinary medicine is a burgeoning area that seeks to address the role that food plays in well-being, disease prevention, and treatment of medical conditions. Specific medical conditions have been found to be responsive to specific diets, such as anti-inflammatory foods for rheumatoid arthritis; ketogenic foods for epilepsy; and the Mediterranean diet for cardiovascular disease, colon cancer, and type 2 diabetes (La Puma 2016). Multiple U.S. medical schools now teach culinary medicine in their curricula, and several hospitals offer culinary medicine programs to clinicians and patients. Tulane University was the first medical school in the United States to offer culinary medicine classes to students in 2012 and has been offering cooking classes to the community since 2013. The Food as Medicine (FAME) culinary medicine class curriculum, directed toward children and parents, is based on Tulane's Health Meets Food community programming (Marshall and Albin 2021).

Often aligned with culinary medicine programs, the subspecialty lifestyle medicine incorporates healthy eating as one of its core pillars, along with physical activity and exercise, effective stress management, restorative sleep, positive social connections, and minimizing risky substances. Academic centers may offer culinary medicine programs as part of lifestyle medicine programs. In New York, the NYC Health + Hospitals system offers comprehensive programs for patients that last 6 months or more and include individual appointments, weekly group classes, exercise classes, recipes and cooking demonstrations, classes on reading Nutrition Facts labels, grocery shopping, meal planning and preparation, and sleep and stress management classes. To name just two others, Columbia University's Institute of Human Nutrition offers a course for clinicians on Cultural Adaptations for the Mediterranean Diet, and Stanford University offers an online course on Food and Health. As the field of culinary medicine has grown, multiple resources now exist, including a culinary medicine curriculum offered by the American College of Lifestyle Medicine (Hauser 2019) and extensive resources at the Teaching Kitchen Collaborative (https://teachingkitchens.org).

Future Research Directions

Many of the studies referenced here were conducted as population-based studies or short-term cooking program interventions. These studies have promising implications for the beneficial effects of home cooking, cooking together, and eating together in diverse populations, ranging from children to older adults. Future research should expand on this work with longer-term cooking interventions embedded in schools or community centers. Many of the participants from prior studies were self-selecting and may have had higher baseline motivation to make dietary changes. It would also be useful to follow up on participants after a year or two to ascertain whether dietary changes persisted and whether there were ongoing, additional significant changes in diet quality and physical health. Studies on eating together have mostly focused on family meals, particularly among parents and children, which are not generalizable to eating with peers or with adult family or friends. More research should explore the impact of cooking and eating together as a social activity and its implications on mental health. Cooking intervention programs primarily focus on whole foods, but such programs are not readily accessible. Meal kits, which offer a compromise between convenience and home cooking, range from boxes of premeasured ingredients with a recipe card to prepre-pared meals. As a more accessible option, meal kits could potentially function as a surrogate for cooking programs. In a qualitative study, primary meal providers viewed meal kits as nutritionally healthy alternatives that allow for enhanced family participation and improved food literacy; however, meal kits may not be as healthy as they appear (Fraser et al. 2022). Future research should include the use of meal kits as a comparison group to home cooking.

Clinical Pearls

- As part of a dietary and lifestyle assessment, clinicians can ask clients about their frequency of home cooking and their past, current, or future interest in home cooking as a form of leisure/recreation and improved diet/nutrition.
- Clinicians seeing children and adolescents can recommend that parents cook with them to promote parent-child bonding and decrease adolescent health risk factors.
- Cooking as a therapeutic intervention can be widely recommended, ranging from children to older adults, and people with a range of mental health conditions, including autism-spectrum disorder and serious mental illness, with appropriate supervision.
- Clinicians can encourage clients to engage in home cooking to reduce depressive symptoms.
- Clinicians can refer clients to therapeutic cooking programs and culinary medicine programs for both physical and mental health benefits.

Key Chapter Points

- Home cooking offers numerous physical health benefits primarily mediated through improved nutrition, such as increased fruit and vegetable intake and increased adherence to healthy diets. These physical health benefits include lower BMI, decreased adiposity, lower blood pressure, and improved cholesterol profiles.
- Home cooking and eating with others offer numerous mental health benefits primarily mediated through social interaction, nutrition, and self-efficacy. These mental health benefits include decreased rates of depression and anxiety, substance use, disordered eating, aggressive behavior, and poor academic performance.
- Children and adolescents derive significant psychosocial benefits from cooking with parents due to greater sense of autonomy, self-esteem, and positive parenting.
- College students and older adults are particularly vulnerable to adverse physical and mental health outcomes associated with poor nutrition in their life stages and would benefit from home cooking, especially with others.
- Culinary medicine and lifestyle medicine are expanding at academic institutions, commonly offering classes to clinicians, health care clients, and the community.

References

Alghamdi MM, Burrows T, Barclay B, et al: Culinary nutrition education programs in community-dwelling older adults: a scoping review. J Nutr Health Aging 27(2):142–158, 2023 36806869

Atomik Research: 2023 Report: Shifting Consumer Eating and Grocery Shopping Habits: National Frozen and Refrigerated Foods Association 2023. Available at: https://nfraweb.org/wp-content/uploads/2018/08/NFRA-2023-Eating-at-Home-Industry-Report.pdf. Accessed December 30, 2024.

Barr-Porter M, Sullivan A, Watras E, et al: Community-based designed pilot cooking and texting intervention on health-related quality of life among college students. Int J Environ Res Public Health 21(3):293, 2024 38541293

Clark A, Bezyak J, Testerman N: Individuals with severe mental illnesses have improved eating behaviors and cooking skills after attending a 6-week nutrition cooking class. Psychiatr Rehabil J 38(3):276–278, 2015 25559077

Cunningham-Sabo L, Lohse B: Cooking with kids positively affects fourth graders' vegetable preferences and attitudes and self-efficacy for food and cooking. Child Obes 9(6):549–556, 2013 24320723

Davis JN, Martinez LC, Spruijt-Metz D, et al: LA sprouts: a 12-week gardening, nutrition, and cooking randomized control trial improves determinants of dietary behaviors. J Nutr Educ Behav 48(1):2–11.e1, 2016 26453367

Eisenberg ME, Olson RE, Neumark-Sztainer D, et al: Correlations between family meals and psychosocial well-being among adolescents. Arch Pediatr Adolesc Med 158(8):792–796, 2004 15289253

Farmer N, Touchton-Leonard K, Ross A: Psychosocial benefits of cooking interventions: a systematic review. Health Educ Behav 45(2):167–180, 2018 29121776

Fraser K, Love P, Campbell KJ, et al: Meal kits in the family setting: impacts on family dynamics, nutrition, social and mental health. Appetite 169:105816, 2022 34801628

Hamad NA, Rahim HFA, Shi Z: Association between dietary patterns and depression symptoms among adults with or without diabetes in Qatar: a population-based study. BMC Public Health 24(1):2260, 2024 39164668

Hari J: Stolen Focus: Why You Can't Pay Attention and How to Think Deeply Again. New York, Crown, 2021.

Hasan B, Thompson WG, Almasri J, et al: The effect of culinary interventions (cooking classes) on dietary intake and behavioral change: a systematic review and evidence map. BMC Nutr 5:29, 2019 32153942

Hauser M: Culinary Medicine Curriculum. American College of Lifestyle Medicine, 2019. Available at: https://lifestylemedicine.org/wp-content/uploads/2022/08/CulinaryMedCourseBook-1.pdf. Accessed May 23, 2025.

Helle C, Hillesund ER, Øverby NC: Maternal mental health is associated with children's frequency of family meals at 12 and 24 months of age. Matern Child Nutr 20(1):e13552, 2024 37596722

Hersch D, Perdue L, Ambroz T, et al: The impact of cooking classes on food-related preferences, attitudes, and behaviors of school-aged children: a systematic review of the evidence, 2003–2014. Prev Chronic Dis 11:E193, 2014 25376015

La Puma J: What is culinary medicine and what does it do? Popul Health Manag 19(1):1–3, 2016 26035069

Maiz E, Urkia-Susin I, Urdaneta E, et al: Child involvement in choosing a recipe, purchasing ingredients, and cooking at school increases willingness to try new foods and reduces food neophobia. J Nutr Educ Behav 53(4):279–289, 2021 33573994

Marshall H, Albin J: Food as medicine: a pilot nutrition and cooking curriculum for children of participants in a community-based culinary medicine class. Matern Child Health J 25(1):54–58, 2021 33200324

Middleton G, Patterson KA, Muir-Cochrane E, et al: The health and well-being impacts of community shared meal programs for older populations: a scoping review. Innov Aging 6(7):068, 2022

Mills S, Brown H, Wrieden W, et al: Frequency of eating home cooked meals and potential benefits for diet and health: cross-sectional analysis of a population-based cohort study. Int J Behav Nutr Phys Act 14(1):109, 2017 28818089

Rees J, Fu SC, Lo J, et al: How a 7-week food literacy cooking program affects cooking confidence and mental health: findings of a quasi-experimental controlled intervention trial. Front Nutr 9:802940, 2022 35369083

Reicks M, Kocher M, Reeder J: Impact of cooking and home food preparation interventions among adults: a systematic review (2011–2016). J Nutr Educ Behav 50(2):148–172.e1, 2018 28958671

Saxe-Custack A, Egan S, Sadler R, et al: Relative impacts of a virtual cooking and nutrition program for children and families. Appetite 191:107041, 2023 37709149

Skeer MR, Ballard EL: Are family meals as good for youth as we think they are? A review of the literature on family meals as they pertain to adolescent risk prevention. J Youth Adolesc 42(7):943–963, 2013 23712661

Tani Y, Fujiwara T, Isumi A, et al: Home cooking is related to potential reduction in cardiovascular disease risk among adolescents: results from the A-CHILD study. Nutrients 12(12):3845, 2020 33339277

Tani Y, Doi S, Isumi A, et al: Association of home cooking with caregiver-child interaction and child mental health: results from the Adachi Child Health Impact of Living Difficulty (A-CHILD) study. Public Health Nutr 24(13):4257–4267, 2021 33722323

Tørslev MK, Bjarup Thøgersen D, Høstgaard Bonde A, et al: Supporting positive parenting and promoting healthy living through family cooking classes. Int J Environ Res Public Health 18(9):4709, 2021 33925145

Utter J, Denny S, Lucassen M, et al: Adolescent cooking abilities and behaviors: associations with nutrition and emotional well-being. J Nutr Educ Behav 48(1):35–41.e1, 2016 26411900

Utter J, Larson N, Berge JM, et al: Family meals among parents: associations with nutritional, social and emotional wellbeing. Prev Med 113:7–12, 2018 29746973

Veneruso M, Varallo G, Franceschini C, et al: Short report. Cooking for autism: a pilot study of an innovative culinary laboratory for Italian adolescents and emerging adults with autism spectrum disorder. Res Dev Disabil 126:104259, 2022 35567827

Zhou S, Ding X, Leung JTY: Healthy aging at family mealtimes: associations of clean cooking, protein intake, and dining together with mental health of Chinese older adults amid Covid-19 pandemic. Int J Environ Res Public Health 20(3):1672, 2023 36767039

14

Gardening, Gardening Together, and Mental Health

Michael T. Compton, M.D., M.P.H.

The glory of gardening: hands in the dirt, head in the sun, heart with nature. To nurture a garden is to feed not just the body, but the soul.

—Alfred Austin, English poet, 1835–1913

Recent years have witnessed a growing interest in the role of natural environments and outdoor activities, including gardens and gardening, for promoting physical health and mental health. Gardening, which involves cultivating and caring for plants—and beautifying and nurturing green spaces—has mental health–promoting therapeutic potential. It involves both physical activity in tasks such as digging, planting, weeding, watering, and harvesting, as well as substantial cognitive activity in terms of planning, problem-solving, and creative thinking. The plants of interest in gardening activities can be highly varied, but here our focus is primarily vegetable gardens; many of the principles naturally convey to nurturing nonedible plants such as cut flowers and those in shade gardens, among others. Gardening can have health benefits when done alone or with others and when done with or without a planned therapeutic intention.

Gardening

Gardening is the activity of planning, cultivating, and tending to a garden, especially as a pastime, although also for one's own food production. The focus is growing plants for their flowers, fruits, vegetables, herbs, and seeds—and for their aesthetically pleasing appearance—within a designated space. People often take part in gardening for its leisurely, recreational, environmental, cultural, spiritual, therapeutic, and health benefits. Gardening encourages mindfulness and relaxation through repetitive and focused tasks while interacting with plants. Gardening also involves diverse cognitive activities such as attention, concentration, planning, reasoning, problem solving, and multiple types of learning and memory, as well as physical activities related to tending to soil, digging, planting, watering, weeding, and harvesting, among other activities.

Gardening and Physical Activity

Gardening tasks provide low- to moderate-intensity physical activity that can improve muscle strength, endurance, and flexibility; regular engagement in such activity can contribute to better physical fitness and functional ability, including among older adults. Physical activity has many health benefits independent of other healthy behaviors like good nutrition. Some of the key points of the Physical Activity Guidelines for Americans are given in Table 14.1. Gardening can be a form of physical activity that provides the same health benefits as other forms of regular physical activity that are known to have positive impacts on physical health and for ameliorating some physical health conditions. Meeting the recommendations in the Physical Activity Guidelines for Americans consistently over time can lead to many long-term health benefits.

For young people, physical activity can help improve cognition, bone health, fitness, and heart health and reduce the risk of depression and other behavioral health disorders. For adults, physical activity helps prevent at least eight types of cancer; reduces the risk of dementia including Alzheimer's disease, all-cause mortality, heart disease, stroke, high blood pressure, type 2 diabetes, and depression; and improves bone

Table 14.1 Beneficial health effects of physical activity and key points from the Physical Activity Guidelines for Americans

Preschool-age children (3–5 years) should be active throughout the day to enhance growth and development. Adults caring for children of this age should encourage active play (light, moderate, or vigorous intensity) and aim for at least 3 hours per day.

Youth ages 6–17 need at least 60 minutes of moderate to vigorous activity daily. Most activity can be aerobic, like walking, running, or anything that makes the heart beat faster. They also need activities that make their muscles and bones strong, like climbing on playground equipment, playing basketball, and jumping rope.

For adults, to attain the most health benefits from physical activity, at least 150–300 minutes (2.5–5 hours) of moderate-intensity aerobic activity are needed each week, like brisk walking or fast dancing.

According to the "talk test," as a general rule, a person doing moderate-intensity aerobic activity is breathing hard but can talk—but not sing—during the activity. One doing vigorous-intensity activity cannot say more than a few words without pausing for a breath.

Adults also need muscle-strengthening activity at least 2 days each week. Muscle-strengthening activities make muscles do more work than they are accustomed to (i.e., they overload the muscles). Examples of muscle-strengthening activities include lifting weights, working with resistance bands, doing calisthenics that use body weight for resistance (like push-ups and pull-ups), and heavy gardening.

Because of the strong relationship between increased sedentary behavior (sitting) and increased risk of heart disease, high blood pressure, and all-cause mortality, all physical activity—but especially moderate to vigorous activity—can help offset these risks.

Any amount of physical activity has some health benefits. We can benefit from small amounts of moderate to vigorous physical activity throughout the day.

Physical activity has immediate health benefits; for example, it can reduce blood pressure and improve quality of sleep and insulin sensitivity.

Walking for exercise, gardening, doing yard work, bicycling, and swimming are among the activities with the lowest injury rates.

Source. U.S. Department of Health and Human Services, Office of Disease Prevention and Health Promotion: Physical Activity Guidelines for Americans. https://odphp.health.gov/sites/default/files/2019-09/Physical_Activity_Guidelines_2nd_edition.pdf. (Accessed May 23, 2025).

health, physical function, and quality of life. For older adults, physical activity also lowers the risk of falls and injuries from falls. For pregnant people, physical activity reduces the risk of postpartum depression. For everyone, physical activity reduces the risk of unhealthy weight gain and helps maintain a healthy weight. In addition to its preventive effects, physical activity can help manage many health conditions that may already be present. For example, physical activity can decrease pain among those with osteoarthritis, reduce disease progression for hypertension and type 2 diabetes, reduce symptoms of anxiety and depression, and improve cognition for those with dementia, multiple sclerosis, ADHD, and Parkinson's disease.

Physical activity is clearly beneficial to physical health and mental health. The physical activity involved in gardening is similar to other forms of physical activity, but also different. Multiple body positions and motions are at play when one is gardening, including gripping, bending, walking, lifting, stretching, and standing, to name a few (Park and Shoemaker 2009). The majority of gardening tasks are classified as low- to moderate-intensity physical activity (Nicklett et al. 2016), although the level of physical activity varies by task and by gardener. Gardening tasks using both the upper and lower body (e.g., digging, weeding, raking, tying plants to stakes) have been shown to require moderate-intensity physical activity; those using the upper body while standing or squatting (e.g., pruning, mixing soil, planting seedlings, sowing seeds, watering using a watering can or hose, harvesting) are low-intensity physical activities; and tasks requiring limited use of the upper body while standing (e.g., filling containers with soil, washing harvested produce) are the least demanding physical activities of the gardening tasks tested by Park and colleagues (2011).

In addition to providing health-beneficial physical activity, gardening can improve balance and coordination, which are crucial for preventing falls and maintaining mobility. Older adults who participate in gardening activities may have better balance and coordination compared with nongardeners. Furthermore, tasks such as bending, reaching, and squatting help maintain joint flexibility and muscle strength, enhancing overall physical health.

Beyond providing physical activity and improving balance and coordination, gardening involves diverse sensory experiences as well—such as the sight of beautiful plants and colorful flowers, the smell of soil and plants, the feel of seeds and plant leaves, the taste of fruit, and the sound of birds and other animals—that can have calming and restorative effects. Imagine being in the garden with flowers blooming, birds chirping, bees buzzing, and vegetables nearing their peak of ripeness; surely all of this is beneficial to one's health in addition to exercising cognition and providing physical activity. The natural environments in which gardening occurs likely have inherent therapeutic benefits, reducing stress and improving mood.

Gardening and Physical Health

As depicted in Figure 14.1, gardening has been associated with various health benefits, including enhanced physical fitness, better nutrition, and reduced risk of chronic diseases. Health-protective effects are likely due to the combined benefits of physical activity, stress reduction through increased exposure to nature, and improved diet quality and nutrition through a greater appreciation of produce and the consumption of home-grown produce. Consuming more fruits and vegetables means having a higher intake of dietary fiber and key vitamins, minerals, and phytonutrients.

Gardening has been shown through research to have health benefits, although more rigorous studies are needed. In a study in Seoul, South Korea, women older than 70 who engaged in a 15-session gardening intervention (as a low- to moderate-intensity form of physical activity) had a significant improvement in their high density lipoprotein level, systolic and diastolic blood pressure, and lab findings related to immunity and oxidative stress (Park et al. 2017). According to cross-sectional data from the 2019 Behavioral Risk Factor Surveillance System, noninstitutionalized U.S. adults 65 and older who engaged in gardening as a form of physical activity ($n = 14{,}903$)—compared with those not reporting physical activity ($n = 45{,}007$)—had better cardiovascular health status (as assessed by cardiovascular disease risks including current or prior cardiovascular disease, stroke, heart attack, high cholesterol, high blood pressure, diabetes, body mass index ≥25, poor physical health status, and poor mental health status); were more likely to consume fruits and vegetables five or more times/day; and had a lower 10-year mortality risk (Veldheer et al. 2023).

The gentle, repetitive movements involved in gardening can provide musculoskeletal benefits, as well; low-impact gardening activities may improve joint flexibility and reduce pain. Additionally, gardening is not associated with osteoarthritis progression and should not be discouraged in those with osteoarthritis (of the knee, as reported in Lo et al. 2024). Gardening may also reduce the risk of osteoporosis and promote bone health.

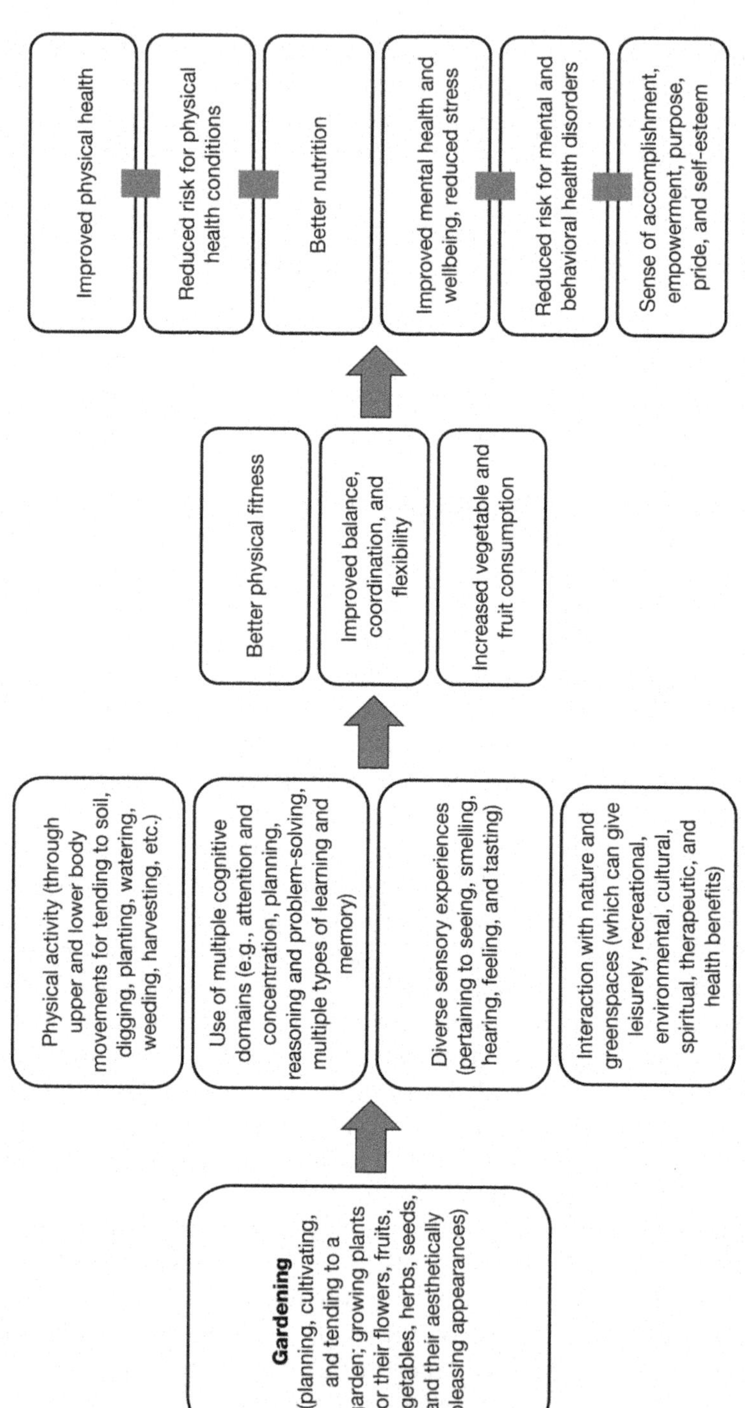

Figure 14.1 Some of the potential beneficial health effects of gardening.

Gardening and Mental Health and Well-Being

Physical activity is widely documented to yield beneficial mental health outcomes. For example, a systematic review of prospective studies found 25 reports demonstrating that baseline physical activity was associated with a lower risk of subsequent depression (Mammen and Faulkner 2013). The majority of the studies were of high methodologic quality, providing consistent evidence that physical activity—at any level, including low levels like walking for less than 150 minutes/week)—may prevent future depression. Given that gardening represents a form of physical activity, health benefits undoubtedly pertain to both physical health and mental health.

The mental health and well-being benefits of gardening extend beyond those stemming from the physical activity involved. Gardening can promote relief from acute stress in terms of both neuroendocrine pathways (e.g., decreased cortisol levels) and self-reported mood (Van Den Berg and Custers 2011). Gardening can bring about enhanced mood and emotional well-being. A meta-analysis including 22 studies published after 2001—comprising 76 comparisons between control and treatment groups (the latter meaning those participating in gardening or identifying as gardeners)—revealed consistent and substantial reductions in depression and anxiety symptoms, stress, and mood disturbance, as well as increases in quality of life, sense of community, and cognitive functioning (Soga et al. 2016).

Lentoor (2024) conducted a systematic review involving 23 studies to evaluate the effect of gardening as a physical activity on promoting neuroplasticity and cognitive functioning. Studies demonstrated that gardening boosts immunity and lowers inflammation, while also increasing levels of neurotrophic factors such as brain-derived neurotrophic factor, vascular endothelial growth factor, and platelet-derived growth factor, which are essential for promoting neuroplasticity and improving cognitive function. The process of learning about plants, planning garden layouts, problem solving, and remembering gardening tasks can stimulate cognitive function and enhance memory.

The act of nurturing plants and witnessing their growth can provide a sense of accomplishment, pride, purpose, and self-efficacy, all of which are critical to mental health. Gardening provides opportunities for individuals to set goals, achieve demonstrable outcomes, and experience a sense of accomplishment. Completing gardening tasks and seeing tangible (if not edible) results, such as a thriving garden and freshly harvested produce, can boost self-esteem and provide a sense of purpose. Developing gardening skills can increase confidence and lend a sense of competence, further enhancing self-esteem and mental health. Nurturing plants and making decisions about gardening activities can empower, give a sense of control over one's environment, and counter negative affect.

Gardening as a mental health–promoting activity is not without its limitations, however. Gardening is often seasonal, and its benefits can be influenced by environmental factors such as weather and climate. These factors can limit the extent to which individuals can engage in gardening activities year-round, potentially affecting the consistency of mental health benefits.

Gardening Together

Gardening can be physically and psychologically beneficial as a solitary activity, but it can also involve social interactions, whether through community gardens, gardening clubs, or simply sharing gardening tips, plants, or produce with neighbors. These social interactions can foster a sense of belonging, community, and connectedness, some of the benefits of which are shown in Figure 14.2.

Community Gardens and Urban Farms

Community gardens—which are different from a private garden in that they are in some sense public gardens in terms of ownership, access, and degree of democratic control (Ferris et al. 2001)—serve as social hubs where individuals from diverse backgrounds can come together, fostering a sense of social cohesion. The shared purpose and cooperative nature of gardening tasks help build social bonds and reduce feelings of isolation or loneliness.

Gardening together often involves people of different ages, promoting intergenerational interaction. Community gardening programs may facilitate interactions between older and younger generations, fostering mutual understanding and respect, reducing age-related stigmatization, and contributing to the psychological well-being of all participants. Ensuring that gardening programs are inclusive and accessible to all individuals, regardless of their physical or socioeconomic status, is crucial. Community gardening activities can be

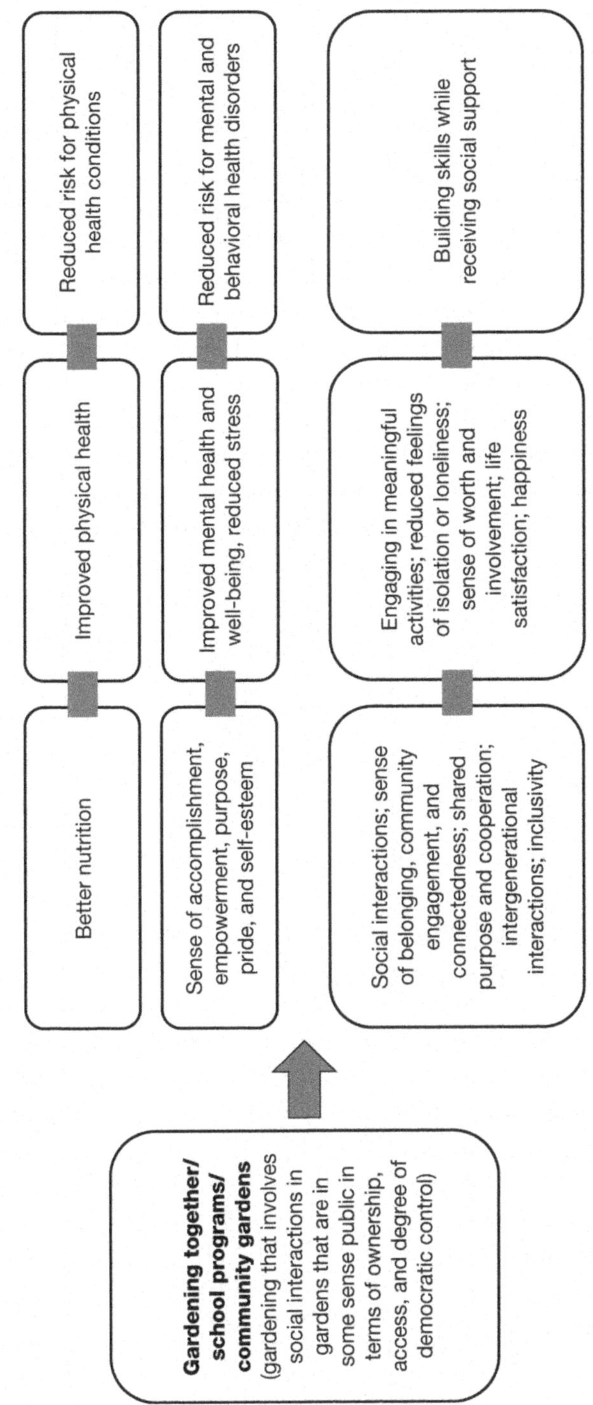

Figure 14.2 Some of the potential beneficial health and social effects of gardening together, with others.

adapted to suit different fitness levels and abilities, making them inclusive of people with varying physical capabilities, as well as individuals facing behavioral health challenges.

Community gardens may be designed as leisure gardens, children's or school gardens, entrepreneurial gardens, crime diversion gardens, work and training gardens, healing and therapy gardens (quiet gardens), neighborhood pocket parks, ecological restoration gardens/parks, or demonstration gardens (Ferris et al. 2001); they all aim to improve well-being, even if not intentionally designed to provide a therapeutic experience. In addition to growing crucial social support networks, community gardens, especially in low-income neighborhoods, can lead to other issues in the neighborhood being addressed—likely owing to the organizing facilitated by the community garden (Armstrong 2000).

Urban farming—the practice of cultivating, processing, and distributing food in or around urban areas—has gained significant attention in recent years because of its potential to improve food security and food justice, foster community engagement, and enhance environmental sustainability. Urban farms can provide mental health support for vulnerable populations, including individuals experiencing homelessness, substance use, and trauma. Urban farm programs tailored for these populations offer safe and supportive environments where individuals can engage in meaningful activities, build skills, and receive social support. Urban farms provide accessible physical activity opportunities for individuals who may face barriers to other forms of physical activity or exercise.

Gardening Together and Mental Health and Well-Being

Community gardens are known to improve both physical health and mental health. For example, like home gardening, community gardening can improve diet quality. In a 2003 survey involving 766 adults in Flint, Michigan (Alaimo et al. 2008), the 15% who participated in a community gardening project in the past 12 months consumed 1.4 times more fruits and vegetables per day than those who did not participate, and they were 3.5 times more likely to consume fruits and vegetables at least five times a day, in keeping with dietary guideline recommendations. In a 2006–2007 survey representing 436 residents across 58 block groups in Denver, Colorado (Litt et al. 2011), urban community gardeners consumed fruits and vegetables 5.7 times per day, an increase compared with home gardeners (4.6 times per day) and nongardeners (3.9 times per day). Some 56% of community gardeners met national recommendations for consuming fruits and vegetables at least five times per day, compared with 37% of home gardeners and 25% of nongardeners. Among 44 families enrolled in a community gardening project designed for migrant seasonal farm worker families in a rural Oregon community (Carney et al. 2012), the frequency of adult vegetable intake of "several times a day" increased from 18.2% to 84.8% ($P < 0.001$), and the frequency of children's vegetable intake of "several times a day" increased from 24.0% to 64.0% ($P = 0.003$). Furthermore, worrying in the past month that food would run out before money was available to buy more (a measure of food insecurity) dropped from 31.2% to 3.1% ($P = 0.006$).

The benefits of participating in gardening programs also extend to children. In a 12-week garden-based nutrition education program designed to promote fruit and vegetable intake among fourth through sixth graders ($n = 93$) attending a YMCA summer camp, increases were observed in the number of fruits and vegetables ever eaten ($P < 0.001$), vegetable preferences ($P < 0.001$), and fruit and vegetable asking behavior at home ($P < 0.002$) (Heim et al. 2009). The intervention consisted of children participating in garden-based activities twice per week, as well as weekly educational activities that included fruit and vegetable taste tests, preparation of fruit and vegetable snacks, and family newsletters sent home to parents. In a systematic review of school gardening programs that included 40 articles (21 quantitative studies, 16 qualitative studies, and three mixed-methods studies), Ohly and colleagues (2016) reported that qualitative research ascribes a range of health and well-being effects and that students who do not excel in classroom activities may particularly benefit. They noted, however, that the quality of quantitative research was generally poor and that more robust research is needed.

For youth and adults alike, qualitative research (e.g., Kingsley et al. 2009) suggests that urban community garden participation allows people to come together and escape daily pressures, provides a source of advice and social support, and offers a place that gives a sense of worth and involvement, while conferring spiritual, fitness, and nutritional benefits. Being engaged in an urban gardening project is positively associated with community involvement and life satisfaction. In a systematic review that included eight studies, Lampert and colleagues (2021) found that community gardeners, irrespective of age, had significantly better health outcomes than their neighbors not engaged in gardening activities in terms of life satisfaction, happiness, general health, mental health, and social cohesion. The authors concluded that community gardens are an affordable and efficient way of promoting physical and mental health and well-being. A systematic review of the literature on the contribution of allotment gardening (a British term for community gardening) to health and well-being revealed benefits in terms of providing a stress-relieving refuge, contributing to a healthier lifestyle, creating social opportunities, providing valued contact with nature, and enabling self-development (Genter et al. 2015). A scoping review of the impacts of urban agriculture—including 51 quantitative, 29 qualitative, and 21 mixed-methods studies from settings ranging from North America to Sub-Saharan Africa—revealed evidence of positive impacts of urban farming on food security, nutritional outcomes, physical and mental health outcomes, and social capital (Audate et al. 2019).

Therapeutic Gardening Programs and Horticultural Therapy

Therapeutic horticulture programs, which use cultivativation of plants and gardening as therapeutic tools, are effective in improving mental health. These programs are designed for various populations, including veterans, older adults, and individuals with physical illnesses or disabilities, mental illnesses, or intellectual/developmental disabilities.

Traditional treatment methods for depression, anxiety, substance use disorders, and other behavioral health disorders include medication, psychotherapy, and evidence-based psychosocial interventions, but there is growing interest in complementary and alternative therapies, including gardening programs. Participating in such programs has been linked to improvements in overall well-being and quality of life. Given the benefits of gardening, it should be no surprise that horticultural therapy can bring about enhanced mood, greater life satisfaction, and a sense of purpose and accomplishment.

Therapeutic Gardening and Horticultural Therapy: Mental Health Effects

Therapeutic gardening and horticultural therapy programs have shown effectiveness across multiple studies in terms of improving mental well-being, reducing symptoms of depression and anxiety, and improving outcomes among those with serious mental illness, among other mental health-related outcomes. The multitude of studies have been summarized in a number of systematic reviews and meta-analyses. A review and meta-analysis involving 40 studies (10 interventional studies, two observational studies, and 28 mixed interventional and observational studies) documented an overall positive impact of gardening activities and horticultural therapy on several measures of mental well-being, quality of life, and general health status (Pantiru et al. 2024). A systematic review and meta-analysis—involving 20 completed and four ongoing trials—evaluated the effectiveness of group-based gardening interventions for increasing well-being and reducing symptoms of poor mental health in adults (Briggs et al. 2023); findings revealed that such interventions may increase well-being and may reduce symptoms of depression. The authors noted, however, that there was uncertainty in the pooled effects due to heterogeneity, small sample sizes, and unclear risk of bias for many of the included studies. In a systematic review of 31 studies of horticultural therapy for stress reduction, Lu and colleagues (2023) found significant improvements in psychological indicators (with a longer duration of participation providing greater effects on stress reduction) but not on physiological indicators such as skin conductance, heart rate, blood pressure, and salivary cortisol levels.

A number of studies have demonstrated the effectiveness of gardening programs in reducing symptoms of depression in particular. Two systematic reviews and meta-analyses pertaining to horticultural therapy for older adults with depression revealed significant effects on reducing depressive symptoms (Xu et al. 2023; Zhang et al. 2022). Positive mental health impacts of horticultural activities extend to older adults in long-term-care facilities (Jueng et al. 2023). Aside from depression per se, gardening programs have also been shown to reduce anxiety and stress. In a review of 10 studies published since 2003 (Clatworthy et al. 2013), all studies reported positive effects of gardening as a mental health intervention, such as reducing symptoms of depression and anxiety, as well as providing a range of benefits across emotional, social, vocational, physical, and spiritual domains. In a systematic review of 14 studies of horticultural therapy for people with mental health conditions from 1992 through 2015, Cipriani et al. (2017) reported statistically significant findings for at least one outcome variable in 11 studies. Beneficial findings were apparent in a variety of settings, across mental health conditions, and in both men and women.

Gardening programs have been implemented for individuals with serious mental illness, including schizophrenia and bipolar disorder. Kam and Siu (2010) evaluated a therapeutic gardening program in Hong Kong for individuals with schizophrenia and other serious mental illnesses. The findings indicated significant improvements in participants' mood, social skills, and overall mental health. The structured nature of the program, combined with the therapeutic effects of gardening, contributed to these positive outcomes. Another study in Hong Kong found horticultural therapy to be effective at increasing mental well-being, engagement, and a sense of meaningfulness and accomplishment among participants (Siu et al. 2020).

In a review of randomized, controlled trials of horticultural therapy—involving target diseases or symptoms of dementia; serious mental illness such as schizophrenia, bipolar disorder, and major depression; frail older adults in nursing homes; and individuals with hemiplegia after stroke—studies showed significant effectiveness in one or more outcomes for mental health and behavior (Kamioka et al. 2014), although higher-quality randomized, controlled trials were recommended. Among older adults, Lin and colleagues (2022) reported—in a systematic review and meta-analysis of 10 studies involving 884 participants—that compared with control conditions, horticultural therapy programs were effective for promoting emotional functioning and well-being, subjective social functioning, and quality of life. No negative effects were found.

Therapeutic Community Gardens

Therapeutic community gardens are specialized garden spaces designed to improve the physical, psychological, and social well-being of individuals. They are laid out to be healing spaces where individuals can participate in gardening activities with an intentional therapeutic aim of improving health and well-being. These gardens provide a unique environment where participants can engage in structured therapeutic horticulture interventions, guided by trained professionals (Genter et al. 2015). Marcus and Sachs (2013) highlighted that such gardens incorporate raised beds for ease of access, shaded areas for comfort, water features for sensory stimulation, and a variety of plants to engage multiple senses.

Therapeutic community gardens are typically designed to facilitate both individual and group activities, providing spaces for solitude as well as social interaction. They cater to a diverse range of populations, including individuals with mental health conditions, older adults, people with disabilities, and those recovering from physical illnesses. In their report on "green care" (a range of activities promoting physical and mental health and well-being through contact with nature by way of farms, gardens, therapeutic horticulture, other outdoor activities, and animal-assisted therapy as therapeutic interventions for vulnerable adults and children), Sempik and colleagues (2010) emphasized that these gardens are particularly beneficial for vulnerable groups that may experience social isolation and have reduced opportunities for physical activity.

Future Research Directions

Although there is growing evidence of the benefits of gardening—and gardening together with others—on mental health, additional large-scale, longitudinal studies to strengthen the evidence base are needed. Many existing studies are small-scale or qualitative, which limits generalizability of findings. Although many observational and quasi-experimental studies exist, a higher level of evidence, including more randomized, controlled trials, are warranted. Such work should also explore ways to make home gardening and community gardening more accessible to a broad range of diverse populations.

Clinical Pearls

- As part of asking about eating patterns, physical activity and exercise, and other lifestyle factors, clinicians can ask clients about their past, current, or future interests in gardening as a form of leisure/recreation or physical activity.
- For clients interested in gardening, clinicians can encourage gardening as a form of physical activity, given its known physical health and mental health benefits.
- Clinicians can recommend gardening with others—in community gardens or on urban farms—for clients interested in gardening or taking up gardening, who would also benefit from social interactions and social connections.
- Clinicians should be aware of the diverse physical health and mental health benefits of gardening, as well as the social benefits of gardening together with others.
- Clinicians can consider referring clients to horticultural therapy—a safe and promising complementary intervention—for adults seeking to reduce stress, improve mental well-being, and decrease psychiatric illness symptoms, or for older adults with cognitive impairment, dementia, or frailty.

Key Chapter Points

- The Physical Activity Guidelines for Americans sets forth recommendations for preschool-aged children, youth ages 6–17, and adults. Any amount of physical activity has some health benefits; adults should strive for 150–300 minutes of moderate-intensity aerobic activity each week.
- Gardening is a form of physical activity that offers numerous physical health benefits. It can improve cardiovascular health, enhance physical fitness, and reduce the risk of chronic diseases, while potentially promoting better nutrition. The physical activity, cognitive tasks, and sensory stimulation provided by gardening contribute to overall physical health, mental health, and well-being.
- Gardening together (with others) offers numerous psychological benefits, in large part by offering social interactions and building social connections. Gardening together can bring about a sense of belonging, community engagement, connectedness, shared purpose, and cooperation.
- Extensive research shows that horticultural therapy can benefit those overcoming physical health challenges, older adults, and individuals living with behavioral health disorders.
- Therapeutic community gardens offer a unique and effective approach to improving physical, psychological, and social well-being. They provide a supportive environment where individuals can engage in meaningful gardening activities in settings specifically designed to promote health and foster social connections.

References

Alaimo K, Packnett E, Miles RA, et al: Fruit and vegetable intake among urban community gardeners. J Nutr Educ Behav 40(2):94–101, 2008 18314085

Armstrong D: A survey of community gardens in upstate New York: implications for health promotion and community development. Health Place 6(4):319–327, 2000 11027957

Audate PP, Fernandez MA, Cloutier G, et al: Scoping review of the impacts of urban agriculture on the determinants of health. BMC Public Health 19(1):672, 2019 31151393

Briggs R, Morris PG, Rees K: The effectiveness of group-based gardening interventions for improving wellbeing and reducing symptoms of

mental ill-health in adults: a systematic review and meta-analysis. J Ment Health 32(4):787–804, 2023 36151719
Carney PA, Hamada JL, Rdesinski R, et al: Impact of a community gardening project on vegetable intake, food security and family relationships: a community-based participatory research study. J Community Health 37(4):874–881, 2012 22194063
Cipriani J, Benz A, Holmgren A, et al: A systematic review of the effects of horticultural therapy on persons with mental health conditions. Occup Ther Ment Health 33(1):47–69, 2017
Clatworthy J, Hinds J, Camic PM: Gardening as a mental health intervention: a review. Ment Health Rev J 18(4):214–225, 2013
Ferris J, Norman C, Sempik J: People, land and sustainability: community gardens and the social dimension of sustainable development. Soc Policy Adm 35(5):559–568, 2001
Genter C, Roberts A, Richardson J, et al: The contribution of allotment gardening to health and well-being: a systematic review of the literature. Br J Occup Ther 78(10):593–605, 2015
Heim S, Stang J, Ireland M: A garden pilot project enhances fruit and vegetable consumption among children. J Am Diet Assoc 109(7):1220–1226, 2009 19559139
Jueng RN, Lin CY, Huang YH: Systematic review on the positive mental health impact of older adults participation in horticultural activities in long term care facilities. Horticulturae 9(10):1076, 2023
Kam MCY, Siu AMH: Evaluation of a horticultural activity programme for persons with psychiatric illness. Hong Kong J Occup Ther 20(2):80–86, 2010
Kamioka H, Tsutani K, Yamada M, et al: Effectiveness of horticultural therapy: a systematic review of randomized controlled trials. Complement Ther Med 22(5):930–943, 2014 25440385
Kingsley J, Townsend M, Henderson-Wilson C: Cultivating health and wellbeing: members' perceptions of the health benefits of a Port Melbourne community garden. Leis Stud 28(2):207–219, 2009
Lampert T, Costa J, Santos O, et al: Evidence on the contribution of community gardens to promote physical and mental health and well-being of non-institutionalized individuals: a systematic review. PLoS One 16(8):e0255621, 2021 34358279
Lentoor AG: Effect of gardening physical activity on neuroplasticity and cognitive function. Explor Neuroprot Ther 4:251–272, 2024
Lin Y, Lin R, Liu W, et al: Effectiveness of horticultural therapy on physical functioning and psychological health outcomes for older adults: a systematic review and meta-analysis. J Clin Nurs 31(15–16):2087–2099, 2022 34694042
Litt JS, Soobader MJ, Turbin MS, et al: The influence of social involvement, neighborhood aesthetics, and community garden participation on fruit

and vegetable consumption. Am J Public Health 101(8):1466–1473, 2011 21680931

Lo GH, Patarini JC, Richard MJ, et al: Gardening/yardwork in people with knee osteoarthritis is not associated with symptom or structural progression over 48 months: data from the Osteoarthritis Initiative. Clin Rheumatol 43(5):1755–1762, 2024 38561590

Lu S, Liu J, Xu M, et al: Horticultural therapy for stress reduction: a systematic review and meta-analysis. Front Psychol 14:1086121, 2023 37564307

Mammen G, Faulkner G: Physical activity and the prevention of depression: a systematic review of prospective studies. Am J Prev Med 45(5):649–657, 2013 24139780

Marcus CC, Sachs NA: Therapeutic Landscapes: An Evidence-Based Approach to Designing Healing Gardens and Restorative Outdoor Spaces. Hoboken, NJ, Wiley and Sons, 2013

Nicklett EJ, Anderson LA, Yen IH: Gardening activities and physical health among older adults: a review of the evidence. J Appl Gerontol 35(6):678–690, 2016 25515757

Ohly H, Gentry S, Wigglesworth R, et al: A systematic review of the health and well-being impacts of school gardening: synthesis of quantitative and qualitative evidence. BMC Public Health 16:286, 2016 27015672

Pantiru I, Ronaldson A, Sima N, et al: The impact of gardening on well-being, mental health, and quality of life: an umbrella review and meta-analysis. Syst Rev 13(1):45, 2024 38287430

Park SA, Shoemaker CA: Observing body position of older adults while gardening for health benefits and risks. Act Adapt Aging 33(1):31–38, 2009

Park S, Lee K, Son K: Determining exercise intensities of gardening tasks as a physical activity using metabolic equivalents in older adults. HortScience 46(12):1706–1710, 2011

Park S, Lee A, Park H, et al: Gardening intervention as a low- to moderate-intensity physical activity for improving blood lipid profiles, blood pressure, inflammation, and oxidative stress in women over the age of 70: a pilot study. HortScience 52(1):200–205, 2017

Sempik J, Hine R, Wilcox D (eds): Green Care: A Conceptual Framework, A Report of the Working Group on the Health Benefits of Green Care, COST Action 866, Green Care in Agriculture. Loughborough, UK, Centre for Child and Family Research, Loughborough University, 2010

Siu AMH, Kam M, Mok I: Horticultural therapy program for people with mental illness: a mixed-method evaluation. Int J Environ Res Public Health 17(3):711, 2020 31979057

Soga M, Gaston KJ, Yamaura Y: Gardening is beneficial for health: a meta-analysis. Prev Med Rep 14(5):92–99, 2016 27981022

Van Den Berg AE, Custers MH: Gardening promotes neuroendocrine and affective restoration from stress. J Health Psychol 16(1):3–11, 2011 20522508

Veldheer S, Tuan WJ, Al-Shaar L, et al: Gardening is associated with better cardiovascular health status among older adults in the United States: analysis of the 2019 behavioral risk factor surveillance system survey. J Acad Nutr Diet 123(5):761–769.e3, 2023 36323395

Xu M, Lu S, Liu J, et al: Effectiveness of horticultural therapy in aged people with depression: a systematic review and meta-analysis. Front Public Health 11:1142456, 2023 36969640

Zhang YW, Wang J, Fang TH: The effect of horticultural therapy on depressive symptoms among the elderly: a systematic review and meta-analysis. Front Public Health 10:953363, 2022 36091570

15

Food Production and Mental Health

Luigi Attademo, M.D.
Francesco Bernardini, M.D.
Michael T. Compton, M.D., M.P.H.

Agriculture is the most healthful, most useful, and most noble employment of man.

—George Washington

Have you ever thought about the mental health impacts of how food is grown? This chapter provides an overview of some of the many issues related to food production and mental health. Although many other topics could be covered, our focus is on large farms and monocultures, genetically modified organism commodity crops, concentrated animal feeding operations, and ultraprocessed foods. Additionally, two healthy eating patterns are described: the local food movement and the slow food movement, as well as the EAT-Lancet Commission's Planetary Health Diet.

Industrial Agriculture and Industrial Food Production

The term *industrial agriculture* refers to large-scale, intensive farming methods focused on maximizing crop and livestock production, often using chemical fertilizers, pesticides, herbicides, genetically modified organism (GMO) crop seeds, antibiotics, and hormones. It involves practices such as monoculture (growing a single crop, such as field corn or soybeans, in a field or across large amounts of acreage), heavy mechanization, and confinement of large numbers of animals in concentrated environments (concentrated animal feeding operations [CAFOs]). These practices and systems have extensive effects on both physical health and mental health (Donham et al. 2007; European Agency for Safety and Health at Work 2024; Mahdizade Ari et al. 2024; McElroy 2010; Tota et al. 2024; Young 2023). Industrial agriculture contrasts with traditional farming methods, which involve smaller farms, diverse crops and livestock, and less intensive and environmentally disruptive practices. The goal of industrial agriculture is to produce vast quantities of food at relatively low cost, often for national or global markets rather than local communities. Rural and agricultural communities have changed dramatically over the past half century, with an overall reduction in the number of farms and a substantial increase in their sizes (Donham et al. 2007).

While encompassing industrial agriculture, the term *industrial food production* can be used to describe further downstream processing, after products leave the farm, and the creation of processed foods and ultraprocessed foods. As just one example among thousands, chicken nuggets are created on a large scale via industrial food production processes: GMO crops such as corn and soybeans are used to feed chickens in CAFOs; after slaughter, a deboning process allows for softer parts of the chicken carcass to be forced through a mesh, resulting in a meat paste that is shaped; the pieces are battered and breaded with industrial techniques that evenly coat all of the pieces, which are then fried in oil until the batter has set and the outside reaches the desired color; and the nuggets are packaged, frozen, and stored for shipping to grocery stores and restaurant chains. Industrial food production refers to that entire process, for countless varieties of processed and ultraprocessed foods.

Rapid population growth, urbanization, rising income, and the consequent changes in food consumption patterns affect food production such that in recent decades we have seen a growing trend toward industrial-scale farming to feed everyone (Young 2023). Beyond impacts on water pollution, air pollution, infectious disease health risks, and community impacts (Merchant and Martin 2024), industrial farming and food production may have largely unrecognized mental health impacts. When analyzing the potential links between industrial agriculture and industrial food production and mental health, several factors must be taken into consideration, including socioeconomic and environmental conditions; large-scale farming and manufacturing practices; and food production, storage, preservation, packaging, and distribution systems. Some potential psychosocial stressors pertaining to the system are shown in Figure 15.1.

Environmental impacts are also substantial. Industrial agriculture and industrial food production pose serious risks to environmental

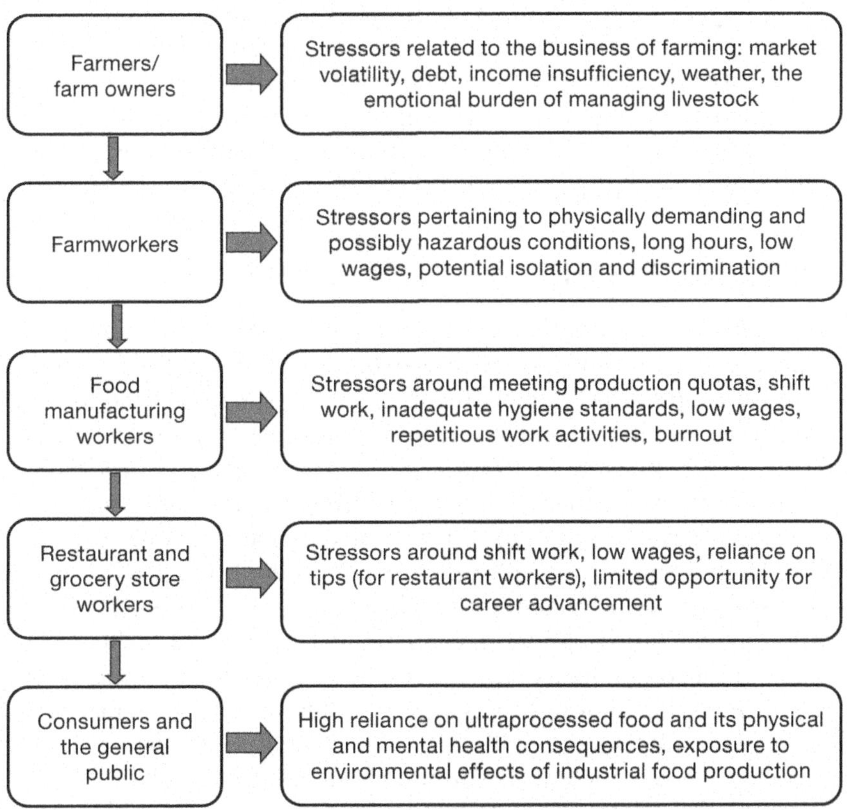

Figure 15.1 **Some of the potential psychosocial stressors pertaining to the industrial food production system.**

health, as they are major contributors to deforestation, greenhouse gas emissions, soil degradation, and water pollution, all of which exacerbate global warming and climate change (Çakmakçı et al. 2023). Climate change and connected extreme weather events, land degradation, and biodiversity loss also affect agricultural and livestock production, with potential impacts on food security (Miraglia et al. 2009). In this complex condition, according to the Food and Agriculture Organization of the United Nations, the future challenge for sustainable agrifood systems will be to deliver food security and nutrition for all in such a way that the economic, social, and environmental bases to generate food security and nutrition for future generations will not be compromised. This means that food production should be profitable throughout, ensuring economic sustainability; have broad-based benefits for society, securing social sustainability; and have a positive or neutral impact on the natural resource environment, safeguarding the sustainability of the environment (Food and Agriculture Organization of the United Nations 2018). Although mental health effects may be less recognized than physical health impacts, pollution, climate change, and biodiversity loss are now thought to significantly affect mental health (Cianconi et al. 2022; Radua et al. 2024).

Large Farms and Monocultures

Monoculture commodity crop farming refers to the agricultural practice of growing a single crop species over a wide area, as either annual monoculture (in which major staples in the food supply such as field corn, soybeans, and wheat are planted each year) or perennial monoculture (which includes, for example, certain types of fruit trees). Monoculture crops are grown for mass production, provide high yields, and in most cases can be easily harvested by mechanized farming practices. In the United States, monoculture farming predominantly takes place in the Midwest, an area commonly referred to as the "Corn Belt." States such as Iowa, Illinois, and Indiana are pivotal in corn and soybean production, reflecting a focus on relatively few species that dominate the agricultural landscape. Other countries worldwide engage in monoculture crop farming, including Brazil, which heavily cultivates soybeans, as well as various regions in China, where rice is a staple. Although the practice allows for streamlined farming techniques and can lead to short-term economic benefits and increased food production, it can foster environmental challenges and it obviously diminishes biodiversity.

The benefits of monoculture commodity crop farming include maximized efficiency in planting and harvesting, reduced labor costs, and increased yield per acre. However, the disadvantages are substantial, including soil nutrient depletion, an elevated need for chemical inputs such as fertilizers, herbicides, and pesticides, and an increased vulnerability to pests and diseases due to limited biodiversity (Balogh 2021). The heavy reliance on chemicals can lead to contamination of water supplies, harming the ecosystem as well as physical and mental health. Additionally, monoculture practices can contribute to poor crop resilience against climate change, making farming more susceptible to variables such as drought and flooding, which are increasingly prevalent in today's changing climate.

Genetically Modified Organism (GMO) Commodity Crops

GMO crops are plants that have been altered at the genetic level using biotechnology to exhibit traits that are not naturally theirs. These modifications typically encompass the introduction of genetic material from different species, offering significant advantages such as increased resistance to pests, enhanced nutritional content, improved tolerance to environmental stresses such as drought or salinity, and the ability to withstand otherwise deadly herbicides (so that entire fields can be sprayed with herbicides such as glyphosate, glufosinate, and dicamba to kill weeds without killing the commodity crop). GMOs can be classified into various types, including herbicide-tolerant crops, insect-resistant crops, and those engineered for improved shelf life or nutritional value. Prominent examples of GMO crops include corn, soybeans, cotton, and canola, widely recognized for their enhanced agricultural capabilities.

Based on U.S. Department of Agriculture survey data (U.S. Department of Agriculture 2025), the percentage of domestic soybean acres planted with herbicide-tolerant genetically engineered seeds rose from 17% in 1997 to 68% in 2001, before plateauing at 94% in 2014. In 2024, herbicide-tolerant genetically engineered soybean acreage reached its highest adoption at 96%. Herbicide-tolerant genetically engineered cotton acreage expanded from approximately 10% in 1997 to 56% in 2001, before reaching a high of 95% in 2019. Herbicide-tolerant genetically engineered cotton acreage stood at 93% in 2024. With regard to herbicide-tolerant genetically engineered field corn, approximately 90%

of acres in 2024 were planted with herbicide-tolerant seeds. Globally, countries such as Brazil and Argentina are also notable for their large-scale production of GMO crops; European nations tend to have stricter regulations regarding GMO cultivation. The rapid adoption of GMOs has been met with various technological advancements, but public sentiment and regulatory frameworks regarding GMO use vary significantly between global regions.

Although the introduction of GMO crops brings several benefits, including higher yield potential, improved farm profits, and reductions in pesticide use, there are notable disadvantages and concerns surrounding their use, particularly regarding potential health impacts of large-scale herbicide application (leading to ecological imbalances and negative impacts on nontarget species and soil health) and the possible development of superweeds and superbugs that evolve resistance to herbicides and pesticides. To the extent that herbicides (like glyphosate, brand name Roundup, which the International Agency for Research on Cancer classifies as a probable human carcinogen) are detrimental to the health of individuals and the population, herbicide-tolerant GMO crops (which inevitably increase herbicide use) are detrimental to the health of individuals and populations. Additionally, environmental concerns arise from the potential for cross-contamination with non-GMO crops and the loss of biodiversity, as monoculture practices might be amplified by the reliance on a limited number of genetically modified varieties. The main uses of GMO food crops in the United States are animal feed (i.e., corn and soybeans are used to feed livestock, poultry, and fish) and ultraprocessed food ingredients (i.e., corn and soybeans are processed to create various ingredients such as cornstarch, corn syrup, corn oil, high fructose corn syrup, soybean oil, soy lecithin, soy protein, and soy protein isolate). Although consumption of GMOs may not pose a threat to human or animal health per se (e.g., the nutritional value of the corn kernel or soybean), to the extent that GMO-derived ingredients are used to drive CAFOs and to create ultraprocessed food, they could not be considered beneficial to health.

Concentrated Animal Feeding Operations

CAFOs are large-scale agricultural facilities designed for the intensive breeding and raising of livestock. These operations are typically defined by their high-density animal confinement and feed aggregation, where animals are kept in close quarters, often indoors, for extended periods. CAFOs can be classified based on the species raised, size, and environmental impact, commonly categorized as large, medium, and small operations. The types of animals often found in CAFOs include poultry (chickens and turkeys), cattle, hogs, and sheep, with the most prevalent being poultry and hogs because of their efficiency in feed conversion and economic viability. In the United States, CAFOs are predominantly situated in regions conducive to large-scale livestock production, such as the Midwest for hogs, southeastern states for poultry, and western states for cattle. This distribution allows for the industrialization of animal farming and meets the growing demand for meat and eggs. Globally, countries such as Brazil, China, and parts of Europe also engage in CAFO practices, adopting similar approaches to meet demand for animal-derived food products. CAFOs increase economies of scale, which can result in reduced consumer prices for meat products.

Despite their potential advantages from the perspective of large-scale food production, the concentration of animals leads to numerous health concerns, including the spread of antibiotic-resistant bacteria due to routine antibiotic use in livestock. Moreover, the environmental impact is significant, with CAFOs contributing to water pollution from runoff, methane emissions, and the destruction of local ecosystems. The association with GMO crops is inherent, as these operations often rely heavily on GMO feed grains, such as field corn and soybeans. This reliance breeds further concerns about herbicide runoff and emphasizes a cycle of industrial agriculture that may harm both human health and the environment. Like the effects of climate change, there are direct and indirect effects of both GMOs and CAFOs on health. The direct effects pertain to eating a diet of poorer quality (more ultraprocessed foods, excess meats and other animal-derived foods that are high in saturated fats, and sugar-sweetened beverages), which is detrimental to both physical health and mental health. The indirect effects might include the discontentment, anxiety, and stress felt by people who are aware of the effects of industrial food production.

Ultraprocessed Foods

Large-scale food production influences what and how we eat. It encourages the consumption of ultraprocessed foods (which comprise a large part of the Western diet or standard American diet, as described in Chapter 4), large amounts of meats, including processed meats, and sugar-sweetened beverages. As the population increasingly follows this eating pattern, the demand encourages expansion of large-scale food production, as depicted in Figure 15.2. Furthermore, large-scale

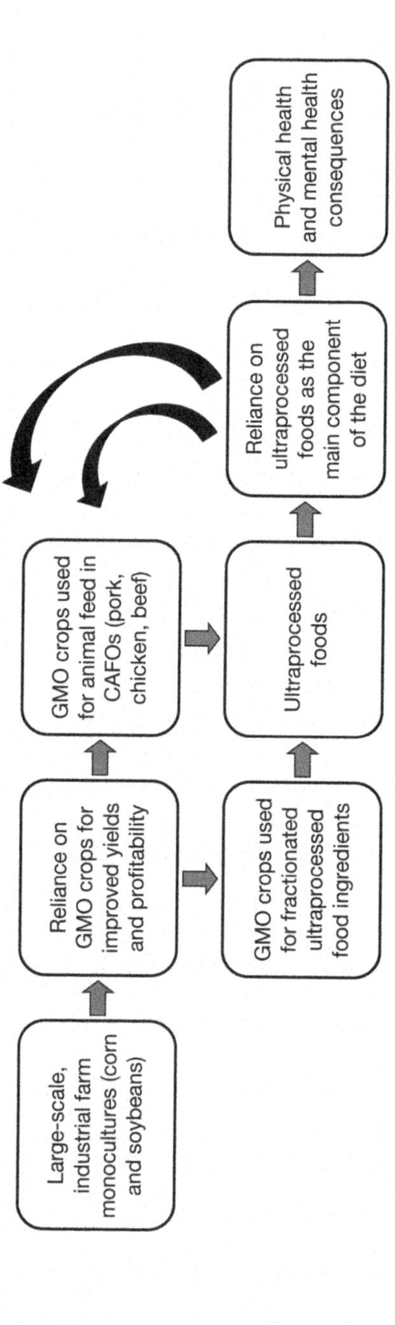

Figure 15.2 Connections between industrial farm monocultures, GMO crops, CAFOs, and ultraprocessed foods.

CAFO = concentrated animal feeding operation; GMO = genetically modified organism. Curved arrows represent feedback loops.

food production also encourages the distribution to consumers of single-use plastic packaged food and beverages. A considerable part of global plastic waste is estimated to come from food and drink packages, which largely contribute to the escalating global environmental problem of plastic pollution (Phelan et al. 2022). Macroplastic pollution is affecting nearly every ecosystem globally (Borrelle et al. 2020) and is degraded to microparticles and nanoparticles of plastic. These can enter the human body by either inhalation or ingestion and may accumulate in different organs and tissues, including the brain (Waring et al. 2018).

Overfishing and Other Sea/Ocean-Related Concerns

Overfishing is defined as the extraction of fish and seafood from aquatic ecosystems at rates that exceed their ability to reproduce, resulting in a depletion of fish stocks. This practice can be classified into various types, including *overfishing of target species*, in which specific fish populations are excessively harvested, and *bycatch*, which involves the accidental capture of nontarget species during fishing activities. Commonly overfished species include cod, tuna, haddock, and various shark species, alongside shellfish like shrimp and crab. Various classifications also consider the fishing methods employed, such as trawling, purse seining, and long-lining, each having distinctive impacts on marine ecosystems. Geographically, overfishing occurs worldwide, affecting different marine regions to varying degrees. In the United States, overfishing is prevalent along both coasts, particularly in the Gulf of Mexico and New England, which are known for their rich fishing opportunities. Globally, regions such as the North Atlantic, East China Sea, and Mediterranean are significantly affected by overfishing. The increasing demand for certain fish and seafood—driven by population growth, dietary shifts favoring seafood, and rising consumer demand—has led to unsustainable fishing practices. Notable examples include the high demand for species such as bluefin tuna and shrimp, which has led to aggressive fishing tactics and declining stock populations.

Overfishing disrupts the balance of aquatic food webs, leading to declines in predator-prey relationships and destruction of habitat, which affects biodiversity. These and other problems represent an urgent challenge for global marine conservation efforts, necessitating sustainable fishing practices, regulatory frameworks, and consumer awareness to ensure the long-term viability of marine resources. Many areas negatively impacted by overfishing are classed by the Food and Agriculture Organization of the United Nations as low-income, food-deficit countries. Massive foreign fishing fleets catch substantial quantities of fish off the coasts of various African countries but with little contribution to the nutritional needs of local populations (most of the catch is destined for Europe and Asia). Such developments widen the gap between rich and poor countries, in terms of health and social conditions, leading to a negative spiral of more poverty, worsening health, and further degradation of ecosystems (Lloret et al. 2024).

In addition to overfishing, other sea/ocean-related concerns could have an impact on health and mental health. For example, the problem of coral reef degradation—as one facet of global warming and climate change—has been described as a potential social determinant of mental health (Attademo, Bernardini, and Compton, unpublished). Gradual endangerment and loss of critical oceanic ecosystems could have substantial adverse mental health impacts for millions of people worldwide.

The Local Food Movement and the Slow Food Movement

One solution to the problems brought about by GMOs, CAFOs, and ultraprocessed food is for people to embrace the local food movement, which typically relies on small farms (farmers in the local community) that produce diverse vegetables and fruits for purchase directly, such as at farm stands, farmers markets, mobile farmers markets, local food cooperatives, and community supported agriculture (CSA) farm shares. A common definition of local food is that which is produced within a certain radius, often defined as 100–250 miles from the consumer (see also Chapter 4). Embracing local food also supports local small farmers and thus one's own community and may considerably reduce the environmental impact of food storage, preservation, packaging, and distribution, which might have positive mental health effects. Supporting small farms and embracing the local food movement can also contribute to the restoration of the landscape of abandoned lands and pastures, as well as sustainable agricultural practices (i.e., reducing the carbon footprint associated with long-distance food transportation and promoting biodiversity through diverse crop cultivation). Related concepts include seasonal eating, farm-to-table restaurants, and urban farming.

In the United States, the *locavore* movement has gained considerable traction over the past two decades, paralleling a growing awareness of health, environmental issues, and food justice and food sovereignty. Many urban centers, such as San Francisco, New York, and Portland, have seen a significant rise in farmers markets and local food initiatives. Elsewhere, regions like Europe and Australia similarly embrace local food movements, with European Union policies supporting local agriculture and sustainable food systems. This shift toward local sourcing is characterized by a resurgence of interest in traditional foods, heirloom varieties, and artisanal production methods, creating a direct connection between producers, consumers, and the food they eat. In sum, the local food movement can contribute to environmental sustainability and represents a holistic approach to food production and consumption that prioritizes health and sustainable community development, further encouraging practices that honor local ecosystems and cultures.

The slow food movement is a global initiative that advocates for the enjoyment of food that is good, clean, and fair. Founded in 1986 in Italy by Carlo Petrini, the movement arose as a response to the rapid industrialization of food production and the threat posed by fast food culture. By prioritizing quality over quantity, the movement seeks to reconnect consumers with the origins of their food and the stories behind it. The types of food involved in the Slow Food movement are diverse, often focusing on locally grown, seasonal, and artisanal products made using traditional methods. The movement is particularly strong in regions throughout Europe, where local culinary practices remain deeply rooted. In the United States as well, the slow food movement has gained substantial traction, with numerous chapters and events dedicated to promoting local foods, sustainable farming, and heritage cooking.

By encouraging consumers to prioritize wholesome, minimally processed foods such as fresh produce, whole grains, and responsibly sourced proteins, the movement promotes a balanced diet that can reduce the risk of chronic health issues like obesity and heart disease. Additionally, the movement fosters community connections and enhances food literacy, encouraging individuals to engage in cooking and food preparation that emphasizes quality ingredients and mindful eating practices.

The EAT-Lancet Commission and the Planetary Health Diet

The EAT-Lancet Commission, established in 2019, is an initiative that combines the expertise of scientists, policymakers, and diverse practitioners to tackle one of the most pressing challenges of our time: how to sustainably nourish a growing global population (Willett et al. 2019). The Commission's report presented a scientific framework for healthy diets from sustainable food systems, emphasizing the need for a radical transformation in how food is produced and consumed, in light of the worldwide population. The commission advocates for a diet, described below, that will both promote better health and minimize environmental degradation. Through this framework, the Commission aims to address the dual urgencies of improved nutrition and environmental sustainability.

Central to the EAT-Lancet Commission's mission is the recognition of the interconnectedness of human health, planetary health, and social equity. The Commission argues that the current food system is responsible for a significant portion of global greenhouse gas emissions and biodiversity loss, while also contributing to rising rates of diet-related chronic diseases. By advocating for a shift toward a food system that embraces sustainability, the Commission emphasizes the importance of collaboration across sectors, including agriculture, health, and environmental policy. The pathway proposed by the commission not only seeks to improve population health and combat climate change but also aims to create a more equitable food system that serves the needs of all individuals, particularly vulnerable communities that are disproportionately affected by food insecurity and health inequities.

The Planetary Health Diet, introduced by the commission, is designed to provide a sustainable approach to global food consumption that promotes both human health and the health of the planet. This diet emphasizes a predominantly plant-based intake, recommending a daily consumption of approximately 2,500 calories that includes a variety of foods, such as whole grains, fruits, vegetables, legumes, nuts, seeds, and unsaturated oils. The Planetary Health Diet advocates for moderate intake of seafood and poultry and lower intake of red meat, processed meat, refined sugar, and refined grains, promoting dietary patterns that are nutrient-dense while simultaneously reducing the environmental impact related to food production. Research using an index on how closely one's diet aligns with the EAT-Lancet Planetary Health Diet suggests that the highest adherence is associated with lower all-cause mortality (HR 0.75; 95% CI 0.67–0.85), cancer mortality (HR 0.76; 95% CI 0.63–0.92), and cardiovascular mortality (HR 0.68; 95% CI 0.54–0.84) than the lowest adherence (Stubbendorff et al. 2022). Adherence to the diet is also associated with lower risk of type 2 diabetes (Zhang et al. 2023). As such, by following this dietary framework, individuals can contribute to a healthier lifestyle while alleviating pressure on Earth's ecosystems (e.g., reducing greenhouse gas emissions associated with meat and dairy production, conserving water resources, and enhancing soil health).

Clinical Pearls

- Direct adverse health effects of both GMOs and CAFOs pertain to eating a diet of poorer quality (more ultraprocessed foods, excess meats and other animal-derived foods that are high in saturated fats, and sugar-sweetened beverages); indirect effects might include the discontentment, anxiety, and stress felt by some who are aware of the impacts of industrial food production.
- A number of psychosocial stressors—including low wages and thus risk for food insecurity—may occur among workers in the industrial food production system, spanning from farm workers to grocery store and restaurant workers.
- The local food movement and the slow food movement foster interpersonal connectedness in addition to a healthier eating pattern with less reliance on ultraprocessed foods and fast food.
- An eating pattern that is more closely aligned to the Planetary Health Diet is associated with lower all-cause mortality, cancer mortality, and cardiovascular mortality, as well as a lower risk of type 2 diabetes.
- The Planetary Health Diet is similar to other healthy eating patterns such as the Mediterranean diet and the Blue Zones diet, with an emphasis on whole foods and plant-predominant food sources—a high reliance on fruits, vegetables, legumes, grains, nuts, and seeds, and a lower reliance on dairy products, eggs, and other animal-based food sources.

Key Chapter Points

- Industrial agriculture—designed to produce vast quantities of food at relatively low cost—contrasts with traditional farming methods that involve smaller farms, diverse crops and livestock, and less intensive and environmentally disruptive practices.

- Industrial food production can be used to describe further downstream processing, after products leave the farm, and the creation of processed foods and ultraprocessed foods.
- Overfishing—caused by increasing demand for fish and seafood—is defined as the extraction of fish and seafood from aquatic ecosystems at rates that exceed their ability to reproduce, resulting in a depletion of fish stocks.
- The local food movement typically relies on small farms in the local community that produce diverse vegetables and fruits for purchase directly, such as at farm stands, farmers markets, mobile farmers markets, local food cooperatives, and community-supported agriculture (CSA) farm shares. The slow food movement is similarly oriented.
- The EAT-Lancet Commission presented a scientific framework for healthy diets from sustainable food systems, emphasizing the need for a radical transformation in how food is produced and consumed by the worldwide population. The Commission advocates for a Planetary Health Diet that will both promote better health and minimize environmental degradation.

References

Balogh A: The rise and fall of monoculture farming. Horizon, 2021. Available at: https://projects.research-and-innovation.ec.europa.eu/en/horizon-magazine/rise-and-fall-monoculture-farming. Accessed May 14, 2025.

Borrelle SB, Ringma J, Law KL, et al: Predicted growth in plastic waste exceeds efforts to mitigate plastic pollution. Science 369(6510):1515–1518, 2020 32943526

Çakmakçı R, Salık MA, Çakmakçı S: Assessment and principles of environmentally sustainable food and agriculture systems. Agriculture 13(5):1073, 2023

Cianconi P, Hirsch D, Chiappini S, et al: Climate change, biodiversity loss and mental health: a global perspective. BJPsych Int 19(4):83–86, 2022

Donham KJ, Wing S, Osterberg D, et al: Community health and socioeconomic issues surrounding concentrated animal feeding operations. Environ Health Perspect 115(2):317–320, 2007 17384786

European Agency for Safety and Health at Work: Mental health in agriculture: preventing and managing psychosocial risks for farmers and farm workers. Luxembourg, Publications Office of the European Union, 2024

Food and Agriculture Organization of the United Nations: Sustainable food systems. concept and framework, 2018. Available at: https://www.fao.org/food-systems/en/. Accessed May 14, 2025.

Lloret J, García-de-Vinuesa A, Demestre M: How human health and well-being depends on healthy marine habitats in the Mediterranean: a review. Heliyon 10(2):e24329, 2024 38293530

Mahdizade Ari M, Dadgar L, Elahi Z, et al: Genetically engineered microorganisms and their impact on human health. Int J Clin Pract 2024 38495751

McElroy KG: Environmental health effects of concentrated animal feeding operations: implications for nurses. Nurs Adm Q 34(4):311–319, 2010 20838176

Merchant J, Martin R (eds): Industrial Farm Animal Production, the Environment, and Public Health. Baltimore, MD, Johns Hopkins University Press, 2024

Miraglia M, Marvin HJP, Kleter GA, et al: Climate change and food safety: an emerging issue with special focus on Europe. Food Chem Toxicol 47(5):1009–1021, 2009 19353812

Phelan AA, Meissner K, Humphrey J, et al: Plastic pollution and packaging: corporate commitments and actions from the food and beverage sector. J Clean Prod 331:129827, 2022

Radua J, De Prisco M, Oliva V, et al: Impact of air pollution and climate change on mental health outcomes: an umbrella review of global evidence. World Psychiatry 23(2):244–256, 2024 38727076

Stubbendorff A, Sonestedt E, Ramne S, et al: Development of an EAT-Lancet index and its relation to mortality in a Swedish population. Am J Clin Nutr 115(3):705–716, 2022 34791011

Tota M, Karska J, Kowalski S, et al: Environmental pollution and extreme weather conditions: insights into the effect on mental health. Front Psychiatry 15:1389051, 2024 38863619

U.S. Department of Agriculture: Adoption of Genetically Engineered Crops in the United States: Recent Trends in GE Adoption. Economic Research Service, 2025. Available at: https://www.ers.usda.gov/data-products/adoption-of-genetically-engineered-crops-in-the-united-states/recent-trends-in-ge-adoption. Accessed April 24, 2025.

Waring RH, Harris RM, Mitchell SC: Plastic contamination of the food chain: a threat to human health? Maturitas 115:64–68, 2018 30049349

Willett W, Rockström J, Loken B, et al: Food in the Anthropocene: the EAT-Lancet Commission on healthy diets from sustainable food systems. Lancet 393(10170):447–492, 2019 30660336

Young J: What should health professions students know about industrial agriculture and disease? AMA J Ethics 25(4):E264–E268, 2023 37014721

Zhang S, Stubbendorff A, Olsson K, et al: Adherence to the EAT-Lancet diet, genetic susceptibility, and risk of type 2 diabetes in Swedish adults. Metabolism 141:155401, 2023 36682448

Index

Page numbers printed in **boldface type** *refer to tables and figures.*